THE COMPLETE GUIDE TO

SPORTS NUTRITION

9TH EDITION

Anita Bean

BLOOMSBURY SPORT
LONDON · OXFORD · NEW YORK · NEW DELHI · SYDNEY

BLOOMSBURY SPORT
Bloomsbury Publishing Plc
50 Bedford Square, London, WC1B 3DP, UK
29 Earlsfort Terrace, Dublin 2, Ireland

BLOOMSBURY, BLOOMSBURY SPORT and the
Diana logo are trademarks of Bloomsbury Publishing Plc

First published in Great Britain 1993
This edition published 2022

Copyright © 2022, 2017, 2013, 2009, 2006, 2003,
2000, 1996, 1993 Anita Bean
Illustrations © David Gardner, 2021
All images © Getty Images
Ninth edition 2022
Eighth edition 2017
Seventh edition 2013; reprinted 2013, 2014 and 2015
Sixth edition 2009; reprinted 2010, 2012
Fifth edition 2006
Fourth edition 2003
Third edition 2000; reprinted 2001
Second edition 1996; reprinted 1997 (twice), 1998,
    1999, 2000
First edition 1993; reprinted 1994, 1995

A catalogue record for this book is available from the
British Library

Library of Congress Cataloguing-in-Publication data has
been applied for

ISBN: PB: 978-1-4729-7694-9;
eBook: 978-1-4729-7696-3

2   4   6   8   10   9   7   5   3   1

Typeset in ITC Galliard Pro by seagulls.net
Printed and bound in China by Toppan Leefung Printing

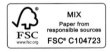

FSC
www.fsc.org
MIX
Paper from
responsible sources
FSC® C104723

To find out more about our authors and books visit
www.bloomsbury.com and sign up for our newsletters

//CONTENTS

Acknowledgements   iv
Foreword   1
Preface to the Ninth Edition   2

Chapter 1   An Overview of Sports Nutrition   4
Chapter 2   Energy for Exercise   16
Chapter 3   Carbohydrate   32
Chapter 4   Protein   65
Chapter 5   Fat   83
Chapter 6   Vitamins and Minerals   92
Chapter 7   Sports Supplements   107
Chapter 8   Hydration   147
Chapter 9   Body Composition   168
Chapter 10   Weight Management   180
Chapter 11   Relative Energy Deficiency in Sport   208
Chapter 12   Gut Health   228
Chapter 13   Immune Health and Recovery from Injury   239
Chapter 14   The Young Athlete   249
Chapter 15   The Plant-based Athlete   262
Chapter 16   The Masters Athlete   277
Chapter 17   Competition Nutrition   289
Chapter 18   Your Personal Nutrition Plan   303
Chapter 19   The Recipes   323

Appendix: Glossary of vitamins and minerals   352
List of abbreviations   362
Symbols used and conversions   363
Further reading   364
References   365
Online resources   405
Index   406

ACKNOWLEDGEMENTS

This book is the culmination of my work as a sports nutritionist and writer for more than 30 years and would not have been possible without the support and help of many brilliant people. First and foremost, thank you to my husband, Simon, for always being there and backing me all the way. Thank you also to my two daughters, Chloe and Lucy, who provide me with inspiration and motivation.

I am very grateful to the many scientists who have provided expert feedback on this book: Professor Graeme Close, Liverpool John Moores University; Professor James Morton, Liverpool John Moores University; Professor Andrew Jones, University of Exeter; Professor Neil Walsh, Liverpool John Moores University; Dr Oliver Witard, Kings College London; Dr Lewis James, Loughborough University; Dr Jamie Pugh, Liverpool John Moores University; Dr Adam Collins, University of Surrey; and James Fern, University of Bath;

Thank you to the wonderful editorial team at Bloomsbury: publisher Charlotte Croft, senior editor Sarah Skipper, copy editor Lucy Doncaster, proof-reader Nicky Gyopari, designer Seagull Design, cover designer Amanda Keyte, head of marketing Lizzy Ewer, senior publicity manager Katherine Macpherson and senior marketing executive Alice Graham.

FOREWORD

Nutrition has always played an important role in my running career and without a doubt has been a key factor in helping me achieve my best performances. In the early days of my career, there was very little reliable information about sports nutrition. Like most runners, I had to work out for myself what to eat before races, the timings of my food intake, how much fluid to drink to prepare for races and also what to take onboard during longer races such as the marathon. This was done mostly by trying out different things rather than having a definite plan. Sometimes I was finding it difficult to get my blood sugar levels right to race well. On occasion I also felt like I'd taken on too much fluid too close to the start of shorter races. Earlier in my career I found it more difficult to recover between tough workouts too. Without some expert advice, it can definitely be very hard to optimise your nutrition strategies.

I've known Anita for many years and have always found her advice invaluable. Learning how to fuel my training has meant that I could train harder and recover quicker – and that was critical at times when I was training up to 100 miles a week or when I was doing intense interval sessions in preparation for championships. Without good nutrition, sports people are much more likely to get injured or pick up illnesses. It's a such a shame when athletes who are motivated to train hard don't achieve their goals due to their nutrition being inadequate.

Anita is absolutely brilliant at translating complex science into easily understandable advice for athletes. This book is such a fantastic resource to me. It contains a huge amount of information that is backed up by science. It is also very practical and displays the wealth of knowledge that Anita has. I've been able to gain fantastic advice from this book and I think it will be an absolute must for all aspiring athletes who want to enjoy their sport and achieve their optimal performances.

Jo Pavey
World, European and Commonwealth
medalist and five-time Olympian

It seems extraordinary that this book is now in its ninth edition. Since the first edition, it has undergone many revisions and updates as the science of sport and exercise nutrition has evolved over the years. When it was first published in 1993, sports nutrition was in its infancy and there was little reliable nutrition information available to athletes, coaches and nutrition practitioners. Since then, our knowledge of how nutrition influences sport and exercise performance has grown enormously, new guidelines have been developed and high-quality research continues to be published. There is now overwhelming evidence that diet significantly influences performance and recovery. Having advised hundreds of athletes over the past 30 years, I have seen first-hand how important diet is in supporting any training programme and helping athletes reach their goals.

The aim of this book has always been to translate the science of sport and exercise nutrition into practical information that athletes can understand and use. It provides evidence-based facts and recommendations in an easy-to-digest format, not opinions or anecdotes. All the information is backed with scientific studies, which are referenced in the text and listed at the back of the book. I am happy to report that, over the years, this book has remained a trusted reference and practical handbook for athletes, trainers, coaches, sports scientists, nutritionists and dietitians.

So, what's new? This ninth edition includes brand new chapters on relative energy deficiency in sport (RED-S), gut health, immunity and recovery from injury. I have added research updates and findings from hundreds of sports nutrition studies around the world. Since the last edition, there has been a huge rise in interest in plant-based diets, with many athletes now reducing meat or switching to a vegan diet for health, ethical, environmental or performance reasons. As a result, research on the benefits of plant proteins has increased dramatically. The thinking around hydration, race fuelling and the management of gut problems has also evolved.

In recent years, research in sports nutrition has focused on new topics such as nutrition periodisation, 'training low', protein timing, low energy availability and optimisation of body composition. There has been a trend towards higher fat intakes and a move away from very low-fat diets once believed beneficial for athletes. However, the controversy surrounding low-carbohydrate diets is ongoing and new research is beginning to provide some interesting insights into the effects of strategic periods of carbohydrate restriction on training adaptations, body composition and performance.

Sports nutrition advice has changed considerably over recent years. For example, guidelines for carbohydrate and protein are now expressed in grams per kg body weight, instead of as a percentage of total energy, and tailored according to the fuel requirements and training goals of specific training sessions. There have been new recommendations on the optimal amount of protein to be consumed after training sessions as well as the timing and type of protein. New concepts such as metabolic efficiency and flexibility have evolved.

It is clear that when it comes to optimal performance, one size doesn't fit all. Athletes should follow a personalised nutrition and hydration plan that takes account of the specific physiological demands of their event, their training and performance goals, practical considerations, food preferences and individual circumstances.

Scientists have also made progress in the quest for giving elite athletes the edge in long-duration competitions, with the development of sports drinks containing 'multiple transportable carbohydrates' that allow the body to absorb higher amounts of carbohydrate per hour. Other changes include the abolition of advice to drink ahead of thirst and a warning against overhydration during long events. There are no longer hard and fast guidelines on fluid intake and, in practice, athletes have to find a compromise between preventing hypohydration (*see* p. 147) and ensuring they don't overhydrate.

I have always taken a 'food first' approach when it comes to optimising nutrition for performance, despite the enormous array of expensive engineered supplements out there! Pills, powders and gels cannot replicate the complex matrix of nutrients and phytochemicals provided by natural food. What's more, food tastes so much nicer and provides a lot more pleasure than any supplement.

If it can improve recovery and performance then this has to be great news for every athlete.

I've watched with equal fascination and scepticism as more and more sports supplements appear on the market. Science continues to disprove the claims of most, which I continue to report in this book. However, there is sound evidence for the benefits of a small handful of supplements, which I have outlined in Chapter 7.

In this book, I have attempted to condense decades of sports nutrition research into practical guidelines and, ultimately, a step-by-step guide to developing a personalised nutrition plan. I hope you will find the information useful and that it will help you reach your sporting potential.

Anita Bean

An Overview of // Sports Nutrition

There is universal scientific consensus that diet affects health, performance and recovery. A well-planned eating strategy will help support any training programme, whether you are training for fitness or for competition; promote efficient recovery between workouts; reduce the risk of illness or overtraining; and help you to achieve your potential in sport.

Of course, everyone has different nutritional needs and there is no single diet that suits all. Some athletes require more calories, protein or vitamins than others; and each sport has its unique nutritional demands. But it is possible to find broad scientific agreement as to what constitutes a healthy diet for sport generally. The following guidelines are based on the Joint Position Statement on Nutrition and Athletic Performance from the American College of Sports Medicine, Academy of Nutrition and Dietetics and Dietitians of Canada (Thomas *et al.*, 2016), the International Olympic Committee Consensus Conference on Sports Nutrition (IOC, 2011) and the International Association of Athletics Federation (IAAF) Consensus Statement (Burke *et al.*, 2019).

These organisations highlight the importance of nutrition strategies in optimising elite perfor-mance. They recognise the advances in sports nutrition research in recent years, including the need for nutrition periodisation, individualisation of nutrition plans to take into account the specific-ity and uniqueness of the event and performance goals, the new concepts of metabolic efficiency and flexibility, and energy availability (energy intake minus the energy cost of exercise); the importance of nutrient timing and optimising the intakes of protein after training to aid long-term maintenance or gain of muscle; greater intakes of carbohydrate (90 g/hr) for exercise over 3 hours; the importance of vitamin D for perfor-mance; and the need for a personalised hydration plan to prevent hypohydration as well as hypona-traemia. They recommend that the requirement for energy, carbohydrate and protein should be expressed using guidelines per kg body weight to take account of a range of body sizes.

The process leading to publication was extremely thorough and drew on the combined expertise of many of the world's leading sports nutrition experts. Of course, these guidelines are only intended to give you an overview of the evidence linking nutrition and performance. Everyone is different and some people respond better or worse to various dietary strategies. So it is important to experiment and find out what works best for you. But, being based on high-quality research, these guidelines are a great place to start.

1. Energy

It is crucial that athletes meet their energy (calorie) needs during hard periods of training in order to achieve improvements in performance and maintain good health. Failure to consume sufficient energy can result in muscle loss, reduced performance, slow recovery, disruption of hormonal function (in females) and increased risk of fatigue, injury and illness. Researchers have recently identified the concept of energy availability (EA), defined as dietary intake minus exercise energy expenditure, or the amount of energy available to the body to perform all other functions after exercise training expenditure is subtracted. In healthy adults, a value of 45 kcal/kg fat-free mass (FFM)/day equates with energy balance and optimum health. It has been suggested that 30 kcal/kg FFM/day should be the lower threshold of energy availability in females. (Fat-free mass includes muscles, organs, fluid and bones.) A low EA may compromise athletic performance in the short and long term. It may occur when energy intake is too low, energy expenditure is too high or a combination of both. The term 'relative energy deficiency in sport (RED-S)' refers to the impaired physiological function, including metabolic rate, menstrual function, bone health, immunity, protein synthesis and cardiovascular health, caused by relative energy deficiency or low EA in male and female athletes. It more accurately describes the clinical syndrome previously known as the Female Athlete Triad.

Your daily calorie needs will depend on your genetic make-up, age, weight, body composition, your daily activity and your training programme. It is possible to estimate the number of calories you need daily from your body weight (BW) and your level of daily physical activity.

STEP 1: ESTIMATE YOUR RESTING METABOLIC RATE (RMR)

Your RMR is an estimate of how many calories you would burn if you were to do nothing but rest for 24 hours. It represents the minimum amount of energy needed to keep your body functioning, including breathing and keeping your heart beating. It can be estimated using the Mifflin-St Jeor equation, which utilises age, weight and height, and is considered more accurate than the more commonly used Harris-Benedict equation.

Men
(10 x weight (kg)) + (6.25 x height (cm)) − (5 x age (y)) + 5

Women
(10 x weight (kg)) + (6.25 x height (cm)) − (5 x age (y)) − 161

STEP 2: WORK OUT YOUR PHYSICAL ACTIVITY LEVEL (PAL)

This is the ratio of your overall daily energy expenditure to your RMR – a rough measure of your lifestyle activity.

- mostly inactive or sedentary (mainly sitting): 1.2
- fairly active (include walking and exercise 1–2 x week): 1.3

- moderately active (exercise 2–3 x weekly): 1.4
- active (exercise hard more than 3 x weekly): 1.5
- very active (exercise hard daily): 1.7

STEP 3: MULTIPLY YOUR RMR BY YOUR PAL TO WORK OUT YOUR TOTAL DAILY ENERGY EXPENDITURE

Daily calorie needs = RMR x PAL

This figure gives you a rough idea of your daily calorie requirement to maintain your weight. If you eat fewer calories, you will lose weight; if you eat more then you will gain weight.

2. Body composition

There is no single or 'optimal' body composition for a particular event or sport. Each individual athlete has an optimal fat range at which their performance improves yet their health does not suffer. However, this should not be achieved at the expense of continual low energy availability, otherwise performance and health are likely to be impaired. Instead, weight and body composition should be periodised in line with the training programme, accepting fluctuations throughout the year. Excessive weight gain should be avoided in the off-season and rapid weight loss strategies avoided in the competition season. The best time to lose weight is in the base training phase or well out from competition to minimise loss of performance. A modest energy deficit of 250–500 kcal/day to achieve a slow rate of weight loss (<1% per week) is recommended along with increasing protein intake to 1.8–2.7 g/kg BW/day to preserve muscle mass.

3. Carbohydrate

Carbohydrate is an important fuel for the brain and central nervous system as well as for muscular work. It is stored as glycogen in your liver and muscles. The size of the body's carbohydrate stores is relatively limited. Approximately 100 g glycogen (equivalent to 400 kilocalories) may be stored in the liver, and up to 400 g glycogen (equivalent to 1600 kilocalories) in muscle cells. It is almost entirely depleted by the end of 90–120 minutes of moderate- to high-intensity

Resting metabolic rate

The resting metabolic rate (RMR) is the amount of energy required to maintain the body's normal metabolic activity, such as respiration, maintenance of body temperature and digestion. Specifically, it is the amount of energy required at rest with no additional activity. The energy consumed is sufficient only for the functioning of the vital organs. It is closely related to the basal metabolic rate (BMR), which can only be measured in an awake but totally rested and post-absorptive state, and in a neutrally temperate environment. It is quite restrictive and only used in clinical or laboratory settings. RMR accounts for 60–75% of the calories you burn daily. Generally, men have a higher RMR than women.

Physical activity includes all activities from doing the housework to walking and working out in the gym. The number of calories you burn in any activity depends on your weight, the type of activity and the duration of that activity.

exercise. The purpose of liver glycogen is to maintain blood sugar levels. When blood glucose dips, glycogen in the liver breaks down to release glucose into the bloodstream. The purpose of muscle glycogen is to fuel physical activity.

Carbohydrate offers advantages over fat as a fuel since it provides more adenosine triphosphate (ATP) (*see* p. 16 'What is ATP?') per volume of oxygen and is therefore considered a more efficient fuel. There is significant evidence that performance of prolonged, sustained or intermittent high-intensity exercise is enhanced by strategies that maintain high carbohydrate availability (i.e. matching glycogen stores and blood glucose to the fuel demands of exercise).

When it is important to train hard or with high intensity, daily carbohydrate intakes should match the fuel needs of training and glycogen replenishment. General guidelines for carbohydrate intake to provide high carbohydrate availability are based on body weight (a proxy for the volume of muscle) and exercise load. These are shown in Table 1.1. The more active you are and the greater your muscle mass, the higher your carbohydrate needs.

While guidelines for carbohydrate intake have been provided in terms of percentage contribution to total dietary energy intake in the past, experts now recommend expressing carbohydrate requirements in terms of grams per kg body weight. Guidelines for daily intakes are 3–5 g to 5–7 g per kg of body weight (BW) per day for low- and moderate-intensity daily training lasting up to 1 hour respectively. Depending on the fuel cost of the training schedule, an endurance athlete may need to consume 8–12 g of carbohydrate per kg body weight each day (560–840 g per day for a 70 kg athlete) to ensure adequate glycogen stores.

To promote rapid post-exercise recovery, experts recommend consuming 1.0–1.2 g carbohydrate per kg BW per hour for the first 4 hours after exercise. If you plan to train again within 8 hours, it is important to begin refuelling as soon as possible after exercise. Moderate and high glycaemic index (GI) carbohydrates (*see* p. 38) will promote faster recovery during this period. When carbohydrate intake is suboptimal for refuelling, adding protein to a meal/snack will enhance glycogen storage. However, for recovery periods of 24 hours or longer, the type and timing of carbohydrate intake is less critical, although you should choose nutrient-dense sources wherever possible.

It is recommended that the pre-exercise meal provides 1–4 g carbohydrate per kg body weight, depending on exercise intensity and duration, and

Table 1.1 GUIDELINES FOR DAILY CARBOHYDRATE INTAKE	
Activity level	**Recommended carbohydrate intake**
Very light training (low-intensity or skill-based exercise)	3–5 g/kg BW daily
Moderate-intensity training (approx. 1 h daily)	5–7 g/kg BW daily
Moderate–high-intensity training (1–3 h daily)	6–10 g/kg BW daily
Very high-intensity training (>4 h daily)	8–12 g/kg BW daily

Source: Burke *et al.*, 2011.

that this should be consumed between 1 and 4 hours before exercise.

During exercise lasting less than 45 minutes, there is no performance advantage to be gained by consuming additional carbohydrates. For intense exercise lasting between 45 and 75 minutes, simply swilling (not swallowing) an energy drink in your mouth ('mouth rinsing') can improve performance. The carbohydrates stimulate oral sensors that act on the central nervous system (brain) to mask fatigue and reduce perceived exertion, thus allowing you to maintain exercise intensity for longer. But for exercise lasting longer than about 1 hour, consuming between 30 and 60 g carbohydrate helps maintain your blood glucose level, spare muscle glycogen stores, delay fatigue and increase your endurance. The amount depends on the intensity and duration of exercise, and is unrelated to body size.

The longer and the more intense your workout or event, the greater your carbohydrate needs. Previously, it was thought that the body could absorb only a maximum of 60 g carbohydrate per hour. However, recent research suggests that it may be higher – as much as 90 g, a level that would be appropriate during intense exercise lasting more than 3 hours. Studies have shown that consuming multiple transportable carbohydrates (e.g. glucose and fructose) increases the rate of carbohydrate uptake and oxidation during exercise compared with glucose alone. A 2:1 mixture of glucose + fructose is generally associated with minimal GI distress. Choose high-GI carbohydrates (e.g. sports drinks, energy gels and energy bars, bananas, fruit bars, cereal or breakfast bars), according to your personal preference and tolerance.

However, recent research has shown that training in a glycogen-depleted state can enhance the adaptive responses to exercise stimulus and increase exercise capacity. The concept of 'training low but competing high' as well as 'carbohydrate periodisation' (integrating short periods of 'training low' into the training programme) has become very popular among elite endurance athletes. Strategies include occasional fasted training, training following an overnight fast, and not replenishing carbohydrate stores after the first of two training sessions of the day. These have been shown to increase muscle adaptation to training by altering signalling and upregulating the metabolic response to

Table 1.2	RECOMMENDATIONS FOR PRE- AND POST-EXERCISE CARBOHYDRATE INTAKE	
Dietary strategy	When	Recommended carbohydrate intake
Pre-exercise fuelling	Before exercise >60 min	1–4 g/kg BW consumed 1–4 h before exercise
Post-exercise rapid refuelling	<8 h recovery between two sessions	$1.0–1.2 \, g \cdot kg^{-1} \cdot h^{-1}$ for first 4 h then resume daily fuel needs
Carbohydrate loading	For events >90 min of sustained/ intermittent exercise	36–48 h of 10–12 g/kg BW/24 h

Source: Burke *et al.*, 2011.

exercise. However, it is important to undertake high-intensity training sessions with high carbohydrate stores. Whether implementing these strategies ultimately improves performance is unclear.

4. Protein

Amino acids from proteins form the building blocks for new tissues and the repair of body cells. They are also used for making enzymes, hormones and antibodies. Protein also provides a (small) fuel source for exercising muscles.

Athletes have higher protein requirements than non-active people. Extra protein is needed to compensate for the increased muscle breakdown that occurs during and after intense exercise, as well as to build new muscle cells. The Thomas *et al.* consensus statement recommends between 1.2 and 2.0 g protein/kg BW/day for athletes, which equates to 84–140 g daily for a 70 kg person, considerably more than for a sedentary person, who requires 0.75 g protein/kg BW daily. These recommendations encompass a range of training programmes and allow for adjustment according to individual needs, training goals and experience.

The timing as well as the amount of protein is crucial when it comes to promoting muscle repair and growth. It is best to distribute protein intake throughout the day rather than consuming it in just one or two meals. Experts recommend consuming 0.25 g protein/kg BW or 15–25 g protein with each main meal as well as immediately after exercise.

Several studies have found that eating carbohydrate and protein together immediately after exercise enhances recovery and promotes muscle building. The types of protein eaten after exercise is important – high-quality proteins, particularly fast-absorbed proteins that contain leucine (such as whey), are considered optimal for recovery. Leucine is both a substrate and a trigger for muscle protein synthesis (MPS). An intake of 2–3 g leucine has been shown to stimulate maximum MPS.

Some athletes eat high-protein diets in the belief that extra protein leads to increased strength and muscle mass, but this isn't true – it is stimulation of muscle tissue through exercise plus adequate – not *extra* – protein that leads to muscle growth. As protein is found in so many foods, most people – including athletes – eat a little more protein than they need. This isn't harmful – the excess is broken down into urea (which is excreted) and fuel, which is either used for energy or stored as fat if your calorie intake exceeds your output.

5. Fat

Some fat is essential – it makes up part of the structure of all cell membranes, your brain tissue, nerve sheaths and bone marrow and it cushions your organs. Fat in food also provides essential fatty acids and the fat-soluble vitamins A, D and E, and is an important source of energy for exercise. The ACSM position statement currently makes no specific recommendation for fat intake. The focus should be on meeting carbohydrate and protein goals with fat making up the calorie balance. It is recommended that athletes' fat intakes are consistent with public health guidelines for fat intake: less than 35% of daily energy intake. The exact amount depends on individual training and body composition goals. However, it is recommended that athletes should consume a minimum of 20% energy from fat, otherwise they risk deficient intakes of fat-soluble vitamins and essential fatty acids (Thomas *et al.*, 2016).

The UK government recommends that the proportion of energy from saturated fatty acids be less than 10%, with the majority coming from unsaturated fatty acids. Omega-3s may be particularly beneficial for athletes, as they help increase the delivery of oxygen to muscles, improve endurance and may speed recovery and reduce inflammation and joint stiffness.

6. Hydration

You should ensure you are hydrated before starting training or competition by consuming 5–10 ml/kg body weight in the 2–4 hours prior to exercise, and aim to minimise hypohydration (see p 147) during exercise. Severe hypohydration can result in reduced endurance and strength, and heat-related illness. The IOC and American College of Sports Medicine advise matching your fluid intake to your fluid losses as closely as possible and limiting hypohydration to no more than 2–3% loss of body weight (e.g. a body weight loss of no more than 1.5 kg for a 75 kg person). Routinely weigh yourself before and after exercise, accounting for fluid consumed and urine lost, to estimate your sweat loss during exercise. A loss of 1 kg body weight equates to 1 litre of sweat lost.

Additionally, experts caution against overhydrating yourself before and during exercise, particularly in events lasting longer than 4 hours. Drinking too much water may dilute your blood so that your sodium levels fall. Although this is quite rare, it is potentially fatal. The American College of Sports Medicine advises drinking when you're thirsty or drinking only to the point at which you're maintaining your weight, not gaining weight.

Sports drinks containing sodium are advantageous when sweat losses are high (more than 1.2 litres/h) – for example, during intense exercise lasting more than 2 hours – because their sodium content will promote water retention and prevent hyponatraemia.

After exercise, both water and sodium need to be replaced to re-establish normal hydration. This can be achieved by normal eating and drinking practices if there is no urgent need for recovery. But for rapid recovery, or if you are severely hypohydrated, it is recommended you drink 25–50% more fluid than lost in sweat. You can replace fluid and sodium losses with rehydration drinks or water plus salty foods.

7. Vitamins and minerals

While intense exercise increases the requirement for several vitamins and minerals, there is no need for supplementation provided you are eating a balanced diet and consuming adequate energy to maintain body weight. The IOC, IAAF and ACSM believe most athletes are well able to meet their needs from food rather than supplements. There's scant proof that vitamin and mineral supplements improve performance, although supplementation may be warranted in athletes eating a restricted diet or when food intake or choices are limited – for example, due to travel. However, athletes should be particularly aware of their needs for calcium, iron and vitamin D, as low intakes are relatively common among female athletes. The role of vitamin D in muscle structure and function, and the risk of deficiency, has been highlighted by the IOC and ASCM/AND/DC. Those who have low vitamin D intakes and get little exposure to the sun may need to take vitamin D supplements.

Similarly, there is insufficient evidence to recommend antioxidant supplementation for

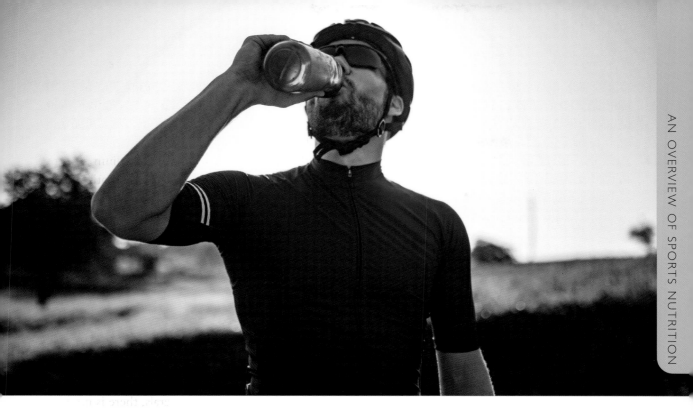

athletes. Caution against antioxidant supplements is currently advised during training, as oxidative stress may be beneficial to the muscles' adaptation to exercise. The IOC also cautions against the indiscriminate use of supplements and warns of the risk of contamination with banned substances. Only a few have any performance benefit; these include creatine, caffeine, nitrate (as found in beetroot juice), beta-alanine and sodium bicarbonate, along with sports drinks, gels and bars and protein supplements. For the majority, there is little evidence to support their use as ergogenic aids (*see* p. 107, 'Definition of sports supplements and ergogenic aids').

8. Competition nutrition

PRE-EVENT
Performance in endurance events lasting longer than 90 minutes may benefit from carbohydrate loading in the 36–48 hours prior to the event (10–12 g carbohydrate/kg BW/24 hours). During the 1–4 hours prior to a race, consume 1–4 g of carbohydrate per kg of body weight. Food choices should be high in carbohydrate and moderate in protein, while low in fat and fibre to reduce risk of gastrointestinal problems.

DURING THE EVENT
In events lasting less than 75 minutes, additional carbohydrate will not benefit performance but rinsing the mouth with an energy drink may reduce perception of fatigue via the central nervous system. In events lasting 1–2½ hours, consuming 30–60 g carbohydrate/h will help maintain blood glucose and liver glycogen, and increase endurance. In events lasting more than 2½ hours, it may be beneficial to increase carbohydrate intake to up to 90 g carbohydrate/h. This may be in the form of dual energy source

drinks or gels, containing a mixture of glucose/maltodextrin and fructose to achieve faster carbohydrate absorption.

AFTER THE EVENT

Replenish glycogen by consuming 1–1.2 g of carbohydrate/kg body weight in the first 4–6 hours after finishing. Consuming protein (in 15–25 g servings) in the recovery period also promotes glycogen recovery and enhances muscle protein resynthesis. Rehydrate with 25–50% more fluid than that lost in sweat.

The 'Athlete's Plate'

A balanced training diet is one that provides enough energy, carbohydrate, protein, fat, fibre, vitamins and minerals to support the physical demands of your training. These nutrients should come from a wide variety of foods. The key is consuming the right amounts and types of different foods that will fuel your workouts and events. To help you do this, I have created the Athlete's Plate, which can be tailored to the day-to-day fuel demands of your training programme. It is based on the Public Health England's EatWell Guide (Public Health England, 2016) and the Athlete's Plate developed by the US Olympic Committee (USOC) dietitians and University of Colorado (UCCS). It gives you a simple guide to the types and proportions of foods you need to achieve a balanced training diet. Each food group supplies a similar profile of nutrients, thus giving you plenty of options and flexibility for planning

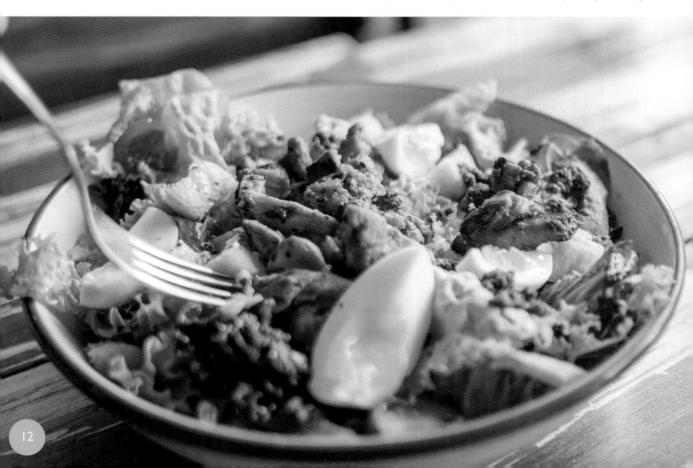

your meals. It is a good idea to vary your meals as much as possible; the wider the variety of foods you eat, the more likely you are to meet your nutritional needs. The Athlete's Plate can be adapted to meet the different fuel demands of your training on different days. Some days may be recovery or easy training days while others may comprise moderate or hard training.

The Athlete's Plate divides foods into four main groups:

1. fruit and vegetables
2. protein-rich foods (including calcium-rich foods)
3. carbohydrate-rich foods
4. healthy fats

Fruit and vegetables – Aim to eat at least five portions a day. A portion is 80 g of any fresh or frozen fruit or vegetable, or 30 g of dried. For example, one small apple, banana or orange, about six strawberries, three broccoli florets or one carrot. Foods in this group are good sources of vitamin C, beta-carotene, folate and potassium, as well as fibre and phytonutrients. At each meal, aim to achieve a rainbow of colours – green, red, purple, yellow, white, and orange – varying them as much as possible. Each colour has its unique set of health-promoting phytonutrients, many of which act as antioxidants that help protect cells from damage and reduce inflammation after exercise.

Protein-rich foods – Include at least one serving of meat, poultry, fish, dairy (e.g. milk, cheese and yoghurt), eggs, beans, lentils, peas or soya products (e.g. soya milk alternative, tofu, tempeh and soya yoghurt alternative) in each meal. These foods should comprise roughly one-quarter of your plate. They also provide fibre, iron, zinc, and magnesium. Athletes need more protein than sedentary people so aim for at least 20 g protein per meal (*see* p. 72).

Calcium-rich foods sub-group – Ensure that you include at least two portions of calcium-rich foods each day: dairy and calcium-fortified plant milk and yoghurt alternatives and calcium-set tofu. These also count towards your protein-rich foods.

Carbohydrate-rich foods – These include pasta, rice, oats, noodles, potatoes, sweet potatoes, bread and cereals. There is no minimum requirement for carbohydrate so adjust your portion size according to your activity level. The more active you are, the bigger the portions you must consume. Whole grains are preferred to refined grains because they contain the entire grain, which means they are richer in fibre, B vitamins and iron.

Healthy fats – These include nuts, seeds, avocados, and olive and rapeseed oil. Aim to include one food from this group in most of your meals. Nuts and seeds also provide protein, magnesium, fibre, iron and zinc.

EASY TRAINING OR RECOVERY DAYS

On recovery and easy training days, your fuel and carbohydrate needs will be relatively low. To ensure you get all the nutrients you need, aim for roughly one-half of your plate to be made up of fruit and vegetables, roughly one-quarter carbohydrate-rich foods, and roughly one-quarter protein-rich and calcium-rich foods. Include some healthy fats such as olive or rapeseed oil, nuts, seeds, nut butter or avocado in each meal.

MODERATE TRAINING DAYS

On moderate training days that comprise 1–2 hours' moderate- or high-intensity endurance exercise your fuel and carbohydrate needs will be higher than on easy training days. Increase your intake of carbohydrate-rich foods. This will allow you to maintain muscle glycogen stores and support your training. Divide your plate into thirds and aim to have roughly one-third of your meal plate made up of carbohydrate-rich foods, roughly one-third protein-rich and calcium-rich foods and roughly one-third fruit and vegetables. Include some healthy fats such as olive or rapeseed oil, nuts, seeds, nut butter or avocado in each meal. You may add extra nutrient-rich snacks to meet your increased energy and nutritional needs.

HARD TRAINING DAYS

On hard training days that comprise more than 2 hours' high-intensity endurance exercise, or two moderate- or high-intensity training sessions or events, your fuel and carbohydrate needs will be very high. Increase your intake of carbohydrate-rich foods. This will allow you to maintain muscle glycogen stores and support your training. Aim to have roughly one-half of your meal plate made up of carbohydrate-rich foods, roughly one-quarter protein-rich and calcium-rich foods and roughly one-quarter fruit and vegetables. Include some healthy fats such as olive or rapeseed oil, nuts, seeds, nut butter or avocado in each meal. You may add extra nutrient-rich snacks to meet your increased energy and nutritional needs.

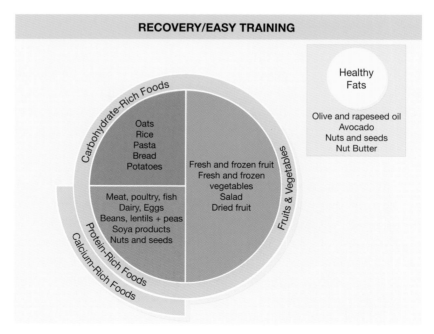

Figure 1.1 The Athlete's Plate for Easy Training or Recovery Days

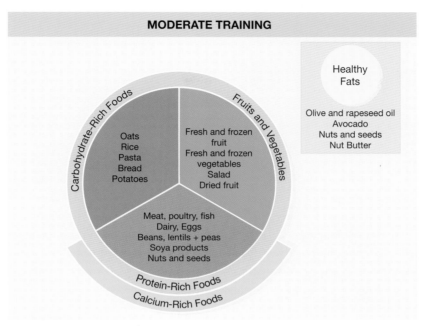

Figure 1.2 The Athlete's Plate for Moderate Training Days

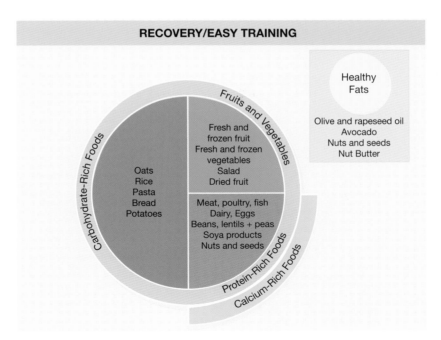

Figure 1.3 The Athlete's Plate for Hard Training Days

Energy for
// Exercise

When you exercise, your body must start producing energy much faster than it does when it is at rest. The muscles start to contract more strenuously, the heart beats faster to pump blood around the body more rapidly, and the lungs work harder. All these processes require extra energy. Where does it come from, and how can you make sure you have enough to last through a training session?

Before we can fully answer such questions, it is important to understand how the body produces energy, and what happens to it. This chapter looks at what takes place in the body when you exercise, where extra energy comes from, and how the fuel mixture used differs according to the intensity of exercise. It explains why fatigue occurs, how it might be delayed, and how you can get more out of training by changing your diet.

WHAT IS ENERGY?

Although we cannot actually see energy, we can see and feel its effects in terms of heat and physical work. But what exactly is it?

Energy is produced by the splitting of a chemical bond in a substance called adenosine triphosphate (ATP). This is often referred to as the body's 'energy currency'. It is produced in every cell of the body from the breakdown of carbohydrate,

fat, protein and alcohol – four fuels that are transported and transformed by various biochemical processes into the same end product.

WHAT IS ATP?

ATP is a small molecule consisting of an adenosine 'backbone' with three phosphate groups attached (*see* Fig 2.1).

Energy is released when one of the phosphate groups splits off. When ATP loses one of its phosphate groups it becomes adenosine diphosphate, or ADP. Some energy is used to carry out work (such as muscle contractions), but most (around three-quarters) is given off as heat. This is why you feel warmer when you exercise. Once this has

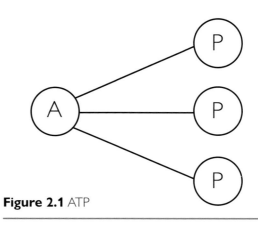

Figure 2.1 ATP

happened, ADP is converted back into ATP. A continual cycle takes place, in which ATP forms ADP and then becomes ATP again (*see* Fig 2.2).

THE INTER-CONVERSION OF ATP AND ADP

The body stores only very small amounts of ATP at any one time. There is just enough to keep up basic energy requirements while you are at rest – sufficient to keep the body ticking over. When you start exercising, energy demand suddenly increases, and ATP is used up within a few seconds. Therefore, more ATP must be produced in order to continue exercising. During intense exercise, muscle ATP production can increase 1000-fold.

HOW DOES THE BODY BURN ENERGY?

Total daily energy expenditure (TDEE) is comprised of four components: 1) resting metabolic rate (RMR, 2) the thermic effect of food (TEF), 3) exercise activity thermogenesis (EAT) and 4) non-exercise activity thermogenesis (NEAT) (*see* Fig 2.3). RMR is the energy burned at rest and makes up the largest component of TDEE, on average between 60 and 75%. TEF is the increase in energy expenditure above RMR that occurs after a meal and is the result of the digestion, absorption, metabolism and storage of food. It represents approximately 10% of TDEE, although the TEF for each macronutrient is different (*see* p. 183). NEAT is the energy burned during all unplanned activity, and may include day-to-day activities such as walking, or involuntary movements such as fidgeting. It typically makes up 15% of TDEE. EAT is the energy burned during planned exercise and is the most variable component of TDEE, ranging from 5% in sedentary people up to 50% in athletes involved in heavy

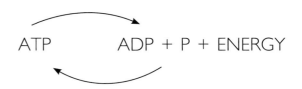

Figure 2.2 The relationship between ATP and ADP

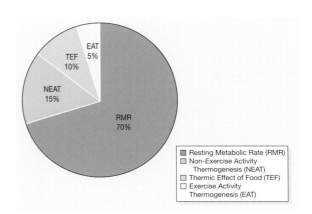

Figure 2.3 The components of total daily energy expenditure (TDEE)

training. EAT and NEAT can both be controlled voluntarily and are therefore extremely important for maintenance of daily energy balance.

WHERE DOES ENERGY COME FROM?

There are four components in food and drink that are capable of providing energy (ATP):

1. carbohydrate
2. protein
3. fat
4. alcohol

When you eat a meal or have a drink, these components are broken down in the digestive system into their various constituents or building blocks. Then they are absorbed into the bloodstream. Carbohydrates are broken down into small, single sugar units, the monosaccharides: glucose (the most common unit), fructose and galactose. Fats are broken down into fatty acids, and proteins into amino acids. Alcohol is mostly absorbed directly into the blood.

The ultimate fate of all of these components is energy production, although carbohydrates, proteins and fats also have other important functions.

Carbohydrates and alcohol are used mainly for energy in the short term, while fats are used as a long-term energy store. Proteins can be used to produce energy either in 'emergencies' (for instance, when carbohydrates are in short supply) or when they have reached the end of their useful life. Sooner or later, all food and drink components are broken down to release energy. But the body is not very efficient at converting this energy into power. For example, during cycling, only 20% of the energy produced is converted into power. The rest becomes heat.

HOW IS ENERGY MEASURED?

Energy is measured in calories or joules. In scientific terms, 1 calorie is defined as the amount of heat required to increase the temperature of 1 gram (or 1 ml) of water by 1 degree centigrade (°C) (from 14.5 to 15.5 °C). The SI (International Unit System) unit for energy is the joule (J). One joule is defined as the work required to exert a force of 1 Newton for a distance of 1 metre.

As the calorie and the joule represent very small amounts of energy, kilocalories (kcal or Cal) and kilojoules (kJ) are more often used. As their names suggest, a kilocalorie is 1000 calories and

a kilojoule 1000 joules. You have probably seen these units on food labels. When we mention calories in the everyday sense, we are really talking about Calories with a capital C, or kilocalories. So, food containing 100 kcal has enough energy potential to raise the temperature of 100 litres of water by 1°C.

To convert kilocalories into kilojoules, simply multiply by 4.2. For example:

- 1 kcal = 4.2 kJ
- 10 kcal = 42 kJ

To convert kilojoules into kilocalories, divide

Metabolism

Metabolism is the sum of all the biochemical processes that occur in the body. There are two aspects: 1) anabolism is the formation of larger molecules; 2) catabolism is the breakdown of larger molecules into smaller molecules. Aerobic metabolism includes oxygen in the processes; anaerobic metabolism takes place without oxygen. A metabolite is a product of metabolism. That means that anything made in the body is a metabolite.

The body's rate of energy expenditure is called the metabolic rate. Your basal metabolic rate (BMR) is the number of calories expended to maintain essential processes such as breathing and organ function during sleep. However, most methods measure the resting metabolic rate (RMR), which is the number of calories burned over 24 hours while lying down but not sleeping.

by 4.2. For example, if 100 g of food provides 400 kJ, and you wish to know how many kilocalories that is, divide 400 by 4.2 to find the equivalent number of kilocalories:

- 400 kJ ÷ 4.2 = 95 kcal

WHY DO DIFFERENT FOODS PROVIDE DIFFERENT AMOUNTS OF ENERGY?

Foods are made of different amounts of carbohydrates, fats, proteins and alcohol. Each of these nutrients provides a certain quantity of energy when it is broken down in the body. For instance, 1 g of carbohydrate or protein releases about 4 kcal of energy, while 1 g of fat releases 9 kcal, and 1 g of alcohol releases 7 kcal.

THE ENERGY VALUE OF DIFFERENT FOOD COMPONENTS

1 g of each of the following provides:

- carbohydrate: 4 kcal (17 kj)
- fat: 9 kcal (38 kj)
- protein: 4 kcal (17 kj)
- alcohol: 7 kcal (29 kj)

Fat is the most concentrated form of energy, providing the body with more than twice as much energy as carbohydrate or protein, and also more than alcohol. However, it is not necessarily the 'best' form of energy for exercise.

All foods contain a mixture of nutrients, and the energy value of a particular food depends on the amount of carbohydrate, fat and protein it contains. For example, one slice of wholemeal bread provides roughly the same amount of energy as one pat (7 g) of butter. However, their composition is very different. In bread, most

energy (75%) comes from carbohydrate, while in butter, virtually all (99.7%) comes from fat.

HOW DOES MY BODY STORE CARBOHYDRATE?

Carbohydrate is stored as *glycogen* in the muscles and liver, along with about three times its own weight of water. Altogether there is about three times more glycogen stored in the muscles than in the liver. Glycogen is a large molecule, similar to starch, made up of many glucose units joined together. However, the body can store only a relatively small amount of glycogen – there is no endless supply! Like the petrol tank in a car, the body can hold only a certain amount.

The total store of glycogen in the average body amounts to about 500 g, with approximately 400 g in the muscles and 100 g in the liver. This store is equivalent to about 2000 kcal – enough to last 1 day if you were to eat nothing and do no activity. This is why a low-carbohydrate diet tends to make people lose quite a lot of weight in the first few days. The weight loss is almost entirely due to loss of glycogen and water.

Glycogen stores can be almost entirely depleted by the end of 90–120 minutes of moderate- or high-intensity exercise and at this point you would experience extreme fatigue. Endurance athletes have higher muscle glycogen concentrations compared with sedentary people. Increasing your muscle mass will also increase your storage capacity for glycogen.

The purpose of liver glycogen is to maintain blood glucose levels both at rest and during prolonged exercise.

Small amounts of glucose are present in the blood (approximately 4 g, which is equivalent to 16 kcal) and the concentration is kept within a

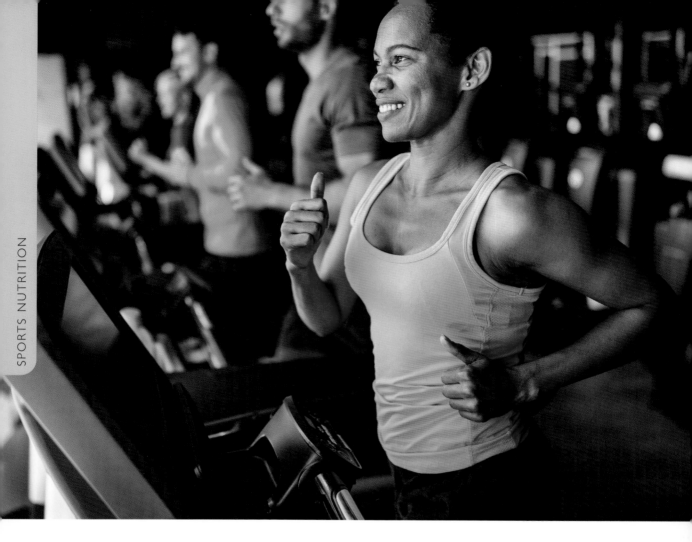

very narrow range (between 4 and 5.5 mmol/ litre, or 70–100 mg/100 ml), both at rest and during exercise. This allows normal body functions to continue. When blood glucose levels rise, the pancreas releases insulin, which causes glucose to move from the blood into the liver and muscle cells. If glucose is not needed for energy immediately it is stored in the form of glycogen, a process known as glycogenesis. Conversely, when blood glucose levels fall, the pancreas releases glucagon, which tells the liver and muscles to break down glycogen and release it back into the bloodstream as glucose, a process known as glycogenolysis.

Once glycogen stores are full, surplus glucose may be converted to fat in a process known as de novo lipogenesis (DNL). However, this process is inefficient and only stores a small amount of fat when you are in positive energy balance (Acheson *et al.*, 1988). Rather than being converted to fat, excessive carbohydrate intake usually leads to fat storage from fat. This is due to oxidative priority: carbohydrate is preferentially oxidised at the expense of fat oxidation (Cronise *et al.*, 2017). Thus, an excessive carbohydrate intake slows or displaces fat oxidation, resulting in fat storage mainly from dietary fat.

HOW DOES MY BODY STORE FAT?

Fat is stored as *adipose* (fat) tissue in almost every region of the body. A small amount of fat, about 300–400 g, is stored in muscles – this is called intramuscular fat – but the majority is stored around the organs and beneath the skin. The amount stored in different parts of the body depends on genetic make-up and individual hormone balance. The average 70 kg person stores 10–15 kg fat. Interestingly, people who store fat mostly around their abdomen (the classic potbelly shape) have a higher risk of heart disease than those who store fat mostly around their hips and thighs (the classic pear shape).

Unfortunately, there is little you can do to change the way that your body distributes fat. But you can definitely change the *amount* of fat that is stored, as you will see in Chapter 9.

You will probably find that your basic shape is similar to that of one or both of your parents. Males usually take after their father, and females after their mother. Female hormones tend to favour fat storage around the hips and thighs, while male hormones encourage fat storage around the middle. This is why, in general, women are 'pear shaped' and men are 'apple shaped'.

HOW DOES MY BODY STORE PROTEIN?

Protein is not stored in the same way as carbohydrate and fat. It forms muscle and organ tissue, so it is mainly used as a building material rather than an energy store. However, proteins *can* be broken down to release energy if need be, so muscles and organs represent a large source of potential energy.

WHICH FUELS ARE MOST IMPORTANT FOR EXERCISE?

Carbohydrates, fats and proteins are all capable of providing energy for exercise; they can all be transported to, and broken down in, muscle cells. Alcohol, however, cannot be used directly by muscles for energy during exercise, no matter how strenuously they may be working. Only the liver has the specific enzymes needed to break down alcohol. You cannot break down alcohol faster by exercising harder, either – the liver carries out its job at a fixed speed. Do not think you can work off a few drinks by going for a jog, or by drinking a cup of black coffee!

Proteins do not make a substantial contribution to the fuel mixture. It is only when carbohydrate availability is low, such as during very prolonged or very intense bouts of exercise, that proteins play a more important role in giving the body energy.

The production of ATP during most forms of exercise comes mainly from broken-down carbohydrates and fats.

Table 2.1 illustrates the potential energy available from the different types of fuel that are stored in the body.

Table 2.1	ENERGY RESERVES IN A PERSON WEIGHING 70 KG		
Fuel stores	**Potential energy available (kcal)**		
	Glycogen	Fat	Protein
Liver	400	450	400
Adipose tissue (fat)	0	135,000	0
Muscle	1600	350	24,000

Source: Cahill, 1976.

WHEN IS PROTEIN USED FOR ENERGY?

Protein is not usually a major source of energy, but it may play a more important role during the latter stages of very strenuous or prolonged exercise as glycogen stores become depleted. For example, during the last stages of a marathon or a long-distance cycle race, when glycogen stores are exhausted, protein in muscles (and organs) may be broken down to make up to 15% of the body's fuel mixture.

During a period of semi-starvation, or if a person follows a low-carbohydrate diet, glycogen would be in short supply, so more proteins would be broken down to provide the body with fuel. Up to half of the weight lost by someone following a low-calorie or low-carbohydrate diet comes from protein (muscle) loss. Some people think that if they deplete their glycogen stores by following a low-carbohydrate diet, they will force their body to break down more fat and lose weight. This is not the case: you risk losing muscle as well as fat, and there are many other disadvantages, too. These are discussed in Chapter 3.

How is energy produced?

The body has three main energy systems it can use for different types of physical activity. These are called:

1. the ATP–PC (phosphagen) system
2. the anaerobic glycolytic, or lactic acid, system
3. the aerobic system – comprising the glycolytic (carbohydrate) and lipolytic (fat) systems

At rest, muscle cells contain only a very small amount of ATP, enough to maintain basic energy

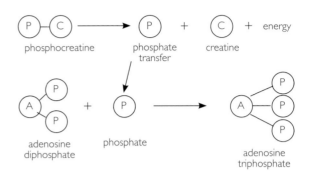

Figure 2.4 PC splits to release energy to regenerate ATP rapidly

needs and allow you to exercise at maximal intensity for about 1 second. To continue exercising, ATP must be regenerated from one of the three energy systems, each of which has a very different biochemical pathway and rate at which it produces ATP.

HOW DOES THE ATP–PC SYSTEM WORK?

This system uses ATP and phosphocreatine (PC) that is stored within the muscle cells to generate energy for maximal bursts of strength and speed that last for up to 6 seconds. The ATP–PC system would be used, for example, during a 20 m sprint, a near-maximal lift in the gym, or a single jump. Phosphocreatine is a high-energy compound formed when the protein, creatine, is linked to a phosphate molecule (*see* p. 23). The PC system can be thought of as a back-up to ATP. The job of PC is to regenerate ATP rapidly (*see* Fig. 2.4). PC breaks down into creatine and phosphate, and the free phosphate bond transfers to a molecule of ADP forming a new ATP molecule. The ATP–PC system can release energy very quickly, but, unfortunately, it is in very

What is creatine?

Creatine is a compound that's made naturally in our bodies to supply energy. It is mainly produced in the liver from the amino acids glycine, arginine and methionine. From the liver, it is transported in the blood to the muscle cells where it is combined with phosphate to make phosphocreatine (PC).

The muscle cells turn over about 2–3 g of creatine a day. Once PC is broken down into ATP (energy), it can be recycled into PC or converted into another substance called creatinine, which is then removed via the kidneys in the urine.

Creatine can be obtained in the diet from fish (tuna, salmon, cod), beef and pork (approx. 3–5 g creatine/kg uncooked fish or meat). That means vegetarians have no dietary sources. However, to have a performance-boosting effect, creatine has to be taken in large doses. This is higher than you could reasonably expect to get from food. You would need to eat at least 2 kg of raw steak a day to load your muscles with creatine.

The average-sized person stores about 120 g creatine, almost all in skeletal muscles (higher levels in fast-twitch muscle fibres, see p. 25). Of this amount, 60–70% is stored as PC, 30–40% as free creatine.

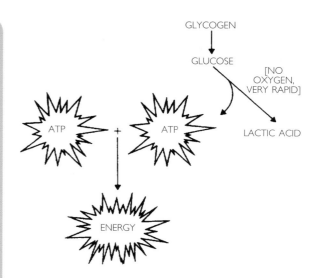

Figure 2.5 Anaerobic energy system

HOW DOES THE ANAEROBIC GLYCOLYTIC SYSTEM WORK?

This system is activated as soon as you begin high-intensity activity. It dominates in events lasting up to 90 seconds, such as a weight training set in the gym or a 400–800 m sprint. In order to meet sudden, large demands for energy, glucose bypasses the energy producing pathways that would normally use oxygen, and follows a different route that does not use oxygen. This saves a good deal of time. After 30 seconds of high-intensity exercise this system contributes up to 60% of your energy output; after 2 minutes its contribution falls to only 35%.

The anaerobic glycolytic system uses carbohydrate in the form of muscle glycogen or glucose as fuel. Glycogen is broken down to glucose, which rapidly breaks down in the absence of oxygen to form ATP and pyruvate, which is then converted into lactate (*see* Fig. 2.5). Each glucose molecule

limited supply and can provide only 3–4 kcal. After this, the amount of energy produced by the ATP–PC system falls dramatically, and ATP must be produced from other fuels, such as glycogen or fat. When this happens, other systems take over.

What happens to the lactate?

Lactate produced by the muscles is not a wasted by-product. It constitutes a valuable fuel. When the exercise intensity is reduced or you stop exercising, lactate has two possible fates. Some may be converted into another substance called pyruvic acid, which can then be broken down in the presence of oxygen into ATP. In other words, lactate produces ATP and constitutes a valuable fuel for aerobic exercise. Alternatively, lactate may be carried away from the muscle in the bloodstream to the liver where it can be converted back into glucose, released back into the bloodstream or stored as glycogen in the liver (a process called gluconeogenesis). This mechanism for removing lactic acid from the muscles is called the lactate shuttle.

This explains why the muscle soreness and stiffness experienced after hard training is not due to lactate or lactic acid accumulation. In fact, the lactate is usually cleared within 15 minutes of exercise.

sity or take a short rest before resuming all-out effort. Once hydrogen ions are removed and the pH rises, you will be able to resume exercising at a high intensity. Contrary to popular belief, it is not lactic acid but the build-up of hydrogen ions (acidity) that causes the 'burning' feeling during or immediately after maximal exercise.

HOW DOES THE AEROBIC SYSTEM WORK?

The aerobic system can generate ATP from the breakdown of carbohydrates (by glycolysis) and fat (by lipolysis) in the presence of oxygen (*see* Fig. 2.6). Although the aerobic system cannot produce ATP as rapidly as can the other two anaerobic systems, it can produce larger amounts. When you start to exercise, you initially use the ATP–PC and anaerobic glycolytic systems, but after a few minutes your energy supply gradually switches to the aerobic system.

Most of the carbohydrate that fuels aerobic glycolysis comes from muscle glycogen. Additional glucose from the bloodstream becomes more important as exercise continues for longer than 1 hour and muscle glycogen concentration dwindles. Typically, after 2 hours of high-intensity exercise (greater than 70% VO_2max), almost all of your muscle glycogen will be depleted. Glucose delivered from the bloodstream is then used to fuel your muscles, along with increasing amounts of fat (lipolytic glycolysis). Glucose from the bloodstream may be derived from the breakdown of liver glycogen or from carbohydrate consumed during exercise.

In aerobic exercise, the demand for energy is slower and smaller than in an anaerobic activity, so there is more time to transport sufficient oxygen from the lungs to the muscles and for glucose to

produces only two ATP molecules under anaerobic conditions, making it a very inefficient system. The body's glycogen stores dwindle quickly, proving that the benefits of a fast delivery service come at a price. The gradual build-up of lactate and the associated hydrogen ions causes the pH in the cell to fall (i.e. an increase in acidity), preventing further muscle contractions. At this point, exercise can no longer be maintained at the same intensity – you'll experience temporary fatigue and will either need to drop your inten-

generate ATP with the help of the oxygen. Under these circumstances, one molecule of glucose can create up to 38 molecules of ATP. Thus, aerobic energy production is about 20 times more efficient than anaerobic energy production.

Anaerobic exercise uses only glycogen, whereas aerobic exercise uses both glycogen and fat, so it can be kept up for longer. The disadvantage, though, is that it produces energy more slowly.

Fats can also be used to produce energy in the aerobic system. One fatty acid can produce between 80 and 200 ATP molecules, depending on its type (*see* Fig. 2.6). Fats are therefore an even more efficient energy source than carbohydrates. However, they can only be broken down into ATP under aerobic conditions when energy demands are relatively low, and so energy production is slower.

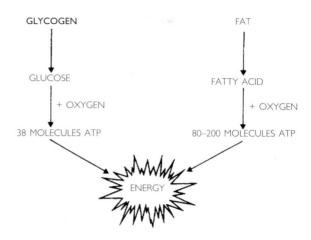

Figure 2.6 Aerobic energy system

MUSCLE FIBRE TYPES AND ENERGY PRODUCTION

The body has several different muscle fibre types, which can be broadly classified into fast-twitch (FT) or type II, and slow-twitch (ST) or type I (endurance) fibres. Both muscle fibre types use all three energy systems to produce ATP, but the FT fibres use mainly the ATP–PC and anaerobic glycolytic systems, while the ST fibres use mainly the aerobic system.

Everyone is born with a specific distribution of muscle fibre types; the proportion of FT fibres to ST fibres can vary quite considerably between individuals. The proportion of each muscle fibre type you have has implications for sport. For example, top sprinters have a greater proportion of FT fibres than average and thus can generate explosive power and speed. Distance runners, on the other hand, have proportionally more

ST fibres and are better able to develop aerobic power and endurance.

HOW DO MY MUSCLES DECIDE WHETHER TO USE CARBOHYDRATE OR FAT DURING AEROBIC EXERCISE?

During aerobic exercise, the use of carbohydrate relative to fat varies according to a number of factors. The most important are:

1. the intensity of exercise
2. the duration of exercise
3. your fitness level
4. your pre-exercise diet

Intensity

The greater the exercise intensity, the greater the rate at which muscle glycogen is broken down (*see* Fig. 2.7). During anaerobic exercise, energy is produced by the ATP–PC and anaerobic glycolytic systems. So, for example, during sprints, heavy weight training and intermittent maximal bursts during sports such as football and rugby,

SPORTS NUTRITION

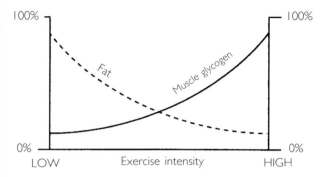

Figure 2.7 Fuel mixture/exercise intensity
Source: Costill, 1986.

muscle glycogen, rather than fat, is the major fuel. As a result, muscle glycogen stores can become quickly depleted even though the total duration of the activity may be relatively short.

During aerobic exercise you will use a mixture of muscle glycogen and fat for energy. Exercise at a low intensity (less than 50% of VO_2max) is fuelled mainly by fat. As you increase your exercise intensity – for example, as you increase your running speed – you will use a higher proportion of glycogen than fat. During moderate-intensity exercise (50–70% VO_2max), muscle glycogen supplies around half your energy needs; the rest comes from fat. When your exercise intensity exceeds 70% VO_2max, fat cannot be broken down and transported fast enough to meet energy demands, so muscle glycogen provides at least 75% of your energy needs.

Duration

Muscle glycogen is unable to provide energy indefinitely because it is stored in relatively small quantities. As you continue exercising, your muscle glycogen stores become progressively lower (*see* Fig. 2.8). Thus, as muscle glycogen

concentration drops, the contribution that blood glucose makes to your energy needs increases. The proportion of fat used for energy also increases but it can never be burned without the presence of carbohydrate.

On average, you have enough muscle glycogen to fuel 90–180 minutes of endurance activity; the higher the intensity, the faster your muscle glycogen stores will be depleted. During interval training, i.e. a mixture of endurance and anaerobic activity, muscle glycogen stores will become depleted after 45–90 minutes. During mainly anaerobic activities, muscle glycogen will deplete within 30–45 minutes.

Once muscle glycogen stores are depleted, protein makes an increasing contribution to energy needs. Muscle proteins break down to provide amino acids for energy production and to maintain normal blood glucose levels.

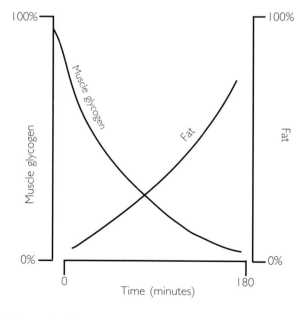

Figure 2.8 Fuel mixture/exercise duration

Fitness level

As a result of aerobic training, your muscles make a number of adaptations to improve your performance, and your body's ability to use fat as a fuel improves. Aerobic training increases the numbers of key fat-oxidising enzymes, such as hormone-sensitive lipase, which means your body becomes more efficient at breaking down fat into fatty acids. The number of blood capillaries serving the muscle increases so you can transport the fatty acids to the muscle cells. The number of mitochondria (the sites of fatty acid oxidation) also increases, which means you have a greater capacity to burn fatty acids in each muscle cell. Thus, improved aerobic fitness enables you to break down fat at a faster rate at any given intensity, thus allowing you to spare glycogen (*see* Fig. 2.9). This is important because glycogen is in much shorter supply than fat. By using propor-

tionally more fat, you will be able to exercise for longer before muscle glycogen is depleted and fatigue sets in.

Pre-exercise diet

A low-carbohydrate diet will result in low muscle and liver glycogen stores. Many studies have shown that initial muscle glycogen concentration is critical to your performance and that low muscle glycogen can reduce your ability to sustain exercise at 70% VO_2max for longer than 1 hour (Bergstrom *et al.*, 1967). It also affects your ability to perform during shorter periods of maximal power output.

When your muscle glycogen stores are low, your body will rely heavily on fat and protein. However, this is not a recommended strategy for fat loss, as you will lose lean tissue. (*See* Chapter 10 for appropriate ways of reducing body fat.)

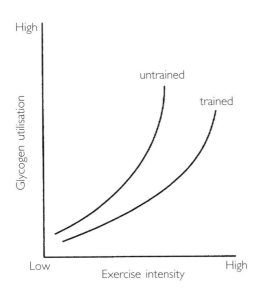

Figure 2.9 Trained people use less glycogen and more fat

Which energy systems do I use in my sport?

Virtually every activity uses all three energy systems to a greater or lesser extent. No single energy system is used exclusively and at any given time energy is being derived from each of the three systems (*see* Fig. 2.10). In every activity, ATP is always used and is replaced by PC. Anaerobic glycolysis and aerobic energy production depend on exercise intensity.

For example, during explosive strength and power activities lasting up to 5 seconds, such as a sprint start, the existing store of ATP is the primary energy source. For activities involving high power and speed lasting 5–30 seconds, such as 100–200 m sprints, the ATP–PC system is the primary energy source, together with some muscle glycogen broken down through anaerobic glycolysis. During power endurance activities such as 400–800 m events, muscle glycogen is the primary energy source and produces ATP via both anaerobic and aerobic glycolysis. In aerobic power activities, such as running 5–10 km, muscle glycogen is the primary energy source producing ATP via aerobic glycolysis. During aerobic events lasting 2 hours or more, such as half- and full marathons, muscle glycogen, liver glycogen, intramuscular fat and fat from adipose tissue are the main fuels used. The energy systems and fuels used for various types of activities are summarised in Table 2.2.

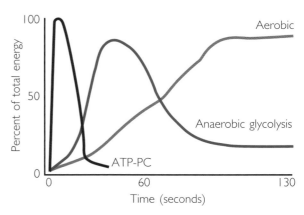

Figure 2.10 Percentage contribution of energy systems during exercise of different durations

Table 2.2	THE MAIN ENERGY SYSTEMS USED DURING DIFFERENT TYPES OF EXERCISE	
Type of exercise	**Main energy system**	**Major storage fuels used**
Maximal short bursts lasting less than 6 sec	ATP–PC (phosphagen)	ATP and PC
High-intensity lasting up to 30 sec	ATP–PC Anaerobic glycolytic	ATP and PC Muscle glycogen
High-intensity lasting up to 15 min	Anaerobic glycolytic Aerobic	Muscle glycogen
Moderate–high-intensity lasting 15–60 min	Aerobic	Muscle glycogen Adipose tissue
Moderate–high-intensity lasting 60–90 min	Aerobic	Muscle glycogen Liver glycogen Blood glucose Intramuscular fat Adipose tissue
Moderate intensity lasting longer than 90 min	Aerobic	Muscle glycogen Liver glycogen Blood glucose Intramuscular fat Adipose tissue

WHAT HAPPENS IN MY BODY WHEN I START EXERCISING?

When you begin to exercise, energy is produced without oxygen for at least the first few seconds, before your breathing rate and heart can catch up with oxygen demands. In effect, the anaerobic system 'buys time' in the first few seconds to minutes of exercise, before the body's slower aerobic system can start to function.

If you continue to exercise aerobically, more oxygen is delivered around the body and fat can be broken down into fatty acids. Carbohydrate (glucose and glycogen) and fatty acids are then broken down with oxygen to produce energy.

For the first 5–15 minutes of exercise (depending on your aerobic fitness level) the main fuel is carbohydrate (glycogen). As time goes on, however, more oxygen is delivered to the muscles, and you will use proportionally less carbohydrate and more fat.

On the other hand, if you begin exercising very strenuously (e.g. by running fast), lactate quickly builds up in the muscles. The delivery of oxygen cannot keep pace with the huge energy demand, so lactate and hydrogen ions accumulate and very soon you will feel fatigue (temporarily). You must then either slow down and exercise more slowly, or stop. Nobody can maintain all-out exercise for very long.

If you start a distance race or training run too fast, you will suffer from fatigue early on and be forced to reduce your pace considerably. A head start will not necessarily give any benefit at all. Warm up *before* the start of a race (by walking, slow jogging, or performing gentle mobility exercises), so that the heart and lungs can start to work a little harder, and oxygen delivery to the muscles can increase. Start the race at a moderate pace, gradually building up to an optimal speed. This will prevent a large 'oxygen debt' and avoid an early depletion of glycogen. In this way, your optimal pace can be sustained for longer.

The anaerobic system can also 'cut in' to help energy production, for instance when the demand for energy temporarily exceeds the body's oxygen supply. If you run uphill at the same pace as on the flat, your energy demand increases. The body will generate extra energy by breaking down glycogen/glucose anaerobically. However, this can be kept up for only a short period of time, because there will be a gradual build-up of hydrogen ions. The lactate and hydrogen ions can be removed aerobically afterwards, by running back down the hill, for example.

The same principle applies during fast bursts of activity in interval training, when energy is produced anaerobically. Lactic acid accumulates and is then removed during the rest interval.

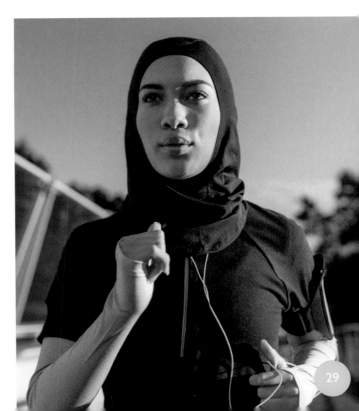

What is fatigue?

In scientific terms, fatigue is an inability to sustain a given power output or speed. It is a mismatch between the demand for energy by the exercising muscles and the supply of energy in the form of ATP. Runners experience fatigue when they are no longer able to maintain their speed; footballers are slower to sprint for the ball and their technical ability falters; in the gym, you can no longer lift the weight; in an aerobics class, you will be unable to maintain the pace and intensity. Subjectively, you will find that exercise feels much harder to perform, your legs may feel hollow and it becomes increasingly hard to push yourself.

WHY DOES FATIGUE DEVELOP DURING ANAEROBIC EXERCISE?

During explosive activities involving maximal power output, fatigue develops due to ATP and PC depletion. In other words, the demand for ATP exceeds the readily available supply.

During activities lasting between 30 seconds and 30 minutes, fatigue is caused by a different mechanism. The rate of lactate removal in the bloodstream cannot keep pace with the rate of lactic acid production. This means that during high-intensity exercise there is a gradual increase in muscle acidity, which reduces the ability of the muscles to maintain intense contractions. It is not possible to continue high-intensity exercise indefinitely because the acute acid environment in your muscles would inhibit further contractions and cause cell death. The burning feeling you experience when a high concentration of hydrogen ions develops is a kind of safety mechanism, preventing the muscle cells from destruction.

Reducing your exercise intensity will lower the rate of lactate production, reduce the hydrogen

ion build-up, and enable the muscles to switch to the aerobic energy system, thus enabling you to continue exercising.

WHY DOES FATIGUE DEVELOP DURING AEROBIC EXERCISE?

Fatigue during moderate- and high-intensity aerobic exercise lasting longer than 1 hour occurs when muscle glycogen stores are depleted. It's like running out of petrol in your car. Muscle glycogen is in short supply compared with the body's fat stores. Liver glycogen can help maintain blood glucose levels and a supply of carbohydrate to the exercising muscles, but stores are also very limited and eventually fatigue will develop as a result of both muscle and liver glycogen depletion and hypoglycaemia (*see* Fig. 2.11).

During low- to moderate- intensity exercise lasting more than 3 hours, fatigue is caused by additional factors. Once glycogen stores have been exhausted, the body switches to the aerobic lipolytic system where fat is able to supply most (not all) of the fuel for low-intensity exercise.

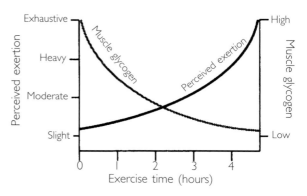

Figure 2.11 The increase in perceived exertion as glycogen stores become depleted
Source: Costill, 1986.

However, despite having relatively large fat reserves, you will not be able to continue exercise indefinitely because fat cannot be converted to energy fast enough to keep up with the demand by exercising muscles. Even if you slowed your pace to enable the energy supplied by fat to meet the energy demand, other factors will cause you to fatigue. These include a rise in the concentration of the brain chemical serotonin, which results in an overall feeling of tiredness, acute muscle damage, and fatigue due to lack of sleep.

HOW CAN I DELAY FATIGUE?

Glycogen is used during virtually every type of activity. Therefore the amount of glycogen stored in your muscles and, in certain events, your liver, before you begin exercise will have a direct effect on your endurance performance. The greater your pre-exercise muscle glycogen store, the longer you will be able to maintain your exercise intensity and delay the onset of fatigue. Conversely, suboptimal muscle glycogen stores can cause earlier fatigue, reduce your endurance, reduce your intensity level and result in smaller training gains.

You may also delay fatigue by reducing the rate at which you use up muscle glycogen. You can do this by pacing yourself, gradually building up to your optimal intensity, and/or by consuming carbohydrate during exercise.

Summary of key points

- The body uses three energy systems: 1) the ATP–PC, or phosphagen, system; 2) the anaerobic glycolytic, or lactic acid, system; 3) the aerobic system, which comprises both glycolytic (carbohydrate) and lipolytic (fat) systems.

- The ATP–PC system fuels maximal bursts of activity lasting up to 6 seconds.
- Anaerobic glycolysis provides energy for short-duration, high-intensity exercise lasting from 30 seconds to several minutes. Muscle glycogen is the main fuel.
- The lacate produced during anaerobic glycolysis is a valuable fuel for further energy production when exercise intensity is reduced.
- The aerobic system provides energy from the breakdown of carbohydrate and fat for submaximal intensity, prolonged exercise.
- Factors that influence the type of energy system and fuel usage are exercise intensity and duration, your fitness level and your pre-exercise diet.
- The proportion of muscle glycogen used for energy increases with exercise intensity and decreases with exercise duration.
- For most activities lasting longer than 30 seconds, all three energy systems are used to a greater or lesser extent; however, one system usually dominates.
- The main cause of fatigue during anaerobic activities lasting less than 6 seconds is ATP and PC depletion; during activities lasting between 30 seconds and 30 minutes, it is hydrogen ion accumulation and muscle cell acidity.
- Fatigue during moderate and high-intensity exercise lasting longer than 1 hour is usually due to muscle glycogen depletion. For events lasting longer than 2 hours, fatigue is associated with low liver glycogen and low blood sugar levels.
- For most activities, performance is limited by the amount of glycogen in the muscles. Low pre-exercise glycogen stores lead to early fatigue, reduced exercise intensity and reduced training gains.

//**Carbohydrate**

Since the beginning of the 20th century, it has been known that carbohydrate is related to performance. In 1924, researchers suggested that low blood glucose concentrations observed at the end of a marathon were associated with fatigue and an inability to concentrate (Levine *et al.*, 1924). In 1939, Christensen and Hansen, demonstrated that a high-carbohydrate diet significantly increased endurance (Christensen and Hansen, 1939). However, it wasn't until the 1960s that scientists discovered that the capacity for endurance exercise is related to pre-exercise glycogen stores and that a high-carbohydrate diet increases glycogen stores. In a pioneering study, Swedish researchers demonstrated that athletes who consumed a high-carbohydrate diet were able to increase their glycogen stores to a greater extent than those consuming a moderate- or low-carbohydrate diet, and were subsequently able to exercise significant longer before reaching fatigue (Bergstrom *et al.*, 1967). Another study in 1967 confirmed the link between glycogen storage in muscles and endurance (Ahlborg *et al.* 1967).

These observations led to the recommendations to carbohydrate load before competition. This was successfully used by runners such as the late Ron Hill who won the 1969 European Athletics championships by undergoing a 3-day glycogen depletion phase followed by a high carbohydrate intake for the final 3 days. In the 1980s, the effects of consuming carbohydrate during exercise on performance were further studied (Coyle and Coggan, 1984; Coyle *et al.* 1986).

This chapter explains the role of carbohydrate intake in exercise performance. More specifically, it looks at the optimal timing of carbohydrate intake in relation to exercise, and provides guidelines for pre-, during and post-exercise carbohydrate intake as well as total daily carbohydrate intake, and shows you how to calculate your daily requirements.

It also gives advice on which types of carbohydrate foods to eat. Finally, it considers the potential benefits and drawbacks of low-carbohydrate diets, training with low carbohydrate availability and carbohydrate periodisation.

Why is carbohydrate important for performance?

Carbohydrate, in the form of glucose, provides a fuel source for every cell in the body. It's the preferred fuel for the brain, nervous system and heart and is used by the muscles to support both aerobic and anaerobic activities. Any glucose that's not needed immediately for energy is converted to glycogen, which is stored in the cells of the liver and muscles (*see* p. 19 'How does my body store carbohydrate?'). The liver can store a maximum of 100 g of glycogen and the muscles a maximum of 400 g, equivalent to a total of 500 g or 2000 kcal worth of energy in an average person. This is sufficient to fuel approximately 90 to 120 minutes of moderate–high-intensity aerobic exercise. The size of your glycogen stores is relatively small compared to your fat stores, which can be several kilos, and can be acutely manipulated by your carbohydrate intake in the preceding hours or days, or even a single session of exercise.

The rate at which muscle glycogen is utilised depends mainly on exercise intensity. At low intensities, your muscles oxidise a mixture of fat and carbohydrate. As the exercise intensity increases, a higher proportion of carbohydrate from muscle glycogen is broken down (*see* pp. 25–26). At very high intensities, muscle glycogen is the dominant fuel as it can be broken down very rapidly to produce energy. During high-intensity

aerobic exercise, carbohydrate offers advantages over fat because it is a more efficient fuel, i.e. it provides more molecules of ATP per volume of oxygen consumed. For this reason, carbohydrate is sometimes referred to as a 'fast' fuel while fat is referred to as a 'slow' fuel because it produces energy relatively slowly. Carbohydrate can produce up to 25–30 kcal per minute; while fat produces only 6 kcal per minute.

How does carbohydrate affect performance?

Carbohydrate availability – the amount of glucose in your bloodstream and glycogen stored in your muscles and liver – has a direct effect on exercise performance. There is plentiful evidence that exercising with 'high carbohydrate availability' (i.e. when muscle glycogen stores and blood glucose are matched to the demands of exercise) enhances endurance and performance during exercise lasting longer than 90 minutes or intermittent high-intensity exercise (Hargreaves *et al.*, 2004; Coyle, 2004; Burke *et al.*, 2004; Thomas *et al.*, 2016; Burke *et al.*, 2011).

In a pioneering study, three groups of athletes were given a low-carbohydrate diet (about 10% of dietary energy), a high-carbohydrate diet (about 70%) or a moderate carbohydrate diet (about 50%) (Bergstrom *et al.*, 1967). Researchers measured the concentration of glycogen in their leg muscles and found that those eating the high-carbohydrate diet stored twice as much glycogen as those on the moderate carbohydrate diet and seven times as much as those eating the low-carbohydrate diet. Afterwards, the athletes were instructed to cycle to exhaustion on a stationary bicycle at 75% of VO_2max. Those on the

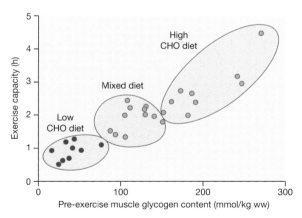

Figure 3.1 The effect of carbohydrate intake on performance

high-carbohydrate diet managed to cycle for 170 minutes, considerably longer than those on the moderate carbohydrate diet (115 minutes) or the low-carbohydrate diet (60 minutes) (*see* Fig 3.1). There was a linear trend between between carbohydrate intake and exercise capacity, suggesting that a high-carbohydrate diet is beneficial for endurance performance (*see* Fig 3.2).

Therefore, for most endurance activities, scientists recommend consuming a high-carbohydrate diet to replenish muscle glycogen stores and promote optimal adaptation to regular training. Depletion of these stores ('low carbohydrate availability') results in fatigue and reduced work rates, impaired skill and concentration and increased perception of effort. In other words, when your glycogen stores become depleted, your capacity for high-intensity exercise will be limited and only low-intensity exercise is possible. This can easily happen if your pre-exercise glycogen stores are low.

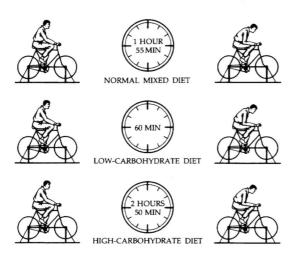

Figure 3.2 The effect of carbohydrate intake on exercise capacity (Bergstrom *et al.*, 1967)

In order to optimise your performance during high-intensity exercise longer than 90 minutes or doing high-intensity intermittent exercise, you should ensure your daily carbohydrate intake matches the fuel needs of your training and that pre-exercise glycogen stores are high. This will help to improve your endurance, delay exhaustion and help you exercise longer and harder (Coyle, 1988; Costill and Hargreaves, 1992).

In a study at Ball State University, Indiana, volunteers ran 16 km on three consecutive days at 80% VO_2max (Costill *et al.*, 1971) while consuming a moderate-carbohydrate diet (40% carbohydrate). A marked decrease in muscle glycogen occurred immediately after the run and although some glycogen was replenished before the next run session the starting glycogen concentrations were lower. Over successive days of training, their glycogen stores became progressively lower, suggesting that they were not consuming enough carbohydrate to fully restore muscle glycogen (*see* Fig 3.3 (b), p. 50).

In another study, volunteers were given a diet containing either 5 g or 10 g carbohydrate/kg of body weight for 7 successive days of training (Sherman *et al.*, 1993). Those consuming 5 g/kg BW experienced a significant decline in muscle glycogen, but those consuming 10 g/kg BW were able to maintain their muscle glycogen stores despite daily training. If you exercise every day then rapid replenishment of muscle glycogen is crucial.

How much carbohydrate should I eat per day?

Previously, researchers recommended a diet providing 60–70% energy from carbohydrate based on the consensus statement from the International Conference on Foods, Nutrition and Performance in 1991 (Williams and Devlin, 1992). However, this recommendation assumes an optimal energy (calorie) intake and does not take into account different training loads on different days. For these reasons, it is no longer considered valid.

Nowadays, scientists recommend calculating your daily carbohydrate requirement from your body weight and also your training volume (Burke *et al.*, 2011; IOC, 2011; Thomas *et al.*, 2016). The ACSM guidelines shown in Table 3.1 express carbohydrate intake in grams per kilogram of body weight. They are intended to provide high carbohydrate availability and enable you to replace your muscle glycogen stores within 24 hours. They assume that your glycogen storage capacity is roughly proportional to your muscle mass and body weight – i.e. the heavier you are, the greater your muscle mass and the greater your glycogen storage capacity. They also allow for daily adjustment according to your training load; the greater your training load, the more carbohydrate you will need to fuel your muscles.

These recommendations are general but most athletes training for up to 1 hour daily are likely to require 5–7 g carbohydrate/kg body weight; however, on heavier training days your requirements may be higher and on lighter training or recovery days your requirements may be lower.

For example, for a 70 kg athlete who trains for 1 hour a day:

- carbohydrate intake = 5–7 g/kg of body weight
- daily carbohydrate intake = $(70 \times 5) - (70 \times 7)$ = 350–490 g

What types of carbohydrate are there?

Carbohydrates are traditionally classified according to their chemical structure. The most simplistic method divides them into two categories: *simple* (sugars) and *complex* (starches and fibres). These terms simply refer to the number of sugar units in the molecule.

Simple carbohydrates are very small molecules consisting of 1 or 2 sugar units. They comprise the *monosaccharides* (1-sugar units): glucose (dextrose), fructose (fruit sugar) and galactose; and the *disaccharides* (2-sugar units): sucrose

Table 3.1	GUIDELINES FOR DAILY CARBOHYDRATE INTAKE	
Training load		**Carbohydrate intake (g/kg body mass)**
Light	Low-intensity or skill-based activities	3–5 g/kg/d
Moderate	Moderate exercise programme (e.g. 1 h/day)	5–7 g/kg/d
High	Endurance programme (e.g. 1–3 h/day of moderate–high intensity)	6–10 g/kg/d
Very high	Extreme commitment (e.g. >4–5 h/day of moderate–high intensity)	8–12 g/kg/d

Source: Thomas *et al.*, 2016.

(table sugar, which comprises a glucose and fructose molecule joined together) and lactose (milk sugar, which comprises a glucose and galactose molecule joined together).

Complex carbohydrates are much larger molecules, consisting of hundreds or thousands of sugar units (mostly glucose) joined together. They include the starches, amylose and amylopectin, and the non-starch polysaccharides (dietary fibre), such as cellulose, pectin and hemicellulose.

In between simple and complex carbohydrates are glucose polymers and maltodextrin, which comprise between 3- and 10-sugar units. They are made from the partial breakdown of corn starch in food processing, and are widely used as bulking and thickening agents in processed foods, such as sauces, dairy desserts, baby food, puddings and soft drinks. They are popular ingredients in sports drinks and meal-replacement products, owing to their low sweetness and high energy density relative to sucrose.

In practice, many foods contain a mixture of both simple and complex carbohydrates, making the traditional classification of foods into 'simple' and 'complex' very confusing. For example, biscuits and cakes contain flour (complex) and sugar (simple), and bananas contain a mixture of sugars and starches depending on their degree of ripeness.

The old notion about simple carbohydrates giving fast-release energy and complex carbohydrates giving slow-release energy is incorrect and misleading. For example, apples (containing mostly simple carbohydrates) produce a smaller and more prolonged rise in blood sugar than potatoes or bread (containing mainly complex carbohydrates), which are digested and absorbed relatively quickly and give a rapid rise in blood sugar.

Nowadays, carbohydrates are more often classified by their nutritional quality or nutrient density. This refers to the presence of other nutrients in the food, such as vitamins, minerals, fibre and phytochemicals (plant compounds). This classifi-

What are the practical difficulties with a high-carbohydrate diet?

For athletes with very high energy needs, eating a high-carbohydrate diet can be difficult. Many carbohydrate-rich foods, such as bread, potatoes and pasta, are quite bulky and filling, particularly if wholegrain and high-fibre foods make up most of your carbohydrate intake. Several surveys have found that endurance athletes often fail to consume the recommended carbohydrate levels (Frentsos and Baer, 1997). This may be partly due to the large number of calories needed and therefore the bulk of their diet, and partly due to lack of awareness of the benefits of a higher carbohydrate intake. It is interesting that most of the studies upon which the carbohydrate recommendations were made used liquid carbohydrates (i.e. drinks) to supplement meals. Tour de France cyclists and ultra-distance athletes, who require more than 5000 calories a day, often consume up to one-third of their carbohydrate in liquid form. If you are finding a high-carbohydrate diet impractical, try eating smaller, more frequent meals and supplementing your food with liquid forms of carbohydrate such as meal replacement products and energy drinks (see pp. 159–60).

cation method gives you a better idea of the food's overall nutritional value. Examples of nutrient-dense carbohydrate foods include whole grains, such as oats, wholemeal bread and brown rice; beans, chickpeas, lentils, fruit and vegetables. Aim to get most of your daily carbohydrate from these foods, while minimising refined carbohydrates. These include sweets, cakes, biscuits, sugar-sweetened drinks, sports drinks, gels, chocolate and refined grains (such as white bread, pasta and rice). While not devoid of nutritional value, these foods generally contain less fibre and fewer vitamins and minerals. You don't have to avoid them completely – simply balance them with nutrient-rich foods.

Is sugar harmful for health?

Sugar is a carbohydrate, which means it is an energy source for the body. Despite the negative press surrounding it, small amounts of sugar are unlikely to cause harm and, provided you time your sugar intake around exercise, it may even aid your performance. During high-intensity exercise lasting longer than an hour, consuming sugar either in the form of solid food (e.g. bananas, dried fruit, gels or energy bars) or drinks can help maintain blood glucose concentration, spare glycogen and increase endurance. Sugar may also be beneficial for promoting rapid glycogen refuelling during the 2-hour period after prolonged intense exercise.

However, one of the main problems with sugar is its ability to cause dental caries. Studies have shown that athletes who consume lots of sports drinks, bars and gels experience significant tooth decay and erosion (Needleman *et al.*, 2015). These products are high in sugar and as they are usually consumed at frequent intervals during exercise, they are particularly damaging to the teeth.

Another problem with sugar is that it has no real nutritional value (apart from providing energy). It makes food and drink more palatable and therefore easy to over-consume. Although sugar is not uniquely fattening, it can contribute towards an over-consumption of calories, especially when combined with lots of fat in the form of cakes, chocolates, biscuits and snacks. Rather than satisfy hunger, sugar can sometimes make us want to eat more! Although high intakes have been linked with obesity and type 2 diabetes, the main contributor to these diseases is excess calories rather than sugar itself.

It is also claimed that high sugar intakes can result in insulin resistance, where the body cells become less responsive to insulin (the hormone responsible for shunting glucose from the bloodstream to the muscles) and more prone to store fat. However, regular exercise blunts the negative effects of sugar, which means the body produces less insulin after consuming sugar. This is one of the many ways the body adapts to exercise: it becomes more sensitive to insulin (Hawley and Lessard, 2008). In other words, you need less insulin to do the same job and your body learns to handle sugar more efficiently.

Claims suggesting that sugar is toxic or addictive relate to studies carried out on mice that were given extremely large amounts of sugar. Such research cannot be extrapolated to humans. It has also been claimed that sugar, specifically the fructose part of the molecule, increases blood triglycerides and cardiovascular disease risk. However, doing regular exercise prevents this because the body increases its production of lipoprotein lipase, an enzyme that removes fats

back of the mouth, rather than swishing around the mouth, and rinsing with water afterwards.

What is the glycaemic index?

The glycaemic index (GI) refers to the increase in blood glucose in response to a standard amount of food. It is a ranking of foods from 0 to 100 based on their immediate effect on blood sugar levels, a measure of the speed at which you digest food and convert it into glucose. It is calculated by a test in which the blood concentration is measured in response to 50 g of carbohydrate over a 2-hour period. Specifically, it is the area under the blood glucose concentration curve. Foods are compared with a reference food, such as glucose or white bread, and are tested in equivalent carbohydrate amounts. The faster the rise in blood glucose and the greater the area under the curve, the higher the GI.

- GI = area under the glucose curve of test food ÷ area under the glucose curve of reference food x 100

Most GI values lie somewhere between 20 and 100. Foods are generally classified as *high GI (71–100)*, *medium GI (56–70)* and *low GI (0–55)*. In a nutshell, the higher the GI, the higher the blood sugar levels after eating that food. The GI of various generic and branded foods can be found at https://glycemicindex.com.

However, the use of GI as a tool for controlling blood glucose concentration is controversial mainly because the GI of a particular food varies considerably between individuals (Dodd *et al.*, 2011). GI values can also be confusing. In general, foods with a high content of sugar have

circulating in the blood and converts them into energy (Seip and Semenkovich, 1998). In a study at the University of Lausanne, Switzerland, when volunteers consumed a high fructose diet (30% fructose) their blood fats concentration increased but when they combined this diet with moderate aerobic exercise there was no increase in blood fat concentration (Egli *et al.*, 2013). In other words, exercise prevents the rise in blood fats caused by a high fructose intake.

On balance, athletes don't need to worry unduly about sugar as it does not have the same effect on blood insulin and blood fats as it does in sedentary people. It may improve endurance during prolonged high-intensity exercise although it would be prudent to mitigate damage to the teeth by, for example, directing sports drinks to the

a higher GI, while complex carbohydrates have a lower GI. However, some complex carbohydrates, e.g. wholemeal bread and baked potato, and vegetables can have a high GI. Similarly, many simple carbohydrates, e.g. apples and oranges, have a low GI. Adding protein or fat to a high-GI food slows the digestion and absorption of glucose, thus lowering the overall glycaemic response (blood sugar rise) e.g. adding cheese, baked beans or tuna to baked potato. Cooking and ripening of fruits tends to increase the GI value.

What is the glycaemic load?

The glycaemic load (GL) is considered a more accurate way to assess the effect of a food on blood glucose concentration than GI as it takes account of portion size as well as the GI. The GI value only tells you how rapidly a food raises blood glucose but does not take into account the amount consumed. GL is calculated by multiplying the GI of a food by the amount of carbohydrate per portion and dividing by 100.

- GL = (GI x carbohydrate per portion) ÷ 100

For example, a slice of watermelon weighing 100 g contains only 6 g of carbohydrate. To get 50 g of carbohydrate you would have to consume 720 g of watermelon. Low GL foods have a value between 1 and 10, medium GL foods between 11 and 19, and high GL foods greater than 20. The GL of various foods can also be found at https://glycemicindex.com.

Glycaemic response in athletes

Scientists have discovered that high-GI foods have a smaller effect on blood glucose and insulin in regular exercisers compared with non-exercisers. That's because regular exercise increases insulin sensitivity and improves glucose uptake by body cells (Hawley and Lessard, 2008). In other words, your body learns to handle glucose more efficiently. Studies at the University of Sydney in Australia have found that when athletes are fed high-GI foods, they produce much less insulin than would be predicted from GI tables. In other words, they don't show the same peaks and troughs in blood glucose and insulin as sedentary people do. This is thought to be related to increased activity of key proteins involved in the regulation of glucose uptake

Carbohydrate timing

CARBOHYDRATE INTAKE BEFORE EXERCISE

Carbohydrate intake in the hours and days prior to a workout or event will affect the size of your glycogen stores and subsequent performance. Numerous studies have concluded that high pre-exercise glycogen levels and/or consuming carbohydrate in the hours before exercise results in improved endurance performance when compared with fasted training (exercising on an empty stomach) (Chryssanthopoulos *et al.*, 2002; Neufer *et al.*, 1987; Sherman *et al.*, 1991; Wright *et al.*, 1991). On the other hand, low pre-exercise glycogen levels or fasted training results in increased perception of effort, reduced training intensity, early fatigue and diminished endurance performance. A pre-exercise meal will also help reduce hunger during exercise.

Fibre and health

Fibre is the term used to describe the complex carbohydrates found in plants that the body cannot digest. Unlike other types of carbohydrate, it provides no calories because it is not absorbed into the body. Fibre helps to keep the gut healthy by encouraging the smooth passage of food through the digestive system as well as feeding the population of healthy microorganisms (microbiota) that live in your large intestine (bowel). A high-fibre diet can help reduce the risk of obesity, type 2 diabetes, heart disease, stroke and constipation. Fibre-rich foods are especially beneficial for weight control as they are more filling, take longer to digest and increase satiety.

Traditionally, fibre was classified as insoluble and soluble. Most plant foods contain both, but proportions vary. Good sources of insoluble fibre include whole grains, such as wholegrain bread, pasta and rice, and vegetables. These help to speed the passage of food through the gut and prevent constipation and bowel problems. Soluble fibre, found in oats, beans, lentils, nuts, fruit and vegetables, reduces LDL cholesterol levels and helps control blood glucose levels by slowing glucose absorption. The UK's Scientific Advisory Committee on Nutrition recommends 30 g of fibre a day for adults.

WHEN IS THE BEST TIME TO EAT BEFORE EXERCISE?

Carbohydrate intake in the 1–4 hours before exercise helps increase liver and muscle glycogen levels and enhances your subsequent performance (Thomas *et al.*, 2016; Hargreaves *et al.*, 2004). Clearly, the exact timing of your pre-exercise meal will depend on your daily schedule and the time of day you plan to train.

Scheduling a pre-exercise meal between 2 and 4 hours before training leaves enough time to digest the food and for your stomach to settle so that you feel comfortable – not too full and not too hungry. Eating a meal too close to exercise may result in stomach discomfort and indigestion, as the blood supply is diverted away from the digestive system to your muscles.

If you have less than 2 hours before your work-out, opt for an easy-to-digest snack. Anything more substantial may result in gut issues and discomfort during exercise. For example, if you work out at 6 p.m. in the evening, either schedule lunch around 2 p.m. (leaving you a 4-hour interval before your workout) or around midday and then eat a snack between 4 and 5.30 p.m. (leaving you a 30 minute –2 hour interval).

Researchers at the University of North Carolina found that performance of moderate-to high-intensity exercise lasting 35–40 minutes was improved after eating a moderately high-carbohydrate, low-fat meal 3 hours before exercise (Maffucci and McMurray, 2000). In this study, the volunteers were able to run significantly longer. Researchers asked the athletes to run on treadmills at a moderate intensity for 30 minutes, with high-intensity 30 second intervals, and then until they couldn't run any longer, after eating a meal either 6 hours or 3 hours beforehand. The

Fasted training

Fasted training means training in a fasted state, i.e. after not eating for 10–14 hours, and is typically done in the morning before breakfast when your liver glycogen (but not muscle glycogen) stores are depleted. Similar to training on a low-carbohydrate, high-fat diet (see p. 55) the idea behind fasted training is: 1) to increase the body's ability to use fat for fuel, training the body to access more efficiently the large amount of energy stored in adipose tissue and conserve glycogen, and 2) to induce greater endurance training adaptations compared to training in the fed state. However, meta-analysis (studies of studies) found that while fasted training increases fat oxidation, it also reduces endurance performance (Aird et al., 2018). People are able to exercise longer when they consume a pre-exercise meal than when they fasted. Additionally, fasting increases perception of effort, which can compromise exercise intensity and volume, resulting in a lower overall calorie expenditure (Terada et al., 2019).

A review of studies concluded that there is little evidence to support the notion of endurance training and fasting-mediated increases in fat oxidation, and recommended that endurance athletes should avoid high-intensity training while fasting (Zouhal et al., 2020). What's more, it may increase protein oxidation and result in a loss of muscle. Despite popular belief, fasted training is not an effective weight loss method. To lose weight, you need to be in a calorie deficit. In other words, you must consume fewer calories than your body needs over the course of several days, not in a single workout. On the other hand, if you prefer training fasted (e.g. first thing in the morning) then that's fine provided you're doing low- or moderate-intensity exercise (as you'll be burning relatively more fat and less carbohydrate). However, if you plan to do high-intensity endurance exercise for longer than an hour then consuming carbohydrate beforehand will help increase your performance.

athletes ran significantly longer if they had eaten the meal 3 hours before training compared with 6 hours.

Furthermore, researchers at Loughborough University found that consuming a high-carbohydrate meal 3 hours before exercise improved endurance running capacity by 9% compared with a no-meal trial (Chryssanthopoulos et al., 2002).

Previously, athletes were advised not to consume carbohydrate in the hour before exercise as this was thought to induce rebound hypoglycaemia (causing blood sugar levels to drop below normal) and negatively affect performance.

However, there is little evidence to support this advice. Instead, you should experiment with different pre-exercise protocols to find the timing that suits you best.

HOW MUCH CARBOHYDRATE SHOULD YOU CONSUME BEFORE EXERCISE?

The size and timing of your pre-training meal are interrelated. The closer you are to the start of your training session, the smaller your meal should be (to allow for gastric emptying), whereas larger meals can be consumed when more time is available before training or competition. Intakes between 1–4 g/kg BW consumed 1–4 hours before exercise have been recommended (Thomas *et al.*, 2016). So, for example, if you weigh 70 kg, this translates to 70–280 g carbohydrate. You may need to experiment to find the exact quantity of food or drink and the timing that works best for you. Some athletes can consume a substantial meal in the 2–4 hours before exercise with no ill effects, while others may experience discomfort and prefer to eat a snack or liquid meal.

WHAT TO EAT BEFORE EXERCISE?

The best foods to eat before exercise depends on your workout goals and individual preference. Your pre-workout meal should be easy to digest and include foods rich in carbohydrate (e.g. rice, oats, pasta or potatoes), with smaller amounts of protein-rich foods and healthy fat. This combination of macronutrients will provide sustained energy to help you get through your workout. Both protein and fat slow the digestion and absorption of carbohydrate, so the closer your meal is to your workout, the less protein or fat you should eat. On the other hand, eating a meal devoid of fat and protein could leave you hungry and lacking in energy. It is usually a good idea to avoid large amounts of fibre-rich foods within 30 minutes of exercise, especially if you are prone to gut issues or feel nervous before an event. Fibre slows stomach emptying, which can make you feel full and uncomfortable. However, moderate amounts of fibre eaten 2–4 hours or longer before exercise should not pose a problem and may even be advantageous for endurance as fibre prevents spikes in blood glucose and insulin during exercise.

Consuming carbohydrate before exercise increases carbohydrate oxidation and reduces fat oxidation during exercise. However, this is not detrimental to performance because increased carbohydrate availability compensates for the greater carbohydrate use (Wee *et al.*, 1999)

Whether to eat high-GI or low-GI foods pre-exercise has long been a controversial area. Many experts recommend a low-GI meal based on the idea that such a meal would supply sustained energy during exercise. One study found that cyclists who ate a low-GI pre-exercise meal of lentils 1 hour before exercise managed to keep going 20 minutes longer than when they consumed high-GI foods (Thomas *et al.*, 1991).

In other studies, the researchers took blood samples at regular intervals from cyclists and found that low-GI meals produce higher blood sugar and fatty acid levels during the latter stages of exercise, which is clearly advantageous for endurance sports (Thomas *et al.*, 1994; DeMarco *et al.*, 1999). In other words, the low-GI meals produce a sustained source of carbohydrate throughout exercise and recovery.

A UK study confirmed that athletes burn more fat during exercise following a low-GI meal of bran cereal, fruit and milk compared with a high-GI meal of cornflakes, white bread, jam and sports drink (Wu *et al.*, 2003). The benefits kick in early during exercise – the difference in fat oxidation is apparent even after 15 minutes.

A 2006 study at the University of Loughborough, found that runners who consumed a low-GI meal 3 hours before exercise were able to run longer (around 8 minutes) than after a high-GI pre-exercise meal (Wu and Williams, 2006). The researchers suggest that the improvements in performance were due to increased fat oxidation following consumption of the low-GI meal, which helped compensate for the lower rates of glycogen oxidation during the latter stages of the exercise trial. In other words, the low-GI meal

allowed the volunteers to burn more fat and less glycogen during exercise, which resulted in increased endurance.

This isn't necessarily a rule of thumb, as other studies have found that the GI of the pre-exercise meal has little effect on performance, with cyclists managing to keep going for the same duration whether they ate lentils (low GI) or potatoes (high GI) (Febbraio and Stewart, 1996). A Greek study also found that ingestion of high-GI or low-GI foods (containing the same quantity of carbohydrate) 30 minutes before exercise did not result in any differences in exercise performance in a group of eight cyclists (Jamurtas *et al.*, 2011).

DURING EXERCISE

For endurance activities lasting less than 45 minutes to 1 hour, consuming anything other than water is unnecessary provided your pre-exercise muscle glycogen levels are high, i.e. you have consumed sufficient carbohydrate during the previous few days and eaten a meal containing carbohydrate 2–4 hours before exercise (Burke *et al.*, 2011; IOC, 2011; Desbrow *et al.*, 2004). Muscle glycogen is generally not a limiting factor to performance during exercise lasting less than 1 hour.

It is well established that consuming carbohydrate during prolonged exercise (more than 1–2 hours) can enhance performance (Stellingworth and Cox, 2014, Smith *et al.*, 2010; Coyle *et al.*, 1986) but research since the late 1990s has suggested that very small amounts of carbohydrate ('mouth rinsing') may be beneficial for high-intensity exercise (>75% VO_2max) lasting 45–75 minutes (Carter *et al.*, 2004; Below, 1995; Jeukendrup *et al.*, 1997). The reasons are quite different.

Exercise lasting 45–75 minutes

Researchers have found that simply rinsing the mouth with an energy drink for 5–10 seconds improves performance even when you do not swallow the drink (Carter, 2004; Burke *et al.*, 2011). The benefits of mouth rinsing may be greater when exercising in a glycogen-depleted state or when fasted rather than after a meal, i.e. when 'training low' (*see* p. 55) as it reduces the perception of effort.

A study at Loughborough University, found that mouth rinsing enabled runners to run faster and cover more distance during a 30-minute treadmill run compared with a placebo (Rollo *et al.*, 2008). In a study at Ghent University, Belgium, cyclists were able to complete a 1-hour high-intensity time-trial 2.4 minutes faster after mouth rinsing compared with a placebo (Pottier *et al.*, 2010). However, ingesting the energy drink did not improve performance compared with the placebo. A systematic review of 11 studies by Brazilian and Australian researchers found that 9 out of 11 showed a significant increase in performance during moderate- to high-intensity exercise lasting approximately 1 hour, ranging from 1.5% to 11.6% (de Ataíde e Silva *et al.*, 2013). Researchers at RMIT University, Australia, found that a carbohydrate mouth rinse improved performance to a greater extent in a fasted compared with a fed state (Lane *et al.*, 2013 (a)).

The performance benefits appear to be even greater when mouth rinsing is combined with caffeine during high-intensity exercise. In a randomised double-blind study at Liverpool John Moores University, glycogen-depleted athletes were given carbohydrate mouth rinse with or without caffeine during a morning 45-minute steady run followed by a high-intensity interval set until they reached the point of exhaustion (Kasper *et al.*, 2015). Those who used a carbohydrate rinse were able to exercise 16 minutes longer than the control (placebo) group but those who *also* took caffeine were able to keep going 29 minutes longer (52 minutes, 36 minutes and 65 minutes respectively).

The ergogenic effects of mouth rinsing are thought to be due to carbohydrate receptors in the mouth signalling to the brain that food is on its way. These sensors activate the brain's pleasure and reward centres and reduce the perception of effort and fatigue, allowing you maintain higher exercise intensity for longer. This strategy may be beneficial for those athletes who find it difficult to consume anything during exercise without experiencing gastrointestinal problems. An effective protocol may comprise swishing an energy drink for 5–10 seconds immediately before exercise and then every 10–15 minutes during exercise. Any home-made or commercial sports drink (containing approximately 6 g carbohydrate/100 ml) would be suitable.

Exercise lasting 1–2½ hours

For moderate–high-intensity exercise lasting longer than 60–90 minutes, where muscle glycogen stores are a limiting factor for performance, consuming carbohydrate can help maintain blood glucose levels and delay fatigue and thus increase exercise capacity and performance (Pöchmüller *et al.*, 2016; Stellingworth and Cox, 2014; Smith *et al.*, 2010; Coyle, 2004; Jeukendrup, 2004; Coggan and Coyle, 1991; Coyle *et al.*, 1986). It may also help you to continue exercising during the latter stages of a workout or event when your muscle glycogen stores are depleted.

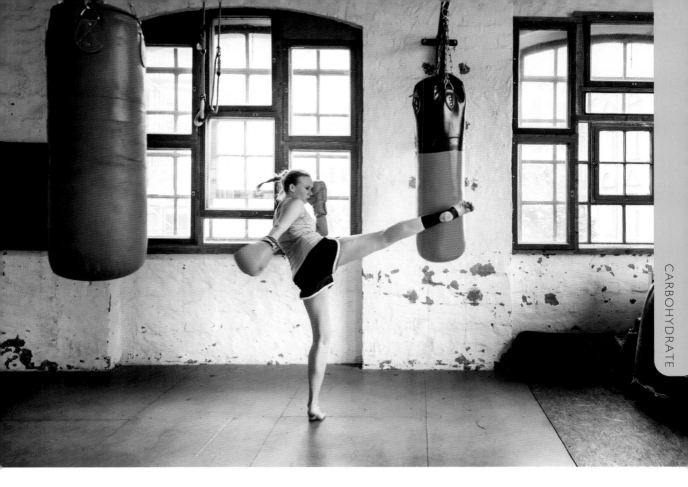

During that first hour of exercise, most of your carbohydrate energy comes from muscle glycogen. After that, muscle glycogen stores deplete significantly, so the exercising muscles must use carbohydrate from some other source. That's where blood glucose comes into its own. As you continue exercising, the muscles take up more and more glucose from the bloodstream. Eventually, after 2–3 hours, your muscles will be fuelled entirely by blood glucose and fat.

This sounds handy, but, alas, you cannot keep going indefinitely because blood glucose supplies eventually dwindle. Some of this blood glucose is derived from certain amino acids and some comes from liver glycogen. When liver glycogen stores run low, your blood glucose levels will fall, and you will be unable to carry on exercising at the same intensity. That's why temporary hypoglycaemia is common after 2–3 hours of exercise without consuming carbohydrate. In this state, you would feel very fatigued and light-headed, your muscles would feel very heavy and the exercise would feel very hard indeed. In other words, the depletion of muscle and liver glycogen together with low blood sugar levels would cause you to reduce exercise intensity or stop completely. This is sometimes called 'hitting the wall' in marathon running.

Clearly, then, consuming additional carbohydrate would maintain your blood sugar levels and allow you to exercise longer. An analysis of 73 previous studies by researchers at Auckland University of Technology, New Zealand, found that carbohydrate consumption during exercise led to an improvement in performance of up to 6% (Vandenbogaerde and Hopkins, 2011).

The consensus recommendation is an intake of *30–60 g carbohydrate/hour*, depending on the exercise intensity (Thomas *et al.*, 2016; IOC, 2011; Burke *et al.*, 2011; Rodriguez *et al.*, 2009; Coggan and Coyle, 1991). If you are exercising at a low intensity then carbohydrate oxidations rates will be relatively low, so an intake towards the bottom of this range would be appropriate. On the other hand, if you are exercising at a high intensity, carbohydrate oxidation rates will be higher and so higher intakes, closer to 60 g/hour, would be appropriate. The maximum amount of a single type of carbohydrate (e.g. glucose) that can be oxidised by the muscles during aerobic exercise is *1 g/min (60 g/h)* because the transporter responsible for carbohydrate absorption in the intestine becomes saturated. Consuming more than 60 g glucose per hour would not increase carbohydrate oxidation, energy output or reduce fatigue. It would remain in the digestive tract and likely cause GI discomfort for many athletes.

Exercise lasting longer than 2½ hours

For high-intensity exercise lasting more than 2½ hours, it would be beneficial to consume greater amounts of carbohydrate. Research at the University of Birmingham has found that consuming a mixture of carbohydrates ('multiple transportable carbohydrates'), such as glucose and fructose, or maltodextrin and fructose in a 2:1 ratio, results in higher absorption and oxidation rates of approximately *1.5 g/min (90 g/hour)* (Jentjens *et al.*, 2004; Wallis *et al.*, 2005). Consuming a combination of carbohydrates overcomes the problems of glucose transporter saturation and

therefore increases the uptake of carbohydrates from the intestines and also the oxidation rate in the muscles (IOC, 2011; Jeukendrup, 2008). It may also increase fluid uptake.

Glucose and fructose are absorbed via different transporter molecules in the small intestine. The transport capacity of each of these carbohydrate molecules is limited. For example, glucose is transported by sodium-dependent glucose transporter 1 (SGLT1) at a maximum rate of 60 g/hour. This means that you will gain no further performance benefit by consuming more than 60 g glucose/hour since the glucose transporters will be fully saturated. The excess glucose will simply stay in the intestine longer. However, by consuming fructose along with glucose, you can make use of the fructose transporters (GLUT5) and thus enhance the amount of carbohydrate absorbed and delivered to the muscles. This is advantageous during high-intensity endurance activities longer than 2½ hours, such as triathlon, long-distance cycling and ultra-distance running. In these events, carbohydrate intakes of *up to 90 g/hour* are recommended from multiple transportable carbohydrates (Jeukendrup, 2014; Thomas *et al.*, 2016). One study found that performance in a cycling time-trial improved by 8% when drinking a glucose-fructose drink compared with a glucose-only drink and 19% when compared with water (Currell and Jeukendrup, 2008).In another study, researchers at Maastricht University found that cyclists were able to absorb and oxidise 46% more carbohydrate when they consumed a glucose-fructose or glucose-sucrose drink compared with a glucose-only drink (Trommelen *et al.*, 2017). Furthermore, they suffered fewer GI symptoms with the combination drinks compared with the glucose-only drink.

WHEN SHOULD I CONSUME CAROHYDRATE DURING EXERCISE?

The timing of carbohydrate intake during exercise affects the rate at which glycogen is oxidised and the onset of fatigue. There are no hard and fast rules but the key is to begin fuelling early, consume carbohydrate little and often and avoid over-consumption. Many athletes prefer to consume fuel approximately every 20–30 minutes, depending on exercise intensity. It takes 15–30 minutes for the carbohydrate you have consumed to reach your muscles, so do not wait until you are exhausted before you begin fuelling.

One study with runners found that consuming carbohydrate from the start of exercise and at frequent intervals (15 x 5 g every 5 minutes) during exercise spared muscle glycogen stores and enabled them to run for longer compared to consuming carbohydrate in one go towards the end of exercise (Menzies *et al.*, 2020).

WHICH FOODS OR DRINKS SHOULD I CONSUME DURING EXERCISE?

The carbohydrate you consume during exercise should be rapidly digested and absorbed. You need it to raise your blood sugar level and reach your exercising muscles rapidly. Thus, high-GI ('fast') carbohydrates (e.g. glucose, sucrose, maltose and maltodextrins) are generally the best choices (*see* Table 3.3 on p. 48). Low-GI ('slow') carbohydrates (e.g. fructose) are poor choices because they are absorbed slower and need to

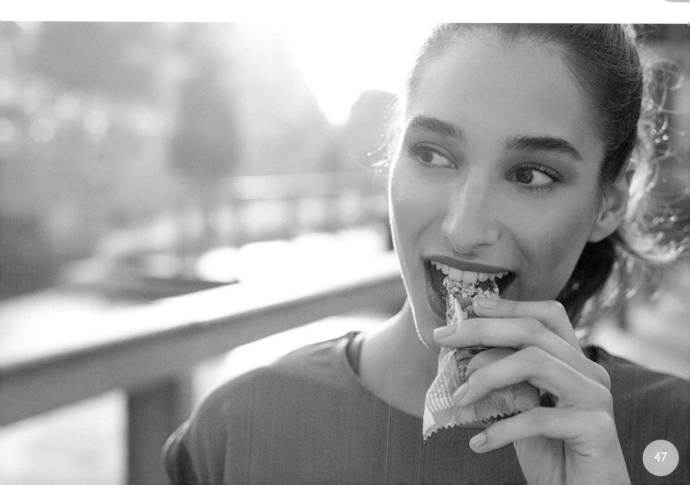

be converted into glucose in the liver first before they can be used by the muscles. This process slows down delivery. Also, consuming large amounts of fructose during exercise can cause GI problems because it cannot be absorbed fast enough and simply stays in the intestine. For this reason, sports drinks, gels and bars (commercial or home-made) that use glucose, sucrose and

Table 3.2	SUMMARY OF RECOMMENDATIONS FOR CARBOHYDRATE INTAKE DURING EXERCISE	
Exercise duration	Recommended amount of carbohydrate	Type of carbohydrate
<45 minutes	None	None
45–75 minutes	Very small amounts (mouth rinse)	Any
1–2½ hours	30–60 g/h	Any
>2½ hours	Up to 90 g/h	Multiple transportable carbohydrates (glucose or maltodextrin + fructose)

Source: Jeukendrup, 2014; Thomas *et al.*, 2016.

Table 3.3	SUITABLE FOODS AND DRINKS TO CONSUME DURING EXERCISE	
Food or drink	Portion size providing 30 g carbohydrate	Portion size providing 60 g carbohydrate
Isotonic sports drink (6 g/100 ml)	500 ml	1000 ml
Banana	1 large (150 g)	2 large (300 g)
Energy bar	1 bar (45 g)	2 bars (90 g)
Diluted fruit juice (1:1)	500 ml	1000 ml
Raisins	40 g	80 g
Medjool dates	2 dates (40 g)	4 dates (80 g)
Fruit and nut bar	2 x 35 g bars	4 x 35 g bars
Energy gel	1 gel (45–55 g)	2 gels (90–110 ml)
Energy chews	4 chews (40 g)	8 chews (80 g)

maltodextrins as their main energy sources (*see* pp. 162–3) are the best options.

Whether you choose solid or liquid carbohydrate makes little difference to your performance, provided you drink water with solid carbohydrate (Pfeiffer *et al.*, 2010 (a); Kennerly *et al.*, 2011; Mason *et al.*, 1993). Most athletes find liquid forms of carbohydrate (i.e. sports drinks) more convenient. Carbohydrate-containing drinks have a dual benefit because they provide fluid as well as fuel, reducing hypohydration and fatigue. Obviously, you do not have to consume a commercial drink; you can make your own from fruit juice, or sugar, or squash, and water (*see* Table 8.2 on p. 163). A study at the University of Birmingham, found that there was no difference in the rates of carbohydrate oxidation (91 g/hour) during 3 hours of cycling after consuming a bar or a drink containing a 2:1 glucose plus fructose mixture (Pfeiffer *et al.*, 2010 (a)). Another study by the same researchers showed there was no difference in carbohydrate oxidation rate when they compared a gel and a drink (Pfeiffer *et al.*, 2010 (b)). The choice, therefore, boils down to individual preference.

A range of commercial sports nutrition products containing a mixture of carbohydrates (energy drinks, bars, gels and chews) is widely available but many wholefoods, including fresh and dried fruit, also supply a similar ratio.

In one study at Appalachian State University, there was no difference in exercise performance when cyclists were given equal amounts of carbohydrate either in the form of a banana or a 6% carbohydrate sports drink (Kennerly *et al.*, 2011). You should experiment with different drinks and foods during training to develop your own fuelling strategy.

It is important to begin consuming carbohydrate *before* fatigue sets in. It takes 30–40 minutes for the carbohydrate to be absorbed into the bloodstream (Coggan and Coyle, 1991). For workouts longer than 60–90 minutes, the best strategy is to begin consuming carbohydrate after about 30–40 minutes.

For long events, you may prefer savoury as well as sweet options to reduce flavour fatigue and the risk of tooth damage. Good options include bite-sized sandwiches, wraps, rolls or pitta filled with yeast extract or nut butter, rice cakes or crackers. Consuming fat-rich foods such as nuts is unlikely to help performance during most activities as fat cannot be turned into energy fast enough, but it may help reduce hunger and slow stomach emptying during ultra-distance events.

AFTER EXERCISE

Depleted glycogen (carbohydrate) stores need to be replaced after exercise if you wish to optimise performance at your subsequent workout or event. Failure to do so will result in cumulative fatigue and under-performance. The length of time that it takes to refuel depends on four main factors:

1. how depleted your glycogen stores are after exercise
2. the extent of muscle damage
3. the amount and the timing of carbohydrate you eat
4. your training experience and fitness level

Depletion

The more depleted your glycogen stores, the longer it will take you to refuel, just as it takes longer to refill an empty fuel tank than one that is half full. This, in turn, depends on the intensity and duration of your workout.

The higher the *intensity*, the more glycogen you use. For example, if your workout or event comprised mainly fast, explosive activities (e.g. sprints, jumps or lifts) or high-intensity aerobic activities (e.g. running), you will have depleted your glycogen stores significantly more than a workout or event comprising low-intensity activities (e.g. walking or slow swimming) of equal duration. The minimum time it would take to refill muscle glycogen stores is 20 hours (Coyle, 1991). After prolonged and exhaustive exercise (e.g. marathon), it may take up to 7 days.

The *duration* of your workout also has a bearing on the amount of glycogen you use. For example, if you run for 1 hour, you will use up more glycogen than if you run at the same speed for half an hour. If you complete 10 sets of shoulder exercises in the gym, you will use more glycogen from your shoulder muscles than

if you had completed only 5 sets using the same weight. Therefore, you need to allow more time to refuel after high-intensity or long workouts.

Muscle damage

Certain activities that involve eccentric exercise (e.g. heavy weight training, plyometric training or hard running) can cause muscle fibre damage. Eccentric exercise is defined as the forced lengthening of active muscle. Muscle damage, in turn, delays glycogen storage and complete glycogen replenishment could take as long as 7–10 days.

Carbohydrate intake

The higher your carbohydrate intake, the faster you can refuel your glycogen stores. Figure 3.3(a) shows how glycogen storage increases with increasing carbohydrate intake.

This is particularly important if you train on a daily basis. For example, in one study, cyclists who consumed a moderate carbohydrate diet

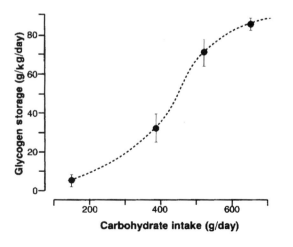

Figure 3.3(a) Glycogen storage depends on carbohydrate intake

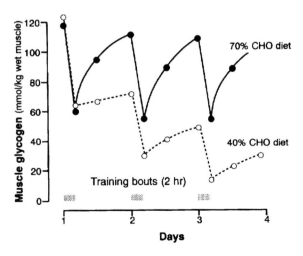

Figure 3.3(b) A low carbohydrate intake results in poor refuelling

Post-exercise snacks

- 500 ml milk or milkshake
- Strained plain Greek yoghurt, banana and nuts
- A wholemeal sandwich/pitta/wrap filled with tuna, chicken, egg, cheese or hummus
- Smoothie or shake – 250 ml milk, 150 g plain yoghurt, one banana, 100 g berries and 1 tbsp nut butter or seeds
- Avocado and egg on toast
- A handful of nuts and dried fruit
- Granola with plain yoghurt and fruit

Post-exercise meals

- Spicy chicken with rice (see p. 329)
- Sweet potato and lentil curry (see p. 334)
- Fish tagine with chickpeas (see p. 326)
- Vegetable tagine with chickpeas (see p. 334)
- Potato and fish pie (see p. 333)
- Vegetarian shepherd's pie with sweet potato mash (see p. 335)
- Salmon and vegetable pasta (see p. 325)
- Vegetarian chilli with rice (see p. 342)

(250–350 g/day) failed to replenish fully their muscle glycogen stores (Costill *et al.*, 1971). Over successive days of training, their glycogen stores became progressively lower. However, in a further study by the same researchers, cyclists who consumed a high-carbohydrate diet (550–600 g/day) fully replaced their glycogen stores in the 22 hours between training sessions (Costill, 1985) (*see* Fig. 3.3(b)).

More recently, a study from the University of Bath highlighted the importance of carbohydrate for short-term recovery when performing two workouts a day (Alghannam *et al.*, 2016). They found that runners who consumed a high-carbohydrate drink (1.2 g/kg body weight) after the first workout were able to run significantly longer (80 min versus 48 minutes) before reaching the point of exhaustion in the second workout than those who drank a low-carbohydrate drink (0.3 g/kg body weight). Muscle biopsies showed that in both cases, exhaustion corresponded to

when their muscles reached a critically low level of glycogen. A high carbohydrate intake is essential for glycogen recovery and subsequent performance for those training twice a day.

Therefore, if you wish to train daily or twice a day, make sure that you consume enough carbohydrate. If not, you will be unable to train as hard or as long, you will suffer fatigue sooner and achieve smaller training gains.

Training experience

Efficiency in refuelling improves with training experience and cardiovascular fitness. Thus, it takes a beginner longer to replace their glycogen stores than an experienced athlete eating the same amount of carbohydrate. That's one reason why elite sportspeople are able to train daily or twice daily while beginners cannot and should not!

Another adaptation to endurance training is an increase in your glycogen storing capacity, perhaps by as much as 20%.

SHOULD I CONSUME CARBOHYDRATE IMMEDIATELY AFTER EXERCISE?

Research has shown that glycogen storage following exercise takes place in three distinct stages. During the first 2 hours, replenishment is most rapid – at approximately 150% (or one-and-a-half times) the normal rate (Ivy *et al.*, 1988). During the subsequent 4 hours the rate slows but remains higher than normal; after this period, glycogen manufacture returns to the normal rate. Therefore, eating carbohydrate during the first few hours post-exercise will promote faster glycogen recovery. This is most important when the recovery period between workouts or events is less than 8 hours, e.g. if you train or compete twice a day. If this is the case, aim to consume carbohydrate as soon as is practical after the first session. It may be more effective to consume several smaller, high-carbohydrate snacks than larger meals during the early recovery phase, according to researchers at the Australian Institute of Sport (Burke *et al.*, 2004). It makes no difference to the glycogen storage rate whether you consume liquid or solid forms of carbohydrate (Keizer *et al.*, 1986).

There are two main reasons why glycogen replenishment is faster during the post-exercise period. First, eating carbohydrate stimulates insulin release, which, in turn, increases the amount of glucose taken up by your muscle cells from the bloodstream, and stimulates the action of the glycogen-manufacturing enzymes, glycogen synthase and hexokinase II. Second, post-exercise, the muscle cell membranes are more permeable to glucose, so they can take up more glucose than normal.

However, for recovery periods of 24 hours or longer, the type and timing of carbohydrate intake is less critical, provided you consume enough energy (calories) and carbohydrate over a 24-hour period.

HOW MUCH CARBOHYDRATE SHOULD I EAT IMMEDIATELY AFTER EXERCISE?

For rapid recovery, researchers recommend consuming 1–1.2 g/kg BW/hour for the 4 hours post-exercise (Burke *et al.*, 2004; Burke *et al.*, 2011; Thomas *et al.*, 2016). This is the maximal rate at which carbohydrate can be absorbed from the intestines. So, for example, if you weigh 70 kg you need to consume 70–84 g carbohydrate/hour. Even if you finish training late in the evening, you still need to start the refuelling process, so do not go to bed on an empty stomach! For efficient glycogen refuelling, you should continue to eat carbohydrate at regular intervals. If you leave long gaps without eating, glycogen storage and recovery will be slower.

WHICH TYPES CARBOHYDRATES ARE BEST FOR RECOVERY?

Since high-GI ('fast') carbohydrates cause a rapid increase in blood glucose levels, it seems logical that they would increase glycogen replenishment during the initial post-exercise period. Indeed, a number of studies have shown that you get faster glycogen replenishment during the first 6 hours after exercise (and, in particular, the first 2 hours) with moderate and high-GI carbohydrates compared with low-GI ones (Burke *et al.*, 2004; Burke *et al.*, 1993).

However, Danish researchers discovered that, after 24 hours, muscle glycogen storage is about the same on a high-GI as on a low-GI diet (Kiens *et al.*, 1990). In other words, high-GI foods post-exercise get your glycogen recovery off to a quick start, but low-GI foods will result in the same level of recovery 24 hours after exercise.

However, there are other performance benefits of a low-GI recovery diet – it may improve your endurance the next day. Researchers at Loughborough University found that when athletes consumed low-GI meals during the 24-hour period following exercise, they were able to exercise longer before exhaustion compared with those who had consumed high-GI meals (Stevenson *et al.*, 2005).

A review of studies found that consuming a mixture of carbohydrates, such as glucose and fructose, increases carbohydrate absorption and glycogen repletion (Gonzalez *et al.*, 2017). It also reduces the likelihood of experiencing GI discomfort and distress, which can occur when consuming more than 1.2 g carbohydrate/hour during the post-exercise period. Many carbohydrate-rich foods (e.g. fresh and dried fruit) naturally contain a mixture of glucose and fructose and, therefore, would be a better option than glucose-only drinks.

The bottom line is that if you perform high-intensity exercise twice a day, consuming high-GI foods during the first 2 hours after exercise will result in more efficient glycogen replenishment. However, if you train once a day (or less frequently), low-GI meals increase your endurance and performance during your subsequent workout.

DOES PROTEIN COMBINED WITH CARBOHYDRATE ENHANCE GLYCOGEN RECOVERY?

You can optimise glycogen recovery either by consuming 1.2g carbohydrate/ kg BW/ h or, if that is not practical by combining a small amount of protein (0.2–0.4 g/kg BW/h) with less carbohydrate (0.8 g/kg BW/h) (Alghannam *et al.*, 2018; Beelen *et al.*, 2010; Betts and Williams, 2010). Protein combined with carbohydrate will stimulate a greater output of insulin than carbohydrate alone, which, in turn, speeds the uptake of glucose and amino acids from the bloodstream into the muscle cells – thereby promoting glycogen synthesis – and blunts the rise in cortisol that would otherwise follow exercise. Cortisol suppresses the rate of protein synthesis and stimulates protein catabolism.

Consuming protein after exercise also stimulates muscle synthesis, inhibits protein breakdown and promotes positive protein balance in the muscle after both resistance and endurance exercise (Howarth *et al.*, 2009).

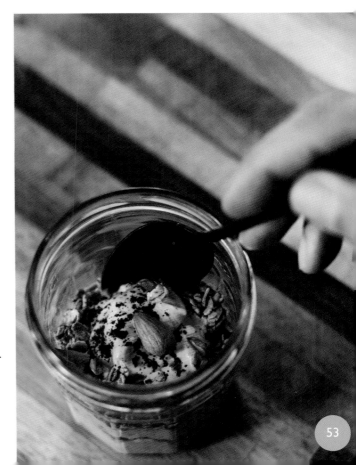

However, if you are able to consume enough carbohydrate, then adding protein will not further increase glycogen synthesis (Craven *et al.*, 2021; Jentjens *et al.*, 2001; Margolis *et al.*, 2021).

Endurance exercise

One of the first studies to demonstrate the advantages of consuming a carbohydrate-protein drink after exercise was carried out at the University of Texas at Austin in 1992 (Zawadski *et al.*, 1992). Researchers found that a carbohydrate-protein drink (112 g carbohydrate, 40 g protein) increased glycogen storage by 38% compared with a carbohydrate-only drink. Other studies subsequently have noted similar results (Ready *et al.*, 1999; Tarnopolsky *et al.*, 1997; Beelen *et al.*, 2010).

Researchers at the University of Texas at Austin measured significantly greater muscle glycogen levels 4 hours after 2½ hours' intense cycling when cyclists consumed a protein-carbohydrate drink (80 g carbohydrate, 28 g protein, 6 g fat) compared with a carbohydrate-only drink (80 g carbohydrate, 6 g fat) (Ivy *et al.*, 2002).

A joint study by researchers at the University of Bath and Loughborough University found that subsequent exercise performance after a carbohydrate-protein recovery drink was greater compared with consumption of a carbohydrate-only drink (Betts *et al.*, 2007). The runners in the study were able to run longer following a 4-hour recovery period during which they consumed a drink containing 0.8 g carbohydrate and 0.3 g protein/kg BW/hour. More recently, Scandinavian researchers found that consuming a mix of carbohydrate and protein in the 2-hour post-exercise window after exhaustive cycling improved endurance performance the following day compared with consuming only carbohydrate (Rustad *et al.*, 2016). Cyclists were able to keep going for 63.5 minutes compared with 49.8 minutes.

Researchers at James Madison University have shown that a carbohydrate-protein drink also reduces post-exercise muscle damage and muscle soreness (Luden *et al.*, 2007).

Resistance exercise

Consuming a protein-carbohydrate drink also appears to enhance recovery and muscle protein synthesis (MPS) following resistance exercise compared with carbohydrate alone. Researchers at the University of Texas Medical Branch measured higher levels of protein retention in athletes after consuming a recovery drink containing a mixture of carbohydrate, protein and amino acids, compared with a carbohydrate-only drink that provided the same number of calories (Borsheim *et al.*, 2004). According to researchers at Ithaca College, New York, consuming a protein-carbohydrate drink immediately after resistance exercise promotes more efficient muscle tissue growth as well as faster glycogen refuelling, compared with a carbohydrate-only drink or a placebo (Bloomer *et al.*, 2000). In this study, the researchers measured higher levels of anabolic hormones such as testosterone and lower levels of catabolic hormones such as cortisol for 24 hours after a weights workout when the volunteers consumed a protein-carbohydrate drink. Canadian researchers measured an increased protein uptake in the muscles after volunteers drank a protein-carbohydrate drink following resistance exercise (Gibala, 2000). A review of studies from Maastricht University in the Netherlands concluded that consuming a protein-carbohydrate drink following resistance exercise helps increase glycogen storage, stimulate protein synthesis and inhibit protein breakdown (Van Loon, 2007). For more information about protein intake after exercise, *see* pp. 70–76.

Putting it together: what, when and how much

Table 3.4 summarises the recommendations on carbohydrate intake before and after exercise. The simplest way to plan your daily food intake is to divide the day into four 'windows': before, during and after exercise, and between training sessions. You can then work out how much and what type of carbohydrate to consume during each 'window' to optimise your performance and recovery.

Low-carbohydrate, high-fat diets

Although it is generally accepted that optimal adaptation to repeated days of endurance training requires a high-carbohydrate diet to replenish muscle glycogen stores, there is also much debate about the possible benefits of consuming a chronic low-carbohydrate, high-fat (LCHF) diet or training with low carbohydrate availability ('training low'), i.e. with low pre-exercise muscle glycogen stores and no additional carbohydrate consumed during exercise.

The thinking behind this strategy is that since our fat stores are considerably greater than our glycogen stores, restricting carbohydrate intake or training with low carbohydrate availability will 1) 'train' the muscles to burn more fat during exercise, conserving precious glycogen and giving muscles greater access to a more plentiful supply of energy in the body, i.e. increase endurance, and 2) enhance metabolic adaptations in muscles.

This innovative approach to training is, of course, in contrast to the traditional advice that every training session should always be done with high carbohydrate availability (i.e. high pre-exercise glycogen levels and carbohydrates consumed during training).

Table 3.4	RECOMMENDATIONS FOR PRE- AND POST-EXERCISE CARBOHYDRATE INTAKE	
Dietary strategy	**When**	**Recommended carbohydrate intake**
Pre-exercise fuelling	Before exercise >60 min	1–4 g/kg BW consumed 1–4 h before exercise
Post-exercise rapid refuelling	<8 h recovery between two sessions	36–48 h of 10–12 g/kg BW/24 h
Carbohydrate loading	For events >90 min of sustained/intermittent exercise	36–48 h of 10–12 g/kg BW/24 h

Source: Burke *et al.*, 2011; Thomas *et al.*, 2016

WHAT ARE THE POTENTIAL ADVANTAGES OF LCHF DIETS OR 'TRAINING LOW'?

A number of studies have shown that restricting carbohydrate intake before and/or during exercise increases the transport, uptake and utilisation of fat during exercise (Spriet, 2014b) and enhances many of the adaptations inherent to endurance training. For example, training in conditions of low carbohydrate availability has been shown to increase mitochondrial biogenesis (formation of new mitochondria), mitochondrial enzyme activity and protein content, and whole-body and intramuscular fat oxidation (Bartlett *et al.*, 2015; Lane *et al.*, 2015; Morton *et al.*, 2009; Hansen *et al.*, 2005; Yeo *et al.*, 2008; Hawley *et al.*, 2011; Muoio *et al.*, 1994; Helge *et al.*, 2001; Lambert *et al.*, 1994). These augmented training responses are thought to be mediated via enhanced activation of cell signalling enzymes (e.g. AMPK, p38MAPK), transcription factors (e.g. p53) and transcription co-activators (Wojtaszewski *et al.*, 2003; Cochran *et al.*, 2010; Bartlett *et al.*, 2013; Yeo *et al.*, 2010).

A 2008 study at RMIT University, Australia, found that cyclists who performed some of their sessions with low glycogen availability had higher levels of fat-oxidising mitochondrial enzymes (Yeo *et al.*, 2008). And a 2010 study at the University of Birmingham found that fat oxidation during steady-state cycling was higher in cyclists when they 'trained low' than when they trained with high glycogen levels (Hulston *et al.*, 2010).

Belgian researchers also found that this protocol resulted in higher levels of fat oxidising enzymes in cyclists compared with non-fasted training (i.e. with high carbohydrate availability) (Van Proeyen *et al.*, 2011).

More recently, a 2015 study by Australian, Swedish and Malaysian researchers found that cyclists who did a fasted 2-hour low-intensity workout in the morning following a high-intensity workout the previous evening ('trained high, slept low', *see* p. 61) had lower muscle glycogen and increased transcription for metabolically adaptive genes than those who performed the same workouts with high glycogen stores (Lane *et al.*, 2015).

Thus, by training with low carbohydrate availability, training adaptations may be amplified and the muscles' ability to use fat as an energy source may be increased. However, these effects are observed only in elite or well-conditioned athletes – and the performance advantage suggested in some of the studies only applies at relatively low exercise intensities below about 65% of VO$_2$max, i.e. moderate, conversational pace. At higher exercise intensities, carbohydrate becomes the principal fuel source. This is sometimes referred to as the 'crossover point' – that intensity at which you start to burn more carbohydrate than fat. Therefore, for less conditioned athletes or untrained individuals, or those exercising above 65% VO$_2$max, chronically training on a LCHF diet would have no performance advantage (Burke *et al.*, 2004).

THEORY TO PRACTICE: HOW TO TRAIN WITH LOW CARBOHYDRATE AVAILABILITY

There are a number of different ways you can 'train low', which are described more fully in the box on p. 61. These include following a chronically low-carbohydrate diet, training after an overnight fast and before breakfast, training high, sleeping low, training twice a day or

Table 3.5	DIET STRATEGIES TO MANIPULATE CARBOHYDRATE AVAILABILITY TO POTENTIALLY ENHANCE PERFORMANCE	
Dietary strategy	**Description**	**Potential benefits**
High carbohydrate availability	High daily carbohydrate intake to fill/replenish muscle glycogen stores, typically 3–12 g/kg BW. Carbohydrate may be consumed before, during and/or after exercise	Optimise high-quality training
Periodised carbohydrate availability	Carbohydrate availability for each session is adjusted according to the structure and goals of the session. May include single sessions of 'train high' and 'train low' strategies	'Training high' enhances training quality/intensity; 'training low' enhances cell signalling and training adaptations
Low-carbohydrate, high-fat (LCHF)	Low daily carbohydrate intake less than muscle needs, typically <2.5 g/kg/day	Induces adaptations to increase the use of fat for fuel during exercise
Ketogenic LCHF diet	Very low carbohydrate intake to induce ketotosis, typically <50 g/day. Very high fat intake, typically 75–80% energy	Induces adaptations to greatly increase the use of fat for fuel (>1 g/min) during exercise

doing a long training session without onsuming carbohydrate

WHAT ARE THE DRAWBACKS OF LCHF DIETS OR TRAINING LOW?

The main drawbacks are the increased perceived exertion and potential reduction in training intensity associated with low carbohydrate availability. A comprehensive analysis of studies concluded that chronically training with low glycogen stores can impair the muscles' ability to store and use carbohydrate during high-intensity exercise (Burke, 2010).

In a landmark study at the University of Guelph, Canada, researchers found that cyclists who consumed a LCHF diet for 5 days followed by a high-carbohydrate diet for 1 day were better able to utilise fat for fuel during aerobic exercise (they burned 45% more fat and 30% less carbohydrate during a 20-minute ride at 70% VO_2max) but they had a reduced ability to use carbohydrate for fuel during a high-intensity time-trial even though they had full glycogen stores prior to the trial (Stellingwerff et al., 2006). The researchers concluded that a LCHF diet results in down-regulation of pyruvate dehydrogenase and other enzymes involved with carbohydrate oxidation. Reduced activity of these enzymes ultimately impairs carbohydrate oxidation and high-intensity performance. This is clearly a disadvantage for many athletes since most competitive events involve high-intensity efforts, sprints or tactical changes in pace.

A study at the University of Cape Town found that a LCHF diet resulted in impaired performance during the sprint stages of a 100 km cycling time-trial (Havemann *et al.*, 2006). Cyclists who consumed a LCHF diet for 6 days followed by 1 day of carbohydrate loading were not able to generate as much power during the sprint stages of a 100 km time-trial compared with those cyclists who consumed a high-carbohydrate diet for 7 days.

Similarly, a study at the University of Birmingham, with well-trained cyclists, found that power output during high-intensity interval training was significantly lower in those training low compared with those those training with high carbohydrate availability (Hulston *et al.*, 2010). A study with competitive mountain bikers found those who followed a LCHF diet experienced a drop in power and performance at high exercise intensities (Zajac *et al.*, 2014).

Another disadvantage of repeatedly 'training low' is the risk of illness, injury and over-reaching (short-term overtraining). The main symptoms of over-reaching are decreased performance, high fatigue rating at rest and during exercise, and altered mood state. A study at the University of Birmingham, found that when runners consumed a high-carbohydrate diet (8.5 g/kg/day) they performed better, experienced less fatigue and maintained a better mood state (i.e. showed fewer symptoms of over-reaching) than train-

Glycogen threshold

The glycogen threshold hypothesis proposes that there are certain concentrations of muscle glycogen that facilitate enhanced training adaptations while allowing completion of required training loads (Impey *et al.*, 2018). In other words, you need to achieve a critical level of glycogen depletion before these adaptations can occur. Studies suggest that the pre-exercise glycogen threshold is likely to be around 300 mmol/kg dry weight.

ing on a 'normal' carbohydrate diet (5.4 g/kg/day) during an 11-day period of intense training (Achten *et al.*, 2004). All athletes experienced a drop in performance with successive days of hard training but those on the high-carbohydrate diet fared significantly better.

In summary, training on a chronic LCHF diet or with low carbohydrate availability impairs the body's ability to use glycogen, reduces the capacity for high-intensity exercise, increases perceived exertion (makes exercise feels harder), and results in a lower power output. Additionally, consuming a LCHF diet in the post-exercise period may impair muscle protein synthesis (Hammond *et al.*, 2019)

WHAT IS THE EVIDENCE THAT LCHF DIETS IMPROVE PERFORMANCE?

Despite increasing the muscles' ability to use fat as an energy source, there is no clear evidence to date that *chronically* consuming a LCHF or ketogenic diet enhances endurance performance (Burke, 2020; Burke and Kiens, 2006; Hawley and Leckey, 2015; Maughan and Shirreffs, 2012; Hawley *et al.*, 2011; Morton *et al.*, 2009).

The first study to examine the effects of LCHF diets on performance was carried out at the University of Connecticut in 1983 (Phinney *et al.*, 1983). Five well-trained cyclists exercised to exhaustion at 63% VO_2 peak after consuming their usual diet (57% energy from carbohydrate) for 1 week, and then after consuming a LCHF diet (<20 g carbohydrate/day, 80% energy from fat) for 4 weeks. Researchers found that although muscle glycogen levels decreased, performance did not decline after consuming a LCHF diet. However, this was a poor-quality study and the average result is somewhat misleading. First, the study involved just five subjects (a very small number), two of whom experienced a significant *drop* in endurance. Two subjects had only a small increase but one subject had a large increase in time to exhaustion, thus skewing the overall study result. Second, exercise was performed at a relatively low intensity, not a race-level effort, which makes the findings irrelevant to the majority of competitive athletes.

An analysis of 20 studies by researchers at Kansas State University, concluded that LCHF diets provide no performance advantage for non-elite athletes but all athletes (especially non-elite) benefited from a high-carbohydrate diet (Erlenbusch *et al.*, 2005).

The most definitive evidence comes from the 'Supernova' study at the Australian Institute of Sport, which compared the performance effects of a high-carbohydrate diet (60–65% carbohydrate), a periodised carbohydrate diet (same macronutrients but periodised within or between days) and a ketogenic LCHF diet (<50 g carbohydrate) in a group of 21 elite race-walkers (Burke *et al.*,

2017). After 3.5 weeks of training, all athletes improved their aerobic fitness (VO_2max) but only those on the high-carbohydrate or periodised carbohydrate diet improved their 10 km race performance. The athletes on the LCHF diet did not make any improvement. Although they were burning a higher proportion of fat during exercise, their muscles became less efficient at producing energy, requiring more oxygen at any given speed. In other words, training on a LCHF diet reduces exercise economy and impairs high-intensity endurance performance.

The results were replicated in the 'Supernova 2' study, which was carried out with a larger number of race-walkers to see whether prior adaptation to a LCHF diet could benefit subsequent race performance after the athletes resumed a high-carbohydrate diet for 2.5 weeks before competition (Burke *et al.*, 2020). Again, fat oxidation was increased after following the LCHF diet, and both exercise economy and performance were reduced. After following the pre-competition high-carbohydrate diet for 2.5 weeks, there was no difference in performance between those previously following the LCHF diet or those following the high- or periodised-carbohydrate diet. In other words, a LCHF diet followed by a pre-competition taper with high carbohydrate availability provided no performance benefit.

It's worth noting that the world's top endurance athletes from Kenya and Ethiopia consume a high-carbohydrate diet containing 9–10 g/kg, well within current ISSN and ACSM recommendations and contrary to the LCHF diet principles (Onywera *et al.*, 2004; Beis *et al.*, 2011).

There is no evidence that ketogenic or LCHF diets benefit power-based athletes. A review of studies looking at the effects of ketogenic diets in CrossFit, gymnasts and power-lifting athletes failed to show any significant performance improvements (Harvey *et al.*, 2019). In fact, researchers have found that the ketogenic diet may even blunt muscle building and reduce muscle mass (Ashtary-Larky *et al.*, 2021).

Nevertheless, there are a few scenarios where chronic LCHF diets may benefit performance or at least not be detrimental. LCHF diets may suit those who do mostly low- to moderate-intensity training (such as ultra-endurance runners) or those who experience GI symptoms when consuming carbohydrate during prolonged exercise.

What is carbohydrate periodisation?

Many elite endurance athletes follow a periodised programme of training and it makes sense to adjust carbohydrate intake to reflect the different training demands of each training cycle. As a result, periodised carbohydrate restriction has become common practice among some endurance athletes.

During the 'base' training cycle, the emphasis is on low-intensity training to build endurance fitness and carbohydrate demands are smaller, so this is the training phase when you can incorporate more 'train low' sessions, perhaps twice a week. Conversely, 'quality' sessions, done at higher intensities later in the training cycle when an athlete is preparing to peak for competition, are best undertaken with high carbohydrate availability. But in any weekly training cycle (microcycle) there will be harder and easier sessions, so your carbohydrate and energy intake should reflect the difference in energy demands. Essentially, low-intensity or steady-state-type training sessions may

be performed with low glycogen stores, and high-intensity sessions with high glycogen stores. The idea is that matching your carbohydrate intake to the structure and aims of your training sessions or 'fuelling for the work required' improves 'metabolic flexibility', i.e. your muscles' ability to switch between both fat and carbohydrate as a fuel, as well as your body composition and performance (Impey *et al.* 2016). The advantage of this day-by-day approach is that you get the dual benefits of 'training low' – namely metabolic flexibility – as well as the performance-enhancing benefits of high-intensity training.

On days when you train low, it is recommended that you increase your protein intake to 2–2.5 kg/kg body weight, which equates to 140–175 g for a 70 kg athlete, and distribute your protein intake evenly across your meals, e.g. 20–30 g every 3 hours (Moore *et al.*, 2014). This will help offset any potential reductions in lean muscle mass that occurs through any chronic periods of energy deficit.

HOW CAN YOU REDUCE FATIGUE WHEN TRAINING LOW?

The downside to training low is that exercise feels much harder and many athletes find they cannot maintain a high exercise intensity. This may be partially overcome by consuming caffeine (1–3 mg/kg body weight, equivalent to 70–210 mg for a 70 kg athlete) before or during exercise. In one study, glycogen-depleted cyclists who consumed caffeine prior to a 4 km cycling time-trial performed better than those who did not consume caffeine but the same as those who were not glycogen depleted (Silva-Cavalcante *et al.*, 2013). Australian researchers also showed that caffeine consumed 1 hour before a high-

'Train low' protocols

There are a number of ways to 'train low'. These include:

A chronically low-carbohydrate diet

This involves consuming a low-carbohydrate diet (i.e. less carbohydrate than you need for fuelling training) and 'training low' for all training sessions. This method may improve fat adaptation but will result in a reduced capacity for high-intensity exercise. It may also reduce immune function and increase the risk of illness.

Training after an overnight fast

This is perhaps the most popular 'train low' protocol and the easiest to adopt. Training is performed in the morning before breakfast following an overnight fast and without consuming carbohydrate during the workout (Van Proeyen et al., 2011).

Train high, sleep low

A high-intensity training session is performed in the evening to deplete muscle glycogen, followed by an overnight fast so muscle glycogen stores are not replenished. The next morning, a light training session is carried out on an empty stomach (i.e. 'train low'). After this, glycogen stores are replenished by consuming normal meals for the rest of the day. Thus, high-intensity sessions are done with high carbohydrate availability and low-intensity sessions are done with low carbohydrate availability (Lane et al., 2015).

Training twice a day

When training twice a day, the first (high-intensity) session is performed with high carbohydrate availability and the second (low-intensity) with low carbohydrate availability (Yeo et al., 2008). This is achieved by limiting carbohydrate consumption after the first session and then consuming a high-carbohydrate meal after the second session.

Prolonged training without consuming carbohydrate

During a long training session lasting more than 90 minutes, no carbohydrate is consumed. This means the latter stages of the session will be performed with low muscle glycogen stores (Morton et al., 2009).

No carbohydrate during recovery

By avoiding carbohydrate for 1–2 hours after exercise, it may be possible to achieve greater training adaptations (Pilegaard et al., 2005). However, post-exercise recovery may take longer.

intensity interval training session improved power output in glycogen-depleted cyclists (Lane *et al.*, 2013(b)). However, power output was still lower than when they performed the same training session with normal glycogen stores. Caffeine is known to reduce perceived exertion and fatigue during exercise (*see* p. 118).

Alternatively, you can practise 'carbohydrate mouth rinsing' (*see* pp. 43–44) during your train-

Fuelling for the work required

Fuelling for the work required is a training model developed by researchers at Liverpool John Moores University in 2016 for elite athletes (Impey *et al.*, 2016). It proposes that carbohydrate availability should be adjusted day to day and meal by meal according to the intensity, duration and goals of specific training sessions to be completed. The aim is to maintain metabolic flexibility and still allow the completion of high-intensity workloads on heavy training days. Essentially, low-intensity or recovery training sessions are completed with low carbohydrate availability ('training low') and high-intensity sessions with high carbohydrate availability ('training high'). In other words, you would consume carbohydrate-rich foods before and during high-intensity sessions, and then low-carbohydrate meals before low-intensity sessions and consume nothing during exercise. A sample eating plan is shown on p. 63. The exact amount of carbohydrate you need at each meal will depend on your body weight and training goals.

ing session to help you maintain your training intensity (or at least avoid too big a reduction) and prevent muscle protein breakdown (Bartlett *et al.*, 2015). Carbohydrate mouth rinsing acts on the central nervous system (brain) to mask fatigue and reduce perceived exertion, thus allowing you to keep going longer. While it may be more beneficial to swallow the drink and thus make use of the calories it contains, it's a useful strategy for improving endurance when 'training low'. A 2015 study at Liverpool John Moores University found that athletes who 'trained low' with a carbohydrate mouth rinse plus caffeine during a high-intensity interval set were able to keep going 13 minutes longer than those who just had a mouth rinse but not caffeine, and 29 minutes longer than those who did neither (placebo) (Kasper *et al.*, 2015).

WHAT IS THE EVIDENCE FOR CARBOHYDRATE PERIODISATION?

Two studies suggest that strategic periodisation of carbohydrate around selected training sessions (i.e. doing your low-intensity sessions with low carbohydrate availability) can not only lead to favourable enhanced metabolic adaptations but can also result in improved performance and body composition.

For example, a multicentre study by French, Australian and UK researchers found that triathletes who employed a carbohydrate periodisation strategy (doing high-intensity evening sessions with high carbohydrate availability, and low-intensity fasted morning sessions with low carbohydrate availability: 'train high, sleep low') for 3 weeks improved their cycling efficiency (power output per calorie) by 11%, 10 km running performance by 2.9%, time to exhaustion during high-intensity

Fuelling for the work required – a sample diet plan

This sample diet shows you how to tailor your eating to your training sessions in a 48-hour period.

Day 1 (high-intensity training session)

- Breakfast: Porridge, bananas, honey
- Snack: Fruit, nuts
- Lunch: Rice, chicken, vegetables
- Snack: Fruit, toast, honey
- Evening training (high-intensity intervals): Sports drink, bananas, gels or dried fruit
- Post-training: Protein recovery drink
- Dinner: Grilled fish, salad

Day 2 (low-intensity session)

- Breakfast (optional): Eggs
- Morning training (long, low-intensity ride): Water
- Post-training: Carbohydrate and protein recovery drink
- Snack: Toast, honey, plain yoghurt, fruit
- Lunch: Pasta, fish, salad
- Snack: Fruit, nuts, granola bar
- Dinner: Sweet potato, chicken, vegetables

exercise by 12.5%, and also cut their body fat (1%) compared with those who did all their training with high carbohydrate availability (Marquet *et al.*, 2016 (a)). A follow-up study with cyclists by the same team found that using a 'sleeping low' strategy for just 1 week resulted in a 3.2% improvement in a 20 km time-trial (Marquet *et al.*, 2016 (b)).

Other studies have not shown such favourable effects on performance when compared to training with high carbohydrate availability. A meta-analysis of nine studies concluded the evidence to support a performance-enhancing effect of carbohydrate periodisation in well-trained endurance athletes is weak (Gejl and Nybo, 2021).

The exact balance between training low and training high depends on many factors, including training goals, frequency and intensity of training, lifestyle and individual make-up. Clearly, everyone responds differently to diet and training regimes and there is no single approach that suits everyone. However, incorporating both glycogen-depleted and glycogen-loaded training sessions in your programme may be beneficial during the 'low' season, i.e. away from competition, when the risk of compromising training intensity is low and the chances of improving your fuel efficiency is higher.

Summary of key points

- Carbohydrate is a major fuel for exercise during almost all exercise intensities.
- Carbohydrate availability in the form of muscle and liver glycogen is an important determinant of performance during prolonged moderate- to high-intensity exercise.
- Glycogen depletion results in fatigue and a reduced capacity for high-intensity exercise.
- Exercising with 'high carbohydrate availability' optimises endurance and performance during high-intensity exercise lasting longer than 90 minutes or intermittent high-intensity exercise.
- High carbohydrate availability is typically achieved with daily carbohydrate intakes of 3–12 g/kg/day.

- Carbohydrates may be classified according to the number of simple sugar units (simple; complex), their nutritional quality or their effect on blood glucose (glycaemic index).
- The GI is a ranking of carbohydrates based on their immediate effect on blood glucose (blood sugar) levels. Carbohydrates with a high GI produce a rapid rise in blood sugar; those with a low GI produce a slow rise in blood sugar.
- Carbohydrate intake in the 1–4 hours before exercise helps increase liver and muscle glycogen levels and enhances your subsequent performance.
- The pre-exercise meal should contain approx. 1–4 g carbohydrate/kg body weight.
- For moderate- to high-intensity exercise lasting 45–75 minutes, mouth rinsing with carbohydrate for 5–10 seconds can improve performance, especially if training in a fasted or glycogen-depleted state.
- For moderate- to high-intensity exercise lasting more than 60 minutes, consuming 30–60 g carbohydrate/h (in solid, semi-solid or liquid form) during exercise can help maintain exercise intensity for longer and delay fatigue.
- For high-intensity exercise lasting more than 2½ hours, higher rates of carbohydrate absorption and oxidation, up to 90 g/h, can be achieved by consuming a mixture of carbohydrates, e.g. glucose and fructose.
- Glycogen recovery takes, on average, 20 hours but depends on the severity of glycogen depletion, the extent of the muscle damage and the amount, type and timing of carbohydrate intake.
- Glycogen replenishment is faster than normal during the 6-hour post-exercise period.
- For rapid recovery where there is <8 hours between sessions, it is recommended to consume 1–1.2 g moderate–high-GI carbohydrate/kg body weight for the 4 hours post-exercise.
- If it is not possible to consume sufficient carbohydrate in the post-exercise period then combining carbohydrate with protein may be equally effective in promoting muscle glycogen recovery.
- Training in conditions of low carbohydrate availability augments fat oxidation and several markers of training adaptation, including mitochondrial biogenesis and mitochondrial enzyme activity.
- Chronically training with low carbohydrate availability can impair the muscles' ability to store and use carbohydrate during high-intensity exercise, increase perceived exertion, reduce power output and increase the risk of illness.
- There is no clear evidence to date that *chronically* consuming a LCHF or ketogenic diet enhances endurance performance.
- Periodising carbohydrate around selected training sessions or 'fuelling for the work required' may improve metabolic flexibility, body composition and performance.

//Protein

The importance of protein – and the question of whether extra protein is necessary – for sports performance is one of the most hotly debated topics among sports scientists, coaches and athletes and has been contended ever since the time of the Ancient Greeks. Protein has long been associated with power and strength, and, as the major constituent of muscle, it would seem logical that an increased protein intake would increase muscle size and strength.

Previously, scientists held the view that athletes do not need to consume more than the Reference Nutrient Intake (RNI) for protein and that consuming anything greater than this amount would produce no further benefit. However, research since the 1980s has cast doubt on this view. There is considerable evidence that the protein needs of active individuals are consistently higher than those of the general population.

This chapter will help to give you a fuller understanding of the role of protein during exercise and enable you to work out how much you need for muscle building and optimising recovery after different types of activities. It explains how individual requirements depend on many factors, including the type of activity, the amount of muscle mass activated during resistance exercise, body mass, age and co-ingestion of other nutrients. It also considers the timing of protein intake throughout the day. Protein supplementation is briefly considered here and discussed in more detail in Chapter 7.

Why do I need protein?

Protein makes up part of the structure of every cell and tissue in your body, including your muscle tissue, internal organs, tendons, skin, hair and nails. On average, it comprises about 20% of your total body weight. Protein is needed for the growth and formation of new tissue, for tissue repair and for regulating many metabolic pathways, and can also be used as a fuel for energy production when carbohydrate availability is low, for example during prolonged high-intensity endurance exercise. It is also needed to make almost all of the body's enzymes as well as hormones (such as adrenaline and insulin), neurotransmitters and antibodies. Protein has a role in maintaining optimal fluid balance in tissues, transporting nutrients in and out of cells, carrying oxygen and regulating blood clotting.

WHAT ARE AMINO ACIDS?

There are 20 types of amino acids, which are the building blocks of proteins. They can be combined in various ways to form hundreds of different proteins in the body. When you eat protein, it is broken down in your digestive tract into smaller molecular units – single amino acids and dipeptides (two amino acids linked together).

Eleven of the amino acids can be made in the body from other amino acids, carbohydrate and nitrogen. These are called non-essential amino acids (NEAAs). The other nine are termed essential amino acids (EAAs), meaning they must be supplied in the diet. All 20 amino acids are listed in Table 4.1. Branched-chain amino acids (BCAAs) include the three EAAs with a branched molecular configuration: valine, leucine and isoleucine. They make up one-third of muscle protein and are a vital substrate for two other amino acids, glutamine and alanine, which are released in large quantities during intense aerobic exercise. Also, they can be used directly as fuel by the muscles, particularly when muscle glycogen is depleted. Strictly speaking, the body's requirement is for amino acids rather than protein.

Table 4.1	ESSENTIAL AND NON-ESSENTIAL AMINO ACIDS
Essential amino acids (EAAs)	**Non-essential amino acids (NEAAs)**
Isoleucine	Alanine
Leucine	Arginine
Lysine	Asparagine
Methionine	Aspartic acid
Phenylalanine	Cysteine
Threonine	Glutamic acid
Tryptophan	Glutamine
Valine	Glycine
Histidine*	Proline
	Serine
	Tyrosine

* Histidine is essential for babies (not for adults)

Table 4.2	THE PROTEIN QUALITY (DIAAS) OF VARIOUS FOODS	
Food		**Protein Quality (DIAAS)**
Animal protein sources		
Milk		114
Egg		113
Plant protein sources		
Soya protein isolate		98
Black beans		59
Green lentils		65
Chickpeas		83
Peanuts		43
White rice		57
White bread		29

Source: Berrazaga *et al.*, 2019

WHAT IS THE DIFFERENCE BETWEEN ANIMAL AND PLANT PROTEINS?

Plant and animal proteins differ in their content of amino acids, as well as their digestibility. Both of these factors dictate how useful the protein will be to the body and how much of it will be converted into body proteins. This is sometimes called 'protein quality' and replaces the outdated notion of complete and incomplete proteins. The idea that plant proteins are incomplete or 'missing' specific amino acids is false. All plant foods contain all 20 amino acids, including the nine essential amino acids, albeit some at low levels – but they do not lack any (Gardner *et al.*, 2019; Mariotti and Gardner, 2019).

Generally speaking, animal protein sources (e.g. dairy and meat) provide EAAs in ratios closely matched to the body's requirements (Berrazaga *et al.*, 2019). Hence, they are considered to be 'high quality'. In contrast, there are only a handful of high-quality plant sources of protein, i.e. that contain all nine EAAs in relatively high amounts, namely soya (e.g. soya milk alternative, soya yoghurt alternative, tofu, tempeh and miso), quinoa, buckwheat, amaranth, chia and hemp seeds. Beans, lentils, peas, grains and nuts contain smaller amounts of one or more EAAs – sometimes called the limiting amino acid – but you can easily compensate by consuming more than one plant food in the same 24-hour period (Gardner *et al.*, 2019; Young and Pellett, 1994). For example, beans are relatively low in methionine, while grains are relatively low in lysine (*see* p. 266) and nuts are low in threonine. Eating beans, rice and nuts will give you all nine EAAs.

The digestibility of proteins can be measured by a score called the digestible indispensable amino acid score (DIAAS), which measures the amount

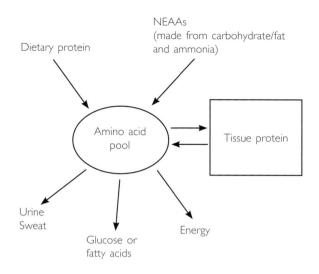

Figure 4.1 Protein metabolism

of protein absorbed from the large intestine and is considered more accurate than the protein digestibility-corrected amino acid score (PDCAAS), which measures the amount of protein absorbed from the small intestine (Rutherfurd *et al.*, 2015). Generally, animal proteins have DIAAS values greater than 100 while plant proteins have DIAAS values less than 75, with the exception of soya protein, which is between 75 and 100 and oats around 75. Table 4.2 shows the DIAAS values of various animal and plant foods. Chapter 15 discusses the protein requirements of vegetarian and vegan athletes in more detail.

HOW DOES EXERCISE AFFECT MY PROTEIN REQUIREMENT?

Endurance training

For endurance athletes, consuming protein in the post-training recovery period is important for optimising the benefits of training (Moore *et al.*, 2014). Following endurance training,

Protein metabolism

Tissue proteins are continually broken down (muscle protein breakdown, MPB), releasing their constituent amino acids into the 'free amino acid pool', which is located in body tissues and the blood. For example, half of your total body protein is broken down and replaced every 150 days. Amino acids absorbed from food and non-essential amino acids made in the body from nitrogen and carbohydrate can also enter the free pool. Once in the pool, amino acids have four fates. They can be 1) used to build new proteins (muscle protein synthesis, MPS), 2) oxidised to produce energy, 3) converted to glucose via gluconeogenesis or 4) converted into fatty acids. During energy production, the nitrogen part of the protein molecule is converted to urea and excreted in urine. MPS and MPB fluctuate over the course of a day, with the difference between the two determining net protein balance (NPB). A positive NPB represents an increase in muscle mass while a negative NPB results in a loss of muscle mass. In sedentary people, protein intake at meals provides the main anabolic stimulus, with transient periods of positive protein balance after meals being offset by periods of negative protein balance between meals. Thus MPS is counterbalanced by MPB and so muscle mass essentially stays the same (see Fig 4.2). Resistance exercise acts as an additional stimulus, increasing both the rate of MPS and MPB for up to 48 hours after exercise.

dietary protein is used for repairing damaged muscle fibres as well as building new mitochondrial proteins, which is where energy production occurs (Churchward-Venne *et al.*, 2020; Wilkinson *et al.*, 2008).

Additional protein is also needed to compensate for the increased breakdown of protein during intense training. When your muscle glycogen stores are low – which typically occurs after 60–90 minutes of high-intensity endurance exercise – certain amino acids, namely glutamate and the BCAAs valine, leucine and isoleucine (*see* p. 66), can be used for energy. The greater the exercise intensity and the longer the duration of exercise, the more protein is broken down for fuel. One of the BCAAs, leucine, is converted into another amino acid, alanine, which is converted in the liver into glucose. This glucose is released back into the bloodstream and transported to the exercising muscles, where it is used for energy. In fact, protein may contribute up to 15% of your energy production when glycogen stores are low. This is quite a substantial increase, as protein contributes less than 5% of energy needs when muscle glycogen stores are high.

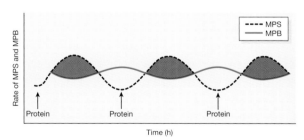

Figure 4.2 Changes in muscle protein synthesis (MPS) and muscle protein breakdown (MPB) in response to protein intake

Source: Burd *et al.*, 2009

Resistance training

Resistance exercise and dietary protein are both potent stimuli for MPS. When they are combined, this results in a synergistic stimulation of MPS, which, over time, results in increased muscle mass (Wilkinson *et al.*, 2008; Burd *et al.*, 2009; Phillips *et al.*, 2011; Phillips, 2012, Biolo *et al.*, 1997) (*see* Fig 4.3).

After resistance training, both the rate of protein breakdown and synthesis increase, although for the first few hours the rate of breakdown exceeds the rate of synthesis. If you consume no or insufficient protein during this post-exercise period then NPB remains negative and you will experience minimal gains in strength, size and mass, or even muscle loss (Phillips *et al.*, 1997; Phillips *et al.*, 1999). Therefore, you need to consume sufficient protein in the post-exercise period to stimulate MPS. A meta-analysis of 18 studies found that consuming more protein than the RDA increases lean mass in people undertaking resistance training (Hudson *et al.*, 2020).

In practice, the body is capable of adapting to slight variations in protein intake. It becomes more efficient at recycling amino acids during protein metabolism if your intake falls over a period of time. It is important to understand that a high-protein diet alone will not result in increased strength or muscle size. These goals can be achieved only when an optimal protein intake is combined with resistance training.

HOW MUCH PROTEIN DO I NEED EACH DAY FOR OPTIMAL PERFORMANCE?

At low–moderate exercise intensities (<50% VO_2max), it appears there is no significant increase in protein requirements above the

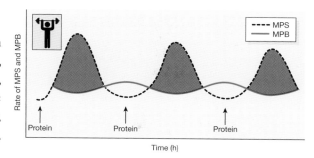

Figure 4.3 Changes in MPS and MPB in response to resistance exercise and protein intake

recommended daily intake for the general population (Hargreaves and Snow, 2001). Thus, for both sedentary people and recreational exercisers, the daily protein requirement is 0.75 or 0.80 g protein/kg BW daily in the UK and US respectively.

For endurance- and resistance-trained athletes, numerous studies have shown that the RDA is inadequate (Thomas *et al.*, 2016; IOC, 2011; Phillips and Van Loon, 2011). The recommendation for athletes generally is 1.2–2.0 g/kg BW/day (Thomas *et al.*, 2016; Phillips *et al.*, 2007; Tipton *et al.*, 2007; Williams, 1998). These recommendations encompass a range of training programmes and allow for adjustment according to the specific goals of your training sessions and body composition goals. For building or maintaining muscle mass, the IAAF recommends an intake in the range of 1.3–1.7 g/kg BW/day (Witard *et al.*, 2019). For example, if you weigh 70 kg then you will need 91–119 g protein a day.

A protein intake at the lower end of the recommended range, around 1.2–1.4 g/kg BW/day, is generally recommended for endurance training (Rodriguez *et al.*, 2009; Phillips *et al.*, 2007; Tipton *et al.*, 2007; Lemon, 1998; Williams and Devlin, 1992; Williams, 1998) but a higher protein intake would also be appropriate when doing more frequent, prolonged or high-intensity endurance sessions, or when training with low glycogen availability (see pp. 55–60).

Guidelines for post-exercise protein intake have moved towards the expression of recommendations on a 'per meal' basis rather than a total daily basis. These are given on pp. 71–72.

During a period of reduced energy availability (weight loss), increasing your dietary protein helps preserve muscle mass (see below 'How much protein should I consume each day if I want to lose weight?'). Also, studies have shown that novices have slightly higher requirements for protein per kg body weight compared with more experienced athletes (Phillips and Van Loon, 2011). One study suggests the requirements per kg body weight of novice bodybuilders can be up to 40% higher than those of experienced bodybuilders (Tarnopolsky, 1988). When you begin a training programme, your protein needs rise due to increases in protein turnover (Gontzea et al., 1975). After about 3 weeks of training, the body adapts to the exercise and becomes more efficient at recycling protein. Muscle protein can be built up again from amino acids released into the amino acid pool. In other words, the body becomes more efficient at conserving protein.

HOW MUCH PROTEIN SHOULD I CONSUME EACH DAY IF I WANT TO LOSE WEIGHT?

When cutting calories to lose body fat, you risk losing muscle mass as well. The more severe the calorie deficit, the greater the losses are likely to be. Also, the leaner you are, the more susceptible you will be to muscle loss. A higher protein intake

can offset some of the muscle wasting effects associated with an energy deficit. Researchers recommend increasing your protein intake to 1.8–2.7 g/kg BW/day (or 2.3–3.1 g/kg fat-free mass), while cutting your daily energy intake by a modest amount (approximately 15%) and including some form of resistance training in order to prevent lean mass losses (Hector and Phillips, 2018; Murphy et al., 2015; Helms et al., 2014 (a); Phillips and Van Loon, 2011). For example, a 70 kg athlete would need to consume 126–189 g protein/day. A study at McMaster University, Ontario, Canada found that volunteers who consumed 2.4 g protein/kg BW in combination with a 40% calorie deficit and an intense resistance training programme lost significantly more body fat (4.8 kg vs. 3.5 kg) and gained significantly more muscle (1.2 kg vs. 0.1 kg) over 4 weeks than a control group who consumed 1.2 g protein/kg BW (Longland et al., 2016). However, the training programme was very hard and may, therefore, not be sustainable for most.

HOW CAN I OPTIMISE MUSCLE PROTEIN SYNTHESIS?

The rate of muscle recovery and muscle protein synthesis after exercise depends on several factors, including the amount of protein you consume before, during and after exercise, the amount of muscle mass activated during exercise, the type of protein consumed, co-ingestion of other nutrients, your age and the distribution of protein intake throughout the day.

Protein before and during exercise

A number of studies suggest that consuming protein plus carbohydrate before and during prolonged, high-intensity exercise stimulates

MPS during exercise, minimises protein break-down, improves recovery from exercise and results in less muscle damage (Beradi *et al.*, 2008; Saunders, 2007; Luden *et al.*, 2007; Romano-Ely *et al.*, 2006).

Researchers at the University of Texas Medical Branch, found that consuming a drink containing protein and carbohydrate before resistance exercise was more effective in stimulating post-exercise MPS than consuming the same drink immediately after exercise (Tipton *et al.*, 2001). Similarly, a study at Maastricht University, found that consuming a drink containing equal amounts of protein plus carbohydrate at regular intervals during a 2-hour resistance workout resulted in significantly increased MPS rates and reduced protein breakdown during exercise compared with a carbohydrate-only drink (Beelen *et al.*, 2008).

While consuming protein during exercise may increase MPS, it has not been shown to provide any performance benefit. For example, one Canadian study found that adding whey protein to an energy drink did not make any difference to the performance of cyclists in a 80 km time-trial (Van Essen and Gibala, 2006). In other words, if carbohydrate is optimal, the addition of protein is unlikely to improve performance.

Amount of protein per meal

A review of studies concluded that protein consumed early in the post-exercise recovery phase increases the rate of MPS, promotes muscle repair and increases muscle adaptation to prolonged exercise (Van Loon, 2014). However, it is not necessary to consume protein immediately after exercise as the post-exercise anabolic window is thought to be as long as 48 hours. One study found no difference in muscle mass, size

Protein and satiety

Protein plays an important role in appetite regulation. It has been shown to promote satiety (the feeling of fullness and reduction in hunger after eating) more than carbohydrate, which is why it is particularly useful when you're trying to lose weight or prevent weight regain (Westerterp-Plantenga et al., 2012). It slows stomach emptying, thus helping you feel full longer. It also triggers the release of appetite-regulating hormones in the gut, such as glucagon-like peptide-1 (GLP-1), peptide YY (PYY) and glucagon; and reduces levels of 'hunger' hormones such as ghrelin. These hormones signal to the appetite control centre in the brain that you are satiated, so you stop eating. Researchers at the University of Copenhagen, Denmark, gave 25 volunteers different amounts of protein and found that there was a dose-dependent effect on levels of appetite hormones and satiety (Belza et al., 2013). Increasing doses of protein stimulated corresponding increases in responses of these hormones after eating, as well as increases in subjective feelings of satiety. The greater the protein intake, the higher the levels of GLP-1, PYY and glucagon and the greater the satiety experienced by the volunteers.

or strength after pre-workout or post-workout protein consumption (Schoenfeld *et al.*, 2017b)).

Several studies suggest that the optimal post-exercise protein intake is 0.24 g/kg BW (or 0.25 g/kg lean body mass), which translates to

20 g for an athlete weighing 80 kg (Thomas *et al.*, 2016; Phillips and Van Loon, 2011; Moore *et al.*, 2009; IOC, 2011; Rodriguez *et al.*, 2009). In a study at McMaster University, volunteers consumed either 5, 10, 20 or 40 g egg protein immediately after resistance training (Moore *et al.*, 2009). Scientists then measured the rate of MPS in the following 4 hours and found there was a dose-response relationship between protein intake and MPS up to a maximum, which occurred with 20 g protein. Higher doses (40 g) produced no further significant increase in MPS. Any excess is simply used as an energy source (oxidised) and the amino nitrogen converted into urea and excreted in the urine.

Following on from this study, researchers measured the increase in the MPS in the 4-hour post-exercise period after consuming different quantities of whey protein (0, 10, 20 or 40 g) (Witard *et al.*, 2014(b)). They, too, found that 20 g of whey protein was the optimal dose for stimulating maximum MPS after resistance training. The average athlete in the studies weighed approximately 80 kg, so it is likely that heavier athletes would require more protein (20–25 g) and lighter athletes would need less (15–20 g) to stimulate maximum MPS (Phillips *et al.*, 2011).

However, most of these studies were done with whey protein supplements, a 'high-quality' rapidly digested protein, so may not be applicable to different protein sources particularly when eaten in combination with other foods. More recent reviews suggest that to maximise MPS, an intake of either 0.31 g/kg high-quality protein (Moore, 2019) or 0.4 g mixed protein/kg/meal across four meals to reach an intake of 1.6 g/kg/day would be more appropriate (Schoenfeld and Aragon, 2018).

Amount of active muscle mass

Most of these studies involved leg-only workouts and subsequent research suggests that when a larger amount of muscle mass is activated, larger amounts of protein may be optimal (Macnaughton *et al.*, 2016). The researchers found that consuming 40 g protein after a whole-body resistance workout (as opposed to a leg-only workout) resulted in 20% greater MPS than 20 g protein. In other words, when a greater muscle mass is activated during resistance training then a higher protein intake may be required to maximise MPS.

Type of protein

Protein sources differ in their ability to stimulate MPS according to their amino acid content (particularly leucine) and how rapidly they are digested. Most studies suggest that 'high-quality' proteins (i.e. those with a high EAA content and that are rapidly digested and absorbed), such as milk and egg, increase MPS more than lower-quality proteins (Phillips *et al.*, 2011; Tipton *et al.*, 2007). EAAs act as a stimulus for MPS in a dose-dependent manner: the greater the concentration of EAAs in the bloodstream, the greater the rate of MPS. Therefore, foods that contain high levels of EAAs would be most effective.

Milk-based proteins (such as whey and casein) have been shown to promote greater protein uptake in the muscle as well as greater MPS compared with soya protein (van Vliet *et al.*, 2015; Wilkinson *et al.*, 2007; Tipton *et al.*, 2004; Tipton *et al.*, 2007). A study at McMaster University found that those who consumed milk after resistance training gained more lean mass after 12 weeks than those who consumed soya drinks containing the same amount of protein (Phillips *et al.*, 2005). This effect is thought to be due to

Leucine and muscle protein synthesis

Studies have shown that of the EAAs, the branched-chain amino acid leucine is largely responsible for the stimulatory effect of MPS (Anthony *et al.*, 2001; Norton and Layman, 2006). Without it, protein synthesis cannot take place. Much of the MPS-enhancing properties of dairy protein are thought to be due to its high content of leucine. Leucine is a branched-chain amino acid (see p. 66) that acts as both a substrate (building block) and a trigger for MPS. It initiates the process of regenerating and building muscle so it is particularly important for those wanting to build strength and muscle mass. Leucine increases MPS by stimulating the mammalian target of rapamycin complex 1 (mTORC1) signalling pathway, which results in the formation of new muscle proteins.

It has been hypothesised that to maximise MPS, a 'leucine threshold' must be surpassed. This is the intake required to achieve maximum MPS and is thought be 2–3 g leucine per meal, perhaps as high as 3.5 g in older athletes (Drummond and Rasmussen, 2008; Katsanos *et al.*, 2006). However, the optimal leucine dose depends on factors such as age and body weight (Burd *et al.*, 2013; Moore *et al.*, 2009; Witard *et al.*, 2014(b)). If leucine concentration is too low, mTORC1 deactivates and no MPS occurs.

In a study at Maastricht University, athletes who consumed a leucine/carbohydrate/protein supplement after resistance training had less muscle protein breakdown and greater MPS than those who consumed a supplement without leucine (Koopman *et al.*, 2005).

Leucine is found widely in animal proteins, including eggs, milk and dairy products, meat, fish and poultry. It is found in particularly high concentrations in whey protein, which explains why whey supplements have been shown to increase MPS more than other sources. Table 4.3 (p. 74) shows the amounts of various foods that you would need to consume to get 2–3 g leucine and 20 g protein.

the greater leucine content of milk. In a study at the University of Connecticut, volunteers gained significantly more muscle when they consumed a daily whey supplement over a 9-month period while following a resistance training programme, compared with soya protein or carbohydrate supplements containing the same calories (Volek *et al.*, 2013). This is thought to be partly because whey is a 'fast' protein, which means it is digested and absorbed relatively quickly, producing a rapid rise in EAAs in the bloodstream, and partly due to its higher content of leucine (Phillips *et al.*, 2011; Tang *et al.*, 2009; Boirie *et al.*, 1997; Dangin *et al.*, 2001). Leucine is an important trigger and substrate for protein synthesis (Phillips and Van Loon, 2011; Burd *et al.*, 2009; Tang *et al.*, 2009) However, the lower analbolic properties of plant proteins may be overcome by consuming greater quantities of plant proteins or consuming a variety of different sources over the day (van Vliet *et al.*, 2015).

Newer research suggests that consuming a mixture of 'fast' and 'slow' proteins may have additional benefits compared with whey protein since different proteins are digested at different rates. A study at the University of Texas

Medical Branch has shown that a supplement containing a 19 g blend of whey, casein and soya protein produced a more sustained rise in blood levels of amino acids and therefore a longer period of increased MPS following resistance exercise compared with the same amount of whey protein (Reidy *et al.,* 2013). Whether this is more effective than consuming protein-rich foods (such as milk) is unclear but given that foods naturally contain a mixture of proteins (milk contains both casein and whey), plus they are sources of many other nutrients, natural food sources may be better options than supplements for most people.

FOODS

It is not clear whether it is advantageous to consume liquid forms of protein, such as milk or whey protein shakes, rather than solid forms of protein (such as meat or eggs). That said, a study at the Australian Institute of Sport found that consuming liquid protein produced a more rapid rise in amino acid levels in the bloodstream

Table 4.3	FOOD PORTIONS SUPPLYING 2–3 G LEUCINE AND 20 G PROTEIN
600 ml milk	
85 g Cheddar cheese	
450 g plain yoghurt	
3 eggs	
85 g meat or poultry	
100 g fish	
17 g whey powder	

following exercise (Burke *et al.,* 2012). While this may increase MPS in the immediate post-exercise period, it does not necessarily mean that MPS is any different over 24 hours or that it results in bigger strength or muscle mass gains.

Food matrix

Most studies on protein intake have used isolated protein sources, such as whey, to eliminate confounding factors and isolate the effects of protein from other nutrients. However, the results may not apply to whole-food protein sources, particularly when consumed with other nutrients as part of a meal. There is very little research on the effects of whole-food protein sources on MPS but a review of studies concluded that whole foods are generally a better option than supplements (Burd *et al.,* 2019). Not only do they supply a range of other nutrients, but the interaction of the other nutrients contained within the food matrix may actually increase the use of protein for muscle repair. For example, a number of studies suggest that milk promotes MPS and may be considered an effective recovery drink (*see* p. 76). Beef has also been shown to support the post-exercise rise in MPS rates (Burd *et al.,* 2015). One study found that consuming whole eggs immediately after resistance exercise resulted in greater MPS than did consumption of egg white despite containing the same amount of protein (van Vliet *et al.,* 2017). Another showed that whole milk is more anabolic than fat-free milk (Elliot *et al.,* 2006). The International Association of Athletic Federations recommends whole-food sources of protein rather than supplements (Burke *et al.,* 2019).

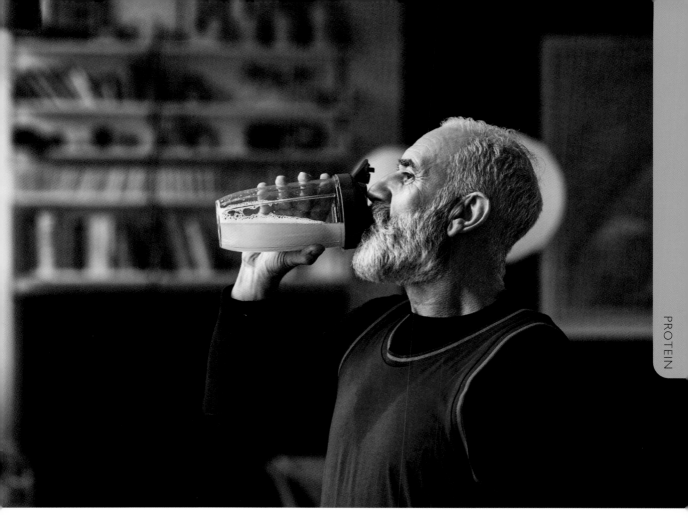

Age

Masters athletes over 65 years old, on the other hand, may need more than 25 g to stimulate maximum MPS. An analysis by Canadian and UK researchers found that in healthy older men, muscles are less sensitive to protein and require a higher protein intake (0.4 g/kg BW per meal) than younger men to stimulate maximum MPS (Moore *et al.*, 2015). In another study of older men, those who consumed a drink containing 40 g whey protein after resistance exercise showed significantly greater MPS than those who consumed 20 g (Yang *et al.*, 2012 (b)).

Distribution of protein intake throughout the day

The window of opportunity to allow MPS to be elevated is not limited to the few hours immediately after exercise. Scientists have shown that this 'anabolic window' extends at least 24 hours (particularly following resistance training), which means it would be beneficial to consume protein throughout the day, not only immediately after exercise (Schoenfeld *et al.*, 2013; Burd *et al.*, 2011). Consuming an optimal amount of protein soon after exercise and then at regular intervals throughout the day results in a more sustained delivery of amino acids to the muscles and promotes increased MPS (Phillips *et al.*, 2016).

A study at RMIT University, Australia, measured the rate of MPS during a 12-hour recovery period following a resistance workout when volunteers consumed 80 g protein either as 2 x 40 g every 6 hours; 4 x 20 g every 3 hours; or 8 x 10 g every 1½ hours (Areta *et al.*, 2013). They found that MPS was 31–48% higher when 20 g protein was consumed every 3 hours compared with the other protocols.

Similarly, researchers at the University of Texas Medical Branch, found that evenly distributing 90 g protein at breakfast (30 g), lunch (30 g) and dinner (30 g) resulted in 25% higher rate of MPS compared with a meal pattern that skewed most of the protein towards dinner (63 g) with small amounts at breakfast (10 g) and lunch (16 g) (Mamerow *et al.*, 2014).

In other words, for maximum MPS, it is advantageous to distribute your protein intake evenly throughout the day. You should also aim to consume 0.25 g/kg BW or 15–25 g protein at each meal or snack. This may mean rethinking your breakfast options to include more protein-rich foods such as milk, yoghurt or eggs, as most people focus on carbohydrates (e.g. cereal, toast) at this meal.

Protein before sleep

The 'anabolic window' probably also extends to overnight recovery during sleep. Scientists have recently evaluated the benefits of consuming protein after an evening resistance training session and before sleep. One study at Maastricht University found that protein synthesis was 22% higher in volunteers who consumed 40 g of protein (in the form of a casein drink) after a resistance workout and before sleep, compared with those who consumed a placebo (Res *et al.*, 2012). Casein was chosen as it is digested and absorbed relatively slowly so produces a sustained rise in amino acids in the bloodstream.

A further study found that consuming 28 g protein (in the form of a drink containing 28 g protein and 15 g carbohydrate) after a resistance workout and before sleep for 12 weeks resulted in significantly greater gains in muscle strength and size compared to a placebo (Snijders *et al.*, 2015). However, the athletes consuming the pre-bed protein drink consumed 1.9 g protein/kg BW/day while the placebo group consumed 1.3 g/kg BW/day. So it is not clear whether consuming protein before sleep is more effective than consuming protein at other times of the day, whether there is an optimal dose or whether there is any advantage of liquid over solid forms of protein.

MILK AS A RECOVERY DRINK

Milk provides a mixture of water, carbohydrate, protein and micronutrients, which makes it uniquely suitable as a post-exercise recovery drink. Research has shown that it promotes key components of the recovery process, including glycogen replenishment, muscle protein synthesis and rehydration (James *et al.*, 2019 (a)).

Muscle protein synthesis

Researchers at the University of Connecticut were among the first to demonstrate that skimmed milk consumed during exercise produces a more favourable hormonal environment in runners immediately following exercise compared with a carbohydrate sports drink or placebo (Miller *et al.*, 2002). Higher levels of anabolic hormones, such as growth hormone and testosterone, were measured after skimmed milk consumption. This, they suggest, may reduce protein breakdown and encourage protein anabolism during recovery.

Since then, milk as a recovery drink has been extensively investigated. University of Texas researchers found that drinking either 237 g whole milk, 237g fat-free milk or 393g fat-free milk containing the same calories as the whole milk after resistance training resulted in increased muscle protein synthesis, with whole milk producing the greatest response (Elliot et al., 2006). Researchers at McMaster University, Ontario showed that skimmed milk increased MPS compared to a soya drink (Wilkinson et al., 2007). In another study, the same researchers measured greater MPS following whey protein compared to soya protein, while MPS following casein protein was lower than either whey or soya (Tang et al., 2009). These studies suggest that milk has the potential to increase muscle mass.

Canadian researchers found that when novice male weight trainers consumed skimmed milk as part of a 12-week resistance training programme, it promoted greater hypertrophy than isoenergetic soya or energy drinks (Hartman et al., 2007). A similar study with women found that drinking skimmed milk after resistance exercise for 12 weeks reduced body fat levels and increased lean mass and strength (Josse et al., 2010). Milk is thought to have a favourable effect on *MPS and body composition* due to its whey content, which is rich in leucine and other branched-chain amino acids.

Rehydration skimmed milk has been shown to be an effective rehydration drink. In 2007, researchers at Loughborough University showed that skimmed milk resulted in more effective post-exercise rehydration than either commercially available sports drinks or water (Shirreffs et al., 2007). Milk contains sodium, carbohydrate and protein, which have all been shown to enhance rehydration (Evans et al., 2017)

Exercise-induced muscle damage

Studies have also shown that consuming milk after training can help alleviate symptoms of exercise-induced muscle damage, including delayed onset muscle soreness (DOMS) and reductions in muscle performance. The original benefits were demonstrated based on drinking quite a large volume of milk (1 litre) but recently, a smaller volume (500 ml) of milk was found to have similar effects on muscle performance, blood measures and muscle soreness in comparison to the larger volume (Cockburn et al., 2012). In this study, 24 men consumed either 500 ml semi-skimmed milk, 1 litre semi-skimmed milk or 1 litre water after performing leg exercises. Those drinking either 500 ml or 1 litre milk experienced less muscle damage than those drinking water, with no difference between the two milk-drinking groups.

Glycogen resynthesis

Many studies have highlighted the benefits of *chocolate milk* as a recovery drink, particularly after endurance exercise. Flavoured milk contains a 3:1 ratio of carbohydrate to protein and is therefore a good option for a recovery drink. In the first of these studies, researchers at Indiana University, showed that cyclists who consumed chocolate milk after an interval workout were able to recover faster and perform better than those consuming energy drink in an endurance workout performed 4 hours later (Karp *et al.,* 2006). A 2008 study by researchers at Northumbria University found that athletes who drank 500 ml of semi-skimmed milk or chocolate milk immediately after training had less muscle soreness and more rapid muscle recovery compared with commercial sports drinks or water (Cockburn *et al.,* 2008). A 2009 study with soccer players from James Madison University, found that chocolate milk promoted faster muscle recovery and resulted in less muscle damage compared with a commercial sports drink containing the same amount of calories (Gilson *et al.,* 2009). University of Texas researchers found that post-exercise chocolate milk consumption not only promoted muscle glycogen recovery but also resulted in greater aerobic capacity and lean body mass and reduced body fat after 4 weeks of aerobic training compared with carbohydrate (sports) drinks (Ferguson-Stegall *et al.,* 2011).

For longer, harder training sessions, extra carbohydrate may be needed to refuel energy stores. Researchers at the University of Texas in Austin found that consuming a bowl of wholegrain cereal plus milk was as effective at refuelling glycogen stores as sports drinks after 2 hours of moderate exercise (Kammer *et al.,* 2009). It also promoted greater MPS compared with the sports drink.

How can I meet my protein needs?

In practice, protein intakes generally reflect total calorie intake, so provided you are meeting your calorie needs from a wide variety of foods, you are likely to be getting enough protein. Dietary surveys show that most athletes already consume diets providing protein intakes above the maximum recommended level without the use of protein supplements.

However, if you reduce your calorie intake or cut out entire food groups (for example, if you eat a vegan diet or you have a dairy allergy), you may find it more difficult to meet your protein needs.

Table 4.4 lists a wide range of foods containing protein. Animal sources generally provide higher levels of essential amino acids, but plant sources can also make a significant contribution to your daily protein intake. The key is to eat a wide variety of foods containing protein. This will not only ensure that you get a better balance of amino acids but also increases your intake of other nutrients such as fibre, vitamins, minerals and carbohydrate. For example, combining rice with pulses gives a better profile of amino acids needed to make new body proteins than eating either of these foods on their own. However, it is not necessary to always combine proteins within a single meal. Our bodies pool the amino acids we need as we eat them over a 24-hour period, and we use them as needed.

IS MORE PROTEIN BETTER?

Although some strength athletes and bodybuilders consume as much as 2–3 g/kg BW/day, there is no evidence that these high daily intakes result in further muscle mass and strength gains (Tipton and Wolfe, 2007).

Consuming more protein than you need certainly offers no advantage in terms of health or physical performance. A meta-analysis of 49 studies concluded that protein intakes beyond a daily total of around 1.6 g/kg BW/day provide no further benefit on gains in muscle mass or strength (Morton *et al.,* 2018). Once your requirements have been met, additional protein

Table 4.4	THE PROTEIN CONTENT OF VARIOUS FOODS		
Food		**Portion size**	**Protein (g)**
Meat and fish	Beef, fillet steak, grilled, lean	2 slices 105 g	31
	Chicken breast, grilled meat only	1 breast 130 g	39
	Turkey, light meat, roasted	2 slices 140 g	47
	Cod, poached	1 fillet 120 g	25
	Mackerel, grilled	1 fillet 150 g	31
	Tuna, tinned in brine	1 small tin (100 g)	24
Dairy products and eggs	Cheese, Cheddar	1 slice (25 g)	6
	Cottage cheese	2 tbsp (100 g)	12
	Milk (all types)	1 glass (250 ml)	8
	Low-fat plain yoghurt	1 carton (125 g)	6
	Low-fat strained plain Greek yoghurt	3 tbsp (150 g)	15
	Eggs	2	12
Nuts and seeds	Peanuts, roasted and salted	1 handful (25 g)	7
	Cashew nuts, roasted and salted	1 handful (25 g)	5
	Walnuts	1 handful (25 g)	4
	Sunflower seeds	2 tbsp (32 g)	6
	Sesame seeds	2 tbsp (24 g)	4
Pulses	Baked beans	1 small tin (205 g)	10
	Red lentils, boiled	4 tbsp (200 g)	18
	Beans, boiled	4 tbsp (200 g)	18
	Chickpeas, boiled	4 tbsp (200 g)	18
Soya products	Plain soya milk	1 glass (250 ml)	8
	Plain soya yoghurt	1 carton (125 g)	51
	Tofu	Half a pack (100 g)	13
Quorn products	Quorn mince	4 tbsp (100 g)	15
	Quorn sausages	3 (100 g)	14
Grains and 'pseudograins'	Wholemeal bread	5 heaped tbsp (80 g)	8
	Wholemeal pasta, boiled	5 heaped tbsp (250 g)	10
	Brown rice, boiled	5 heaped tbsp (180 g)	7
	Quinoa, cooked	5 heaped tbsp (250 g)	11
	Oats	4 tbsp (50 g)	7

will not be converted into muscle, nor will it further increase muscle size, strength or stamina. What's more, resistance training was shown to be a much more potent anabolic stimulus than protein, accounting for the majority of strength and muscle mass gains.

The nitrogen-containing amino group of the protein is converted into a substance called urea in the liver. This is then passed to the kidneys and excreted in the urine. The remainder of the protein is converted into glucose and used as an energy substrate. It may either be used as fuel immediately or stored as glycogen. If you are already eating enough carbohydrate to refill your glycogen stores, excess glucose may be converted into fat. However, in practice this does not occur to a great extent. Fat gain is usually the result of excessive calorie consumption. Recent studies have shown that eating protein increases the metabolic rate, so a significant proportion of the protein calories are oxidised and given off as heat

(*see* p. 68 'Protein metabolism'). Thus, a slight excess of protein is unlikely to be converted into fat.

In a study carried out at McMaster University, Ontario, strength athletes were given either a low-protein (0.86 g/kg BW/day – similar to the RNI), medium-protein (1.4 g/kg BW/day) or high-protein diet (2.3 g/kg BW/day) for 13 days (Tarnopolsky *et al.,* 1992). The low-protein diet, which was close to the RNI for sedentary people, caused the athletes to lose muscle mass. Both the medium- and high-protein diets resulted in an increased muscle mass, but the amount of the increase was the same for the two groups. In other words, no further benefits were gained by increasing the protein intake from 1.4 g to 2.4 g/kg BW/day.

Similar findings were reported at Kent State University, Ohio. Researchers gave 12 volunteers either a protein (total daily protein was 2.62 g/ kg BW) or a carbohydrate supplement (total

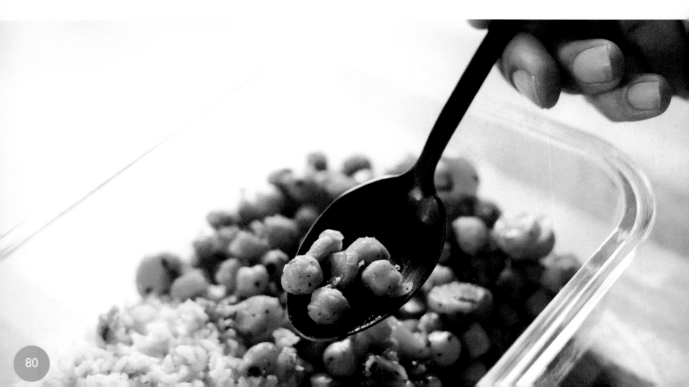

daily protein was 1.35 g/kg BW) for 1 month, during which time they undertook intense weight training 6 days a week (Lemon *et al.*, 1992). Nitrogen balance measurements were carried out after each diet and the researchers found that an intake of 1.4–1.5 g/kg BW/day was needed to maintain nitrogen balance, although strength, muscle mass and size were the same with either level of protein intake.

The researchers concluded two main points. First, strength training approximately doubles your protein needs (compared with sedentary people). Second, increasing your protein intake does not enhance your strength, mass or size in a linear fashion. Once your optimal intake has been reached, additional protein is not converted into muscle.

IS TOO MUCH PROTEIN HARMFUL?

It has been proposed that high protein intakes might cause kidney damage through increased pressure and hyperfiltration in the blood capillaries of the kidneys. However, this has never been demonstrated in healthy people, so it remains only a theoretical possibility (Tipton and Wolfe, 2007; Martin *et al.*, 2005). A review of 26 studies found no evidence for an adverse effect of high protein intakes on kidney function in healthy individuals (Van Elswyk *et al.*, 2018) and a meta-analysis of 40 studies found no difference in kidney function between those consuming a higher- or normal-protein diet (Devries *et al.*, 2018). On the other hand, excessive protein intake is a concern for those with pre-existing kidney disease, for whom a low-protein diet is advised.

It has also been claimed that eating too much protein leads to hypohydration (*see* p. 147) because extra water is drawn from the body's fluids to dilute and excrete the increased quantities of urea. The only evidence for this comes from a study reported at the 2002 Experimental Biology meeting in New Orleans, which found that a high-protein diet (246 g daily) consumed for 4 weeks caused hypohydration in trained athletes. Their blood urea nitrogen – a clinical test for proper kidney function – reached abnormal levels and they produced more concentrated urine. According to the researchers at the University of Connecticut, this could have been avoided by increasing their fluid intake. This is unlikely to be a problem if you drink enough fluids.

Fears that high-protein diets cause more acid to be produced in the body (due to the breakdown of sulphur-containing amino acids) leading to an excessive excretion of calcium and increased risk of osteoporosis, are largely unfounded, too. A systematic review of studies found no evidence of any detrimental effect of protein intake on calcium status (Darling *et al.*, 2019).

In conclusion, while consuming protein in excess of your requirement offers no health or performance advantages, is unlikely to be harmful either. For this reason, there is no official upper limit for protein intake in healthy individuals.

Summary of key points

- Protein is needed for the maintenance, replacement and growth of body tissues. It is used to make the enzymes and hormones that regulate the metabolism, maintain fluid balance, and transport nutrients in and out of cells.
- Proteins are made up of amino acids, of which 11 can be made in the body (non-essential amino acids) and nine must be supplied in the diet (essential amino acids).

- Proteins are constantly being broken down into amino acids (muscle protein breakdown) and amino acids are constantly incorporated into proteins (muscle protein synthesis).

- After exercise, both muscle protein breakdown and synthesis increase. MPS increases more than breakdown following the consumption of protein. The balance between MPS and MPB determines whether the muscle mass stays the same, increases (hypertrophy) or decreases (atrophy).

- All animal protein sources, and certain plant protein sources (soya, chia and hemp seeds, buckwheat and amaranth) provide EAAs in ratios closely matched to the body's requirements, and are therefore considered to be 'high quality'. However, both animal and plant proteins can contribute towards daily intake.

- Endurance training increases protein requirements. Protein is needed to compensate for the increased breakdown of protein during intense training, repairing muscle tissue and for building mitochondrial proteins.

- Resistance training and protein consumption are both potent stimuli for MPS. Strength and power athletes have additional protein needs to facilitate muscle protein synthesis.

- Current guidelines recommend a protein intake in the range 1.2–2.0 g/kg BW/day. For building muscle mass and strength gains, an intake in the range of 1.4–2.0 g/kg BW/day is recommended; while 1.2–1.4 g/kg BW/day is recommended for endurance training.

- During weight loss, a higher protein intake of 1.8–2.7 g/kg BW/day (or 2.3–3.1 g/kg fat-free mass), in conjunction with an energy deficit plus resistance training, may help prevent lean mass losses.

- The rate of MPS depends on the amount of protein consumed before, during and after exercise, the amount of muscle mass activated during exercise, the type of protein consumed, co-ingestion of other nutrients, age and the distribution of protein intake throughout the day.

- Consuming protein plus carbohydrate before and during prolonged, high-intensity exercise increases MPS during exercise and minimises protein breakdown.

- To optimise MPS, consume 0.25–0.4 g protein/kg BW (or a minimum of 20 g) in each meal and distribute your protein intake evenly throughout the day.

- Older athletes may need as much as 0.4 g/kg BW per meal to stimulate maximum MPS.

- When a greater muscle mass is activated during resistance training, a higher protein intake (40 g) may be required to maximise MPS.

- 'High-quality' proteins with a high EAA and leucine content are the best type of protein to consume after exercise. Leucine acts as both a substrate (building block) and a trigger for MPS.

- Consuming protein (casein) after resistance training and before sleep may increase MPS.

- Milk is a particularly valuable recovery food and has been shown to increase MPS, reduce symptoms of exercise-induced muscle damage, and promote rehydration, muscle repair and glycogen resynthesis.

- Protein intake above your requirement will not result in further muscle mass or strength gains; instead, it will be used as an energy substrate. However, there is no evidence that excess protein is harmful for healthy people.

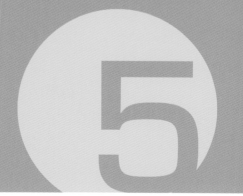

//**Fat**

Fat provides fuel for the body. One gram of dietary fat provides 9 calories, which means it has the highest calorie density of all nutrients. This, along with our seemingly unlimited storage capacity for fat, makes it our largest reserve of energy. Fat also makes up part of the structure of cell membranes, brain tissue, nerve sheaths and bone marrow and it cushions your organs. Fat in food also provides essential fatty acids and helps the body absorb and transport the fat-soluble vitamins A, D, E and K in the bloodstream. It is also needed for making the hormones oestrogen and testosterone and ensuring normal menstrual function in women. This chapter explains how fat is burned during exercise and its roles in health. It gives guidance on recommended fat intakes and explains the health effects of different types of fats found in the diet. Finally, it summarises the research on omega-3 supplementation and athletic performance.

HOW DOES THE BODY BURN FAT DURING EXERCISE?

Fat is an important source of energy for exercise. During aerobic exercise, you will oxidise a mixture of carbohydrate and fat. The relative proportions of each fuel oxidised depends on the intensity and duration of exercise, your level of fitness, and your pre-exercise diet (*see* pp. 25–27). During low-intensity exercise, fat is the main fuel, while carbohydrate is the main fuel during high-intensity exercise. However, total fat oxidation in grams increases as exercise intensity increases from low to high, even though the percentage contribution of fat decreases. That's because total energy expenditure increases, i.e. you burn more calories per minute. On average, the highest rates of fat oxidation ('fat max') occur at 62–63% of VO_2max.

Fat oxidation increases as exercise duration increases. This is due to the decrease in glycogen stores, i.e. as glycogen becomes depleted your muscles will break down more fat for fuel (*see* p. 26). Your level of fitness also affects the fuel mixture. As your fitness increases with training, your muscles become more efficient at using fat for fuel at any given exercise intensity (*see* p. 27). Pre-exercise diet also affects the fuel mixture. Generally, a low-carbohydrate, high-fat diet increases the percentage of fat oxidised while a high-carbohydrate, low-fat diet reduces fat oxidation (*see* p. 27). Additionally, consuming carbohydrate in the hours before exercise increases the proportion of carbohydrate oxidised in the muscles and reduces the proportion of fat oxidised.

HOW MUCH FAT SHOULD I EAT?

The ACSM position statement, IOC and IAAF currently make no specific recommendation for fat intake. The focus should be on meeting carbohydrate and protein goals with fat making up the calorie balance. It is suggested that athletes follow the public health guidelines for fat intake, which are less than 35% of daily energy intake, but also adapt their intake according to individual training and body composition goals (Thomas *et al.*, 2016). The emphasis should be on obtaining adequate energy, essential fatty acids and fat-soluble vitamins.

For example, an athlete consuming 3000 kcal a day and meeting their requirement for carbohydrate and protein may consume 66–117 g fat:

- (3000 x 20%) ÷ 9 = 66 g
- (3000 x 35%) ÷ 9 = 117 g
- Dietary fat intake = 66–117 g fat a day

Although athletes need to focus on obtaining adequate carbohydrate and protein, this does not necessarily mean eating a low-fat diet. There is evidence that restricting fat too severely may reduce your performance. Conversely, eating more than the recommended maximum of 35% calories from fat intake does not appear to have any adverse effect on heart disease risk factors in athletes. In one study, runners who consumed a 42% fat diet had higher levels of HDL ('good') cholesterol and lower cardiovascular risk factors than those consuming a 16% fat diet (Leddy *et al.*, 1997). Another study by New Zealand researchers found that during periods of hard endurance training when energy requirements are high, increasing the percentage of fat in the diet to 50% of energy did not have an adverse

Popular high-fat diets

Popular low-carbohydrate, high-fat diets (LCHF), such as the ketogenic diet and Paleo diet, all work on the same premise. The theory is that a lower carbohydrate intake, coupled with high fat intake, leads to burning body fat as the main fuel source while exercising. However, despite increasing the muscles' ability to use fat as an energy source, there is no clear evidence to date that *chronically* consuming a LCHF or ketogenic diet enhances endurance performance. Furthermore, it can impair the muscles' ability to store and use carbohydrate during high-intensity exercise, increase perceived exertion, reduce power output and increase the risk of illness (see pp. 57–58). In terms of weight loss, ketogenic diets are not superior to other dietary approaches for weight loss and, while they may have advantages related to appetite control, are difficult to maintain in the long term (Ashtary-Larky *et al.*, 2021) (see p. 185).

effect on blood fats or cardiovascular risk (Brown and Cox, 1998).

Diets containing moderate amounts of fat (such as the traditional Mediterranean diet) may be more effective than low-fat diets for protecting against heart disease, stroke and type 2 diabetes (Estruch *et al.*, 2013). Researchers suggest it's the *type* of fat you eat that is more important than the *amount* you eat when it comes to cardiovascular risk. Artificial trans fatty acids appear to raise cardiovascular risk; unsaturated fatty acids (especially omega-3s) lower the risk; while the majority of saturated fatty acids are thought to increase risk.

What are fats?

Fats and oils found in food consist mainly of *triglycerides*. These are made up of a unit of glycerol and three fatty acids. Each fatty acid is a chain of carbon and hydrogen atoms (a hydrocarbon chain) with a carboxyl group (–COOH) at one end and a methyl group at the other end (–CH3) – chain lengths between 14 and 22 carbon atoms are most common. These fatty acids are classified in three different groups, according to their chemical structure: saturated, monounsaturated and polyunsaturated. In food, the proportions of each group determine whether the fat is hard or liquid, how it is handled by the body and how it affects your health.

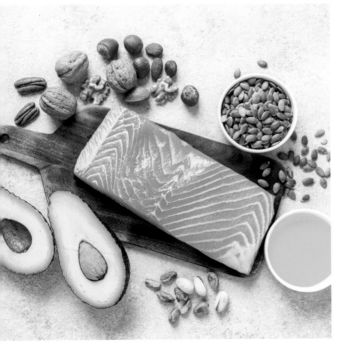

WHAT ARE SATURATED FATS?

Saturated fatty acids have no double bonds in their carbon chains so are said to be fully saturated with the maximum amount of hydrogen; in other words, all of their carbon atoms are linked with a single bond to hydrogen atoms. Fats containing a high proportion of saturates are hard at room temperature and mostly come from animal products such as butter, lard, cheese and meat fat, as well as processed foods made from these fats (biscuits, cakes and pastries). Palm oil and coconut oil are also highly saturated, and are commonly used in spreads, as well as in biscuits and bakery products.

Saturated fats and health

The population recommendation for saturated fat in the UK is an intake of less than 10% of total calorie intake (SACN, 2019). Additionally, the UK government recommends that the reduction in saturated fat intake should be achieved by replacing some of the saturated fat in your diet with unsaturated fat found in vegetable oils, nuts, seeds and oily fish. This advice is in line with the recommendations of the US and the World Health Organization, both of which recommend limiting saturated fat to no more than 10% of total calorie intake (Sacks *et al.*, 2017; Astrup *et al.*, 2019).

The link between saturated fatty acids and cardiovascular disease stems from Ancel Keys's Seven Countries study (Keys, 1980). This study, combined with others, led to the development of the diet-heart hypothesis, which suggests that saturated fat raises LDL cholesterol levels and thus increases the risk of heart disease. Since then, numerous studies have shown high LDL cholesterol levels to be a major cause of cardiovascular disease (Ference *et al.*, 2017; WHO, 2016; Kannel *et al.*, 1986).

However, not all types of saturated fats increase LDL-cholesterol (Chowdhury *et al.*, 2014; de Oliveira Otto *et al.*, 2012; German *et al.*, 2009). For example, those found in dairy foods have not been shown to increase blood cholesterol or cardiovascular disease and may even have a protective effect (Alexander *et al.*, 2016; Drouin-Chartier *et al.*, 2016; Mensink, 2003; Toth, 2005). The fat in milk, cheese and yoghurt (but not butter) is encased in a spherical structure called the milk fat globule membrane, which prevents it raising blood cholesterol levels. Additionally, the high calcium content of dairy binds some of the saturated fat, stopping it from being absorbed.

Subsequently, many studies have shown that reducing saturated fat intake leads to a reduction in cardiovascular disease risk (Ference *et al.*, 2017). A meta-analysis of 15 randomised control trials showed a 21% reduced risk of cardiovascular events in people who reduced their saturated fat intake over 2 years compared to those who consumed their usual diet (Hooper *et al.*, 2020). Crucially, this analysis found that replacing saturated fat with unsaturated fat was more effective than replacing it with refined carbohydrate.

What you replace saturated fats with is important. If you replace saturated fats with highly refined carbohydrates, LDL cholesterol levels and heart disease risk increase. This may explain why some studies have found little benefit to reducing saturated fat since most people tend to replace them with refined carbohydrates.

Instead, it is recommended to replace some of the saturated fats in your diet with unsaturated fats (Hooper *et al.*, 2020; Hooper *et al.*, 2015 (b); Astrup *et al.*, 2010; Jakobsen *et al.*, 2009).

Unsaturated fats raise HDL and lower LDL levels. They also improve the ratio of total cholesterol to HDL cholesterol, lowering the risk of cardiovascular disease. A review of studies from the Cochrane Collaboration found that people who did this for at least 2 years reduced their risk of heart attacks, angina and stroke by 14% (Hooper *et al.*, 2012).

Scientists from Harvard T.H. Chan School of Public Health analysed data from two large populations: 84,628 women in the Nurses' Health Study and 42,908 men in the Health Professionals Follow-Up Study, who were followed from the 1980s to 2010 (Li *et al.*, 2015). People who ate more saturated fat had a higher risk of heart disease compared to those who ate less. Also, people who ate more unsaturated fats and more wholegrain carbohydrates lowered their risk of heart disease compared to people who included less of these nutrients in their diet. They estimated that replacing 5% energy intake from saturated fats with an equivalent energy intake from either polyunsaturated fats, monounsaturated fats or carbohydrates from whole grains was associated with a 25%, 15% and 9% lower risk of heart disease, respectively.

WHAT ARE MONOUNSATURATED FATS?

Monounsaturated fatty acids have slightly less hydrogen because their carbon chains contain one double or unsaturated bond (hence 'mono'). Oils rich in monounsaturates are usually liquid at room temperature, but may solidify at cold temperatures. The richest sources include olive, rapeseed, groundnut, hazelnut and almond oil, avocados, olives, nuts and seeds.

Monounsaturated fatty acids are thought to have the greatest health benefits. They can reduce total cholesterol, in particular LDL cholesterol, without affecting the beneficial high density lipo-protein (HDL) cholesterol. The UK government recommends a monounsaturated fatty acid intake of up to 12% of total calorie intake.

WHAT ARE POLYUNSATURATED FATS?

Polyunsaturated fatty acids have the least hydrogen – the carbon chains contain two or more double bonds (hence 'poly'). Oils rich in polyunsaturates are liquid at both room and cold temperatures. Rich sources include most nut and seed oils, nuts, seeds and oily fish.

Numerous studies have found that eating polyunsaturated fatty acids can reduce LDL blood cholesterol levels and lower the risk of heart disease (Mozaffarian *et al.*, 2011). However, they can also lower HDL cholesterol slightly. It is a good idea to replace some with monounsaturates, if you eat a lot of them. For this reason, the UK government recommends a maximum intake of 10% of total calorie intake (SACN, 2019).

What are essential fatty acids?

A subcategory of polyunsaturated fats, called essential fatty acids, cannot be made in your body, so they have to come from the food you eat. They are grouped into two families: the omega-3 (n-3) family, derived from alpha-linolenic acid (ALA); and the omega-6 (n-6) family, derived from linoleic acid.

The families are called omega-3 and omega-6 because the last double bond is 3 and 6 carbon atoms from the last carbon in the chain respectively.

The omega-3 fatty acids can be further divided into two groups: long chain and short chain. The long chain omega-3 fatty acids are eicosapentaenoic acid (EPA) and docosahexaenoic acid

(DHA). They are found in oily fish but can also be formed in the body from ALA, the short chain omega-3 fatty acid. However, this conversion of ALA to DHA is very inefficient, less than 10% on average. Fig 5.1 shows how the body converts the two series of fatty acids

EPA and DHA are then converted into hormone-like substances called prostaglandins, thromboxanes and leukotrienes. These control many key functions, such as blood clotting (making the blood less likely to form unwanted clots), inflammation (improving the ability to respond to injury or bacterial attack), the tone of blood vessel walls (widening and constriction of blood vessels) and the immune system.

The omega-6 fatty acids include linoleic acid, gamma-linolenic acid (GLA) and docosapentaenoic acid (DPA) (*see* Fig. 5.1) and are important for healthy functioning of cell membranes. They are especially important for healthy skin. People on very low-fat diets, who are deficient in linoleic acid,

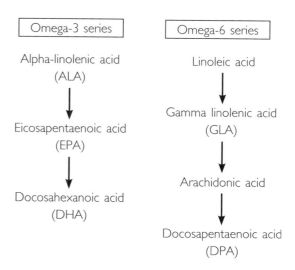

Figure 5.1 How the body uses and converts the omega-3 and omega-6 fatty acids

can develop extremely dry, flaky skin. Omega-6 fatty acids reduce LDL cholesterol, but a very high intake may also reduce HDL cholesterol and increase oxidative damage (*see* p. 231) and, therefore, cancer risk. A moderate intake is recommended. Food sources of omega-6 fatty acids include vegetable oils, such as sunflower, soybean, safflower and corn oil, spreads or margarine and a wide range of foods made from these oils.

WHAT ARE THE HEALTH BENEFITS OF OMEGA-3 FATTY ACIDS?

Omega-3s are incorporated into cell membranes and therefore affect the functioning of many tissues and body systems, including muscle tissue, the brain, the cardiovascular and immune systems. Omega-3s also help to reduce inflammation. Studies show that people with a high intake of omega-3 fatty acids have a lower risk of cardio-

vascular disease, type 2 diabetes, certain cancers, arthritis, dementia and depression than those with low intakes (Shahidi and Ambigaipalan, 2018).

WHAT ARE THE BEST FOOD SOURCES OF OMEGA-3 FATTY ACIDS?

Oily fish such as mackerel, fresh tuna (not tinned), salmon and sardines are the richest sources of DHA and EPA. Vegetarians can obtain long chain fatty acids from the conversion of ALA that takes place in the body. The richest plant sources include flaxseeds, flaxseed oil, pumpkin seeds, walnuts, chia seeds, rapeseed oil and soybeans. The dark green leaves of leafy vegetables (e.g. spinach, kale) also contain small amounts. There is an increasing range of omega-3-fortified foods, including omega-3 eggs (achieved by feeding hens on omega-3-enriched feed), bread and spreads. However, the conversion of ALA into long chain

Table 5.1 THE OMEGA-3 FATTY ACID CONTENT OF FOODS			
Food	g ALA	g DHA	g EPA
1 tbsp flaxseed oil	7.26	0	0
25 g chia seeds	5.06	0	0
25 g walnuts	2.57	0	0
1 tbsp flaxseeds	2.35	0	0
85 g farmed salmon	0	1.24	0.59
85 g wild salmon	0	1.22	0.35
1 tbsp rapeseed oil	1.28	0	0
85 g mackerel	0	0.59	0.43
85 g tinned salmon	0.04	0.63	0.28
85 g trout	0	0.44	0.40
½ cup edamame beans	0.28	0	0
85 g tinned tuna	0	0.17	0.02

Source: The USDA database, FoodData Central

fatty acids isn't very efficient as the body can only convert around 5–10% of the ALA you eat into EPA and 2–5% into DHA. The omega-3 content of various foods is shown in Table 5.1.

HOW MUCH DO I NEED?

The UK government recommends a minimum consumption of 450 mg EPA + DHA per day, which can be met through eating at least two portions of fish a week, one of which should be oily fish (SACN, 2019). Additionally, it recommends that linoleic acid (omega-6) provides at least 1% of total energy and ALA provides at least 0.2% total energy. The Academy of Nutrition and Dietetics and Dietitians of Canada recommends 500 mg EPA + DPA per day, whereas the European Food Safety Authority recommends 250 mg EPA + DPA per day (European Food Safety Authority, 2009). The World Health Organization advises one to two servings of oily fish per week, equivalent to 200–500 mg of omega-3s per day (World Health Organization, 2003).

However, these recommendations are for the general population, not athletes, and are primarily for the reduction of heart disease risk. The requirement for athletes is likely to be higher. Many athletes, though, are likely to have suboptimal levels. One study of 1,500 US college athletes showed that less than 10% met the omega-3 guidelines and less than 40% ate fish twice weekly (Ritz et al., 2020). The best way to correct this is to eat more omega-3-rich foods (see Table 5.1) or take supplements. When choosing a supplement, check the EPA + DHA content rather than the 'omega-3' or 'fish oil' content. A daily dose of 1–3 g EPA + DHA, including both dietary sources and supplements, has been suggested for athletes (Ritz and Rockwell, 2021).

We need both omega-3s and omega-6s to be healthy, but our diets are more often deficient in omega-3s. Most people have a far greater intake of omega-6 compared with omega-3; we tend to get most of our omega-6s from spreads and vegetable oils. Experts recommend shifting this balance in favour of omega-3s.

The right balance between omega-3 and omega-6 fatty acids is the most important factor if you are to get enough EPA and DHA. That's because both ALA (omega-3) and linoleic acid (omega-6) compete for the same enzymes to metabolise them. A high intake of LA interferes with the conversion process of ALA to EPA and DHA.

HOW CAN OMEGA-3 FATTY ACIDS HELP ATHLETIC PERFORMANCE?

It is thought that omega-3s may enhance performance by reducing post-exercise inflammation and/or by improving the functional capacity of muscle cell membranes. However, there is relatively little research to support the use of omega-3s as ergogenic aids. One review concluded that omega-3 supplements may promote recovery from eccentric (muscle-damaging) exercise but will not enhance muscle growth following resistance exercise (Philpott et al., 2019). Early studies suggested that omega-3s 'switch on' the mTORC1 pathway (see p. 73) and increase muscle protein synthesis (MPS) following protein intake (Smith et al., 2011 (a); Smith et al., 2011 (b)). However, subsequent studies found that omega-3 supplementation did not confer any muscle anabolic advantage (McGlory et al., 2016).

Another review of 32 studies showed a positive association between omega-3 supplementation and reaction time, skeletal muscle recovery, inflammatory markers and cardiovascular dynamics but no effect on endurance performance, lung function, muscle function or training adaptation (Lewis *et al.*, 2020). There is some evidence, though, that they may help prevent and treat sports-related concussion and mild traumatic brain injuries (Oliver *et al.*, 2018; Barrett *et al.*, 2014).

What are trans fatty acids?

Small amounts of trans fatty acids are found naturally in meat and dairy products, but most come from processed fats. These are produced by hydrogenation, a process that changes liquid oils into solid or spreadable fats. During this highly pressurised heat treatment, the geometrical arrangement of the atoms changes. Technically speaking, one or more of the unsaturated double bonds in the fatty acid are altered from the usual *cis* form to the unusual *trans* form. This means the two hydrogen atoms are on opposite sides of the double bond.

Artificially produced trans fats may be found in foods made from hydrogenated vegetable oils such as certain snack products, bakery products, fried foods and takeaway foods. The exact effect of trans fatty acids on the body is not certain, but it is thought that they may be worse than saturates: they could lower HDL and raise LDL levels. They may also increase levels of a substance that promotes blood clot formation and stops your body using essential fatty acids properly. A US meta-analysis of 41 previous studies by researchers at McMaster University, Canada, found that people eating more trans fats had a 34% higher risk of dying from any cause compared with those eating less, a 28% higher risk of dying from heart disease, and a 21% greater risk of having heart-related health issues (De Souza *et al.*, 2015). In a review of prospective studies, for every 2% increase in calorie intake from trans fats, a person's heart disease risk increases by 23% (Mozaffarian *et al.*, 2006). Adverse effects were observed when trans fats contributed as little as 3% of total calories.

This is why all major public health organisations are trying to phase trans fats out of the food supply. The World Health Organization recommends 'virtual elimination' of trans fats from the food supply (Uauy *et al.*, 2009). The UK Scientific Advisory Committee on Nutrition recommends that trans fatty acids make up no more than 2% of total calorie intake – roughly 5 g per day. The average intake is estimated to be around 0.7% of calories, so most people are within the recommended maximum.

As there is no law requiring trans fats to be listed on food labels, the best advice is to avoid any foods that list hydrogenated or partially hydrogenated oils on the label. Reformulation in recent years means that hydrogenated fats have been removed from many foods and replaced with palm oil and other fats. For example, they are no longer used in major brands of fat spreads.

What is cholesterol?

Cholesterol is an essential part of our bodies; it makes up part of all cell membranes and helps produce several hormones. Some cholesterol comes from our diet, but most is made in the liver from saturated fats. In fact, the cholesterol we eat has only a small effect on our LDL cholesterol; if we eat more cholesterol (from meat, offal, eggs, dairy products, seafood) the liver compensates by making less, and vice versa. This keeps a steady level of cholesterol in the bloodstream.

Several factors can push up blood cholesterol levels. The major ones are obesity (especially

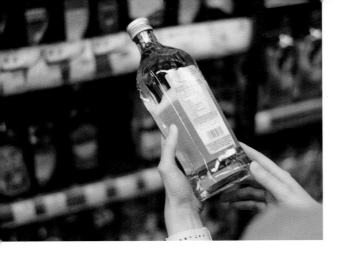

central obesity, where fat is stored mainly around the abdomen), lack of exercise and the amount of saturated fatty acids we eat. Studies have shown that replacing saturated fatty acids with unsaturated fatty acids can lower total and LDL cholesterol levels.

So, which are the best types of fats to eat?

For cooking and salad dressings, choose oils that are high in omega-3 fatty acids or monounsaturated fatty acids – olive, rapeseed, flaxseed and nut oils are good choices for health as well as taste. These are healthier than oils rich in omega-6 fats, such as sunflower and corn oil, which, in high quantities, may disrupt the formation of EPA and DHA. Include avocados, nuts, seeds and nut butters in your daily diet; they provide many valuable nutrients apart from omega-3 fatty acids and monounsaturates. If you eat fish, include one to two portions of oily fish (e.g. mackerel and salmon) per week. Vegetarians should make sure they include plant sources of omega-3 fatty acids in their daily diet (*see* p. 272).

Butter has a relatively high content of saturated fat so it should be used in moderation. Alternatively, opt for a spread with a high content of olive oil. Hard margarines and vegan spreads (or butter substitutes) made with palm oil and coconut oil tend to have the highest content of saturated fatty acids.

Summary of key points

- Fat is an important fuel for exercise. The relative proportions of fat and carbohydrate oxidised depends on the intensity and duration of exercise, your level of fitness and your pre-exercise diet.
- Public health recommendations advise a fat intake of less than 35% of daily energy intake; athletes should adapt their intake according to individual training and body composition goals.
- Unsaturated fatty acids should make up the majority of your fat intake, with saturated fatty acids making up no more than 10% energy and trans fatty acids kept as close to zero as possible.
- High LDL cholesterol levels have been shown to be a major cause of cardiovascular disease. Replacing some of your saturated fat intake with unsaturated fats will help lower LDL cholesterol and cardiovascular disease risk.
- Omega-3 fatty acids have been shown to reduce inflammation and the risk of cardiovascular disease and other chronic diseases.
- Omega-3 supplementation has been shown to improve muscle adaptation, energy metabolism, muscle recovery and injury prevention.
- Dietary recommendations for omega-3 range from 250–500 mg EPA + DPA daily; the requirement for athletes is likely to be higher.
- Omega-3 supplementation may be required for athletes to achieve optimal omega-3 status; a daily dose of 1–3 g EPA + DHA, including both dietary sources and supplements, has been suggested.

Vitamins
//and Minerals

Vitamins and minerals are often equated with vitality, energy and strength. Many people think of them as health enhancers, a plentiful supply being the secret to a long and healthy life.

In fact, vitamins and minerals do not in themselves provide energy. They are nutrients that are required in tiny amounts and are essential for health as well as for physical performance. It is tempting to think that extra vitamins and minerals lead to better performance, but consuming too much can sometimes be just as harmful as consuming too little.

This chapter explains what vitamins and minerals do, where they come from, and how exercise affects requirements. It considers whether athletes need more than the recommended daily intakes and whether they need to take supplements.

The functions, sources, requirements and safe upper limits (SULs) of vitamins and minerals are given in the glossary of vitamins and minerals (*see* pp. 352–61). The glossary also examines the evidence for the claims made for supplementation of vitamins and minerals.

WHAT ARE VITAMINS?

Vitamins are required in tiny amounts for growth, health and physical well-being. There are 13 vitamins that your body cannot make (or which are only made in small amounts), so they must be supplied in your diet. Many form the essential parts of enzyme systems that are involved in energy production and exercise performance. Others are involved in the functioning of the immune system, the hormonal system and the nervous system.

WHAT ARE MINERALS?

Minerals are inorganic elements that have many regulatory and structural roles in the body. There are about 20 minerals and trace elements that are essential for health. Some (such as calcium and phosphorus) form part of the structure of bones and teeth. Others are involved in controlling the fluid balance in tissues, muscle contraction, nerve function, enzyme secretion and the formation of red blood cells. Like vitamins, they cannot be made in the body and must be obtained in the diet.

HOW MUCH DO I NEED?

Everyone has different nutritional requirements. These vary according to age, size, level of physical activity and individual body chemistry. It is, therefore, impossible to state an intake that would be right for everyone. To find out your exact requirements, you would have to undergo a series of biochemical and physiological tests.

However, scientists have studied groups of people with similar characteristics, such as age and level of physical activity, and have come up with some estimates of requirements. The Reference Nutrient Intake (RNI) is the measure used in the UK, but the RNI value for a nutrient can vary from country to country. European Union (EU) regulations require Nutrient Reference Values (NRVs) to be shown on food and supplement labels. In the US, labels show the Daily Value (DV). RNIs are said to apply to 'average adults' and are only very rough guides.

RNI values are derived from studies of the physiological requirements of healthy people. For example, the RNI for a vitamin may be the amount needed to maintain a certain blood concentration of that vitamin. The RNI is not the amount of a nutrient recommended for optimum health or athletic performance.

WHAT ARE DIETARY REFERENCE VALUES (DRVS)?

In 1991, the Department of Health published *Dietary Reference Values for Food Energy and Nutrients for the United Kingdom* (Department of Health, 1991). A Dietary Reference Value (DRV) is a generic term for various daily dietary recommendations and covers three values that have been set for each nutrient:

1. The **Estimated Average Requirement** (**EAR**) is the amount of a nutrient needed by an average person, so 50% of the population will need more and 50% will need less.
2. The **Reference Nutrient Intake** (**RNI**) is the amount of a nutrient that should cover the needs of 97.5% of the population. It is more than most people require, and only a very few people (2.5%) will exceed it.
3. The **Lower Reference Nutrient Intake** (**LRNI**) is the amount of a nutrient that is enough for the small number of people who have low needs (about 2.5% of the population). Most people will need more than this amount.

Individual nutritional requirements vary widely and these values are based on population groups, not individuals. Athletes and sportspeople may exceed the upper limits because they have the highest requirements. EARs are used for energy, RNIs are often used as a reference amount for population groups.

The RNI is not a target intake to aim for – it is only a guideline. It should cover the needs of most people but, of course, it is possible that many athletes may need more than the RNI, due to their higher energy expenditure.

In practice, if you are eating consistently less than the RNI, you may be lacking in that particular nutrient.

How are DRVs set?

First of all, scientists have to work out what is the minimum amount of a particular nutrient that a person needs to be healthy. Once this has been established, scientists usually add on a safety margin, to take account of individual variations. No two people will have exactly the same requirement. Next, a storage requirement is assessed. This allows for a small reserve of the nutrient to be kept in the body.

Unfortunately, scientific evidence of human vitamin and mineral requirements is fairly scanty and contradictory. A lot of scientific guesswork is inevitably involved, and results are often extrapolated from animal studies.

In practice, DRVs are arrived at through a compromise between scientific data and good judgement. They vary from country to country and are always open to debate.

CAN A BALANCED DIET PROVIDE ALL THE VITAMINS AND MINERALS I NEED?

Most athletes eat more food than the average sedentary person. With the right food choices, this means you should automatically achieve a higher vitamin and mineral intake. However, in practice many athletes do not plan their diets well enough, or they may restrict their calorie intake so it can be difficult to obtain sufficient amounts of vitamins and minerals from food. Vitamin losses occur during storage, food processing, preparation and cooking, thus reducing your actual intake. Intensive farming practices and the use of agro-chemicals mean that certain plants may have a lower nutrient content than previously.

Eating a balanced diet may not always be easy in practice, particularly if you travel a lot for training, competition or business, work shifts or long hours, train and eat at irregular times, eat on the move or are unable to purchase and prepare your own meals. Planning and eating a well-balanced diet requires considerably more effort under these circumstances, so you may not be getting all the vitamins and minerals you need. A deficient intake is also likely if you are on a restricted diet (e.g. eating less than 1500 calories a day for a period of time or excluding a food group from your regular diet).

A number of surveys have shown that many sportspeople do not achieve an adequate intake of vitamins and minerals from their diet (Short and Short, 1983; Steen and McKinney, 1986; Bazzare et al., 1986). Low intakes of certain minerals and vitamins are more common among female athletes compared with males. A study of 60 female athletes found that calcium, iron and zinc intakes were less than 100% of the RNI (Cupisti et al., 2002). US researchers also measured low intakes of vitamin E, calcium, iron, magnesium, zinc and phosphorus in US national figure skaters (Ziegler, 1999). This was correlated with lower than recommended intakes of fruit, vegetables, dairy and high-protein foods. Study of US elite female heptathletes by researchers at the University of Arizona found that while average nutrient intakes were greater than 67% of the RNI, vitamin E intakes fell below this minimum level (Mullins, 2001). However, more than half of the athletes were taking vitamin and mineral supplements, which would boost their overall intake. A study of 58 swimmers found that 71% of males and 93% of females did not meet the recommended intakes for at least one of the anti-oxidant vitamins (Farajian et al., 2004).

All these results suggest that athletes do not consume a well-balanced diet, with not enough fruit and vegetables in particular.

HOW DOES EXERCISE INCREASE MY REQUIREMENTS OF VITAMINS AND MINERALS?

Regular intense exercise places additional demands on your body, which means the requirement for many micronutrients is likely to be higher than the RDAs for the general population. Micronutrients play an important role in energy production, haemoglobin synthesis, bone health, immune function and protection of the body against oxidative damage. They help with synthesis and

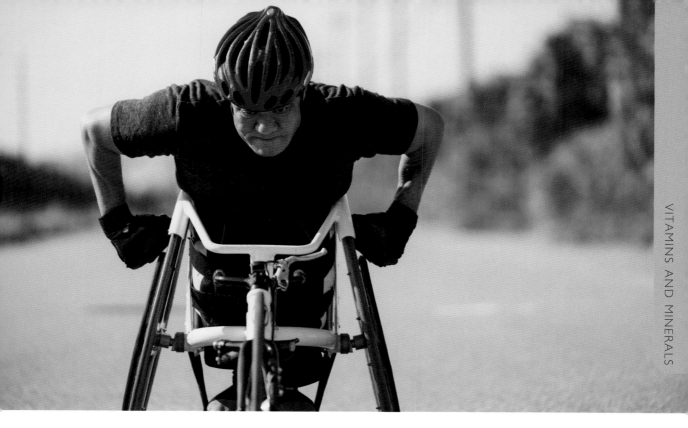

repair of muscle tissue during recovery. As a result, greater intakes of micronutrients may be required to cover increased needs for building, repair and maintenance of lean body mass in athletes. Failure to get enough micronutrients could leave you lacking in energy and susceptible to minor infections and illnesses.

Vitamin E

Vitamin E is a fat-soluble vitamin found in nuts, seeds, plant oils, oily fish, avocados and egg yolk, as well as a powerful antioxidant, which helps prevent the oxidation of fatty acids in cell membranes and protects the cell from damage. Early studies suggested that vitamin E supplementation reduced the amount of oxidative damage following prolonged intense cycling to exhaustion, compared with a placebo (Rokitzki *et al.*, 1994).

However, more recent studies have shown that supplementation may reduce training adaptations and result in decreased performance. For example, triathletes who took vitamin E supplements (800 IU) daily for 2 months performed no better than those who took a placebo (Nieman *et al.*, 2004). Although blood levels of vitamin E were higher, this did not reduce markers of oxidative stress or translate into any improvement in performance. Similarly, another study found that 8 weeks of vitamin E supplementation did not reduce markers of oxidative stress or improve exercise performance (Gaeini *et al.*, 2006). And more recently, Norwegian researchers showed that supplementation with vitamins E and C did not improve endurance performance compared with a placebo (Paulsen *et al.*, 2013). This is because the vitamin supplements interfered with exercise-induced cell-signalling in cell muscle fibres.

Taking high doses of vitamin E supplements above the RDA will not confer any performance advantage and may blunt training adaptations (*see* below 'Vitamin C'. Aim to get your vitamin E from food rather than supplements.

Vitamin C

Vitamin C has several exercise-related functions. It is required for the formation of connective tissue and certain hormones (e.g. adrenaline), which are produced during exercise; it is involved in the formation of red blood cells, which enhances iron absorption; it is a powerful antioxidant, which, like vitamin E, can also protect against exercise-related cell damage. It also enhances immune cell function (*see* p. 243).

However, there is little evidence that vitamin C supplementation improves performance in athletes who are not deficient in the vitamin. In fact, rather than improving exercise performance, high doses (more than 1000 mg) of vitamin C may have detrimental effects. In a double-blind randomised study, athletes who took vitamin C supplements (1000 mg/day) experienced a reduction in endurance capacity after 8 weeks (Gomez-Cabrera *et al.*, 2008). That's because supplements prevented muscle cell adaptations (e.g. an increase in enzyme production) to exercise, resulting in no improvement in aerobic capacity.

Norwegian researchers found that people who took high-dose supplements of vitamins C (1000 mg) and E (235 mg) for 11 weeks gained no performance benefit compared with those taking a placebo (Paulsen *et al.*, 2013). Those taking the supplements produced fewer mitochondria than those taking a placebo. The researchers concluded that vitamins C and E

should be used with caution as they may 'blunt' the way muscles respond to exercise.

A review of studies concluded that vitamin C supplementation reduced the benefits of training and resulted in slower recovery and strength gains (Adams *et al.*, 2014).

Lower doses of vitamin C (<1000 mg/day) may be useful if you are involved in prolonged high-intensity training because it may stabilise cell membranes and protect against viral attack. One study (Peters *et al.*, 1993) found a reduced incidence in upper respiratory tract infections in ultra-marathon runners after taking 600 mg vitamin C for 21 days prior to the race. Another study at the University of North Carolina, found that vitamin C supplementation before and after resistance exercise reduced post-exercise muscle soreness and muscle damage and promoted recovery (Bryer and Goldfarb, 2006). However, you should aim to get your vitamin C from food before considering supplements.

Vitamin D

The role of vitamin D in maintaining bone health is well-recognised but following the discovery of a vitamin D receptor in many tissues, including muscle tissue, recent sports science research has focused on its role in muscle structure and function.

Several studies suggest that vitamin D deficiency is widespread among athletes, particularly those in northern latitudes who train mainly indoors or get little sun exposure, or who do not consume vitamin D-rich foods (Owens *et al.*, 2015; Larson-Meyer and Willis, 2010; Lovell, 2008; Meier *et al.*, 2004). One study measured inadequate serum vitamin D levels (25(OH)D <50 nmol/litre) in 38 out of 61 (62%) UK athletes (Close *et al.*,

2013 (a)), while another found that more than half (57%) of club-level athletes were deficient (Close *et al.*, 2013 (b)). Another study of male cyclists found that the majority had suboptimal levels of vitamin D (Keay *et al.*, 2018).

This is an area of concern because there is increasing evidence that low levels reduce muscle function, strength and performance (Hamilton, 2011). Low levels can also have a negative effect on the immune system, increasing the risk of upper respiratory tract infection (URI), which will have a detrimental effect on your training and performance (Halliday, 2011; He *et al.*, 2013). An inadequate vitamin D status may also affect injury risk and the risk of stress fractures (*see* pp. 241–2).

Several studies have observed a correlation between vitamin D status and athletic performance (Larson-Meyer and Willis, 2010). Inadequate levels are associated with reduced performance while adequate levels are associated with optimal performance. A review of studies has highlighted a seasonal variation in performance (Cannell, 2009). The latter found that performance peaks in the summer months (when vitamin D levels peak), and declines in winter months (when vitamin D levels decline), reaching its lowest point when vitamin D levels are at their lowest. Peak athletic performance seems to occur when vitamin D levels approach those obtained by natural, full-body, summer sun exposure, which is above 50 ng/ml. The National Academy of Medicine (formerly called the Institute of Medicine) classifies blood serum vitamin D3 (25(OH)D) <30 nmol/litre as deficient, 30–50 nmol/litre as inadequate (Heaney, 2011) and >50 nmol/litre as adequate. The optimal level of vitamin D for performance is not established but researchers recommend a blood concentration >75 nmol/litre (Owens *et al.*, 2015; He *et al.*, 2013; Heaney, 2013).

Getting adequate levels of vitamin D, whether from sunlight exposure (ultraviolet B radiation) or diet, is therefore important for optimal performance. In the summer months, most of us can get all the vitamin D we need from sunlight exposure, but in winter getting adequate vitamin D becomes harder to accomplish. For this reason, Public Health England recommends everyone take a 10 mcg (400 IU) supplement from October to April. Those at high risk of deficiency (e.g over-65s, with dark skin or with little outdoor access) are advised to take a supplement all year round. Because vitamin D is found only in a small number of foods (oily fish, egg yolk, liver and some fortified breakfast cereals, yoghurts and spreads), it may be difficult to get enough from food alone.

Supplementation for performance is a controversial area and scientific opinion is divided. Some researchers believe that vitamin D supplements may not benefit athletic performance (Powers *et al.,* 2011). However, others propose that it would be beneficial for athletes who get little sun exposure or perhaps during the winter months (IOC, 2011; Halliday, 2011). The idea is to ensure vitamin D levels >50 nmol/litre. One study showed that supplementation for 8 weeks improved performance in athletes who had baseline vitamin D levels <50 nmol/litre (Close *et al.,* 2013 (a)). Another found that supplementation improved muscle recovery following exercise-induced muscle damage (Owens *et al.*, 2015). Supplementation may also improve immunity. One study showed a linear relationship between vitamin D status and URT infection, and for each 10 nmol/litre increase in 25-hydroxyvitamin D

(25(OH) D, the best indicator of vitamin D status in the blood), there was an associated 7% lower risk of infection (Berry *et al.*, 2011). A review of studies recommends a supplement containing 50–100 ug (2000–4000 IU) (Owens *et al.*, 2018). Since vitamin D is a fat-soluble vitamin, it can be stored and at high levels result in toxicity. The tolerable upper intake level (UL) set by Public Health England is 100 mcg (4000 IU)/ day. If you think you may be at risk of vitamin D deficiency, you should consult your doctor and/or sports nutritionist, who may recommend a simple blood test to determine whether you would benefit from vitamin D supplements.

B vitamins

The B vitamins, thiamin (B_1), riboflavin (B_2) and niacin (B_3) are involved in releasing energy from food. Since requirements for these are based on the amount of carbohydrate and calories consumed, athletes are likely to need more than sedentary people. Food sources of B vitamins include wholegrain bread, breakfast cereals, oatmeal and brown rice. If you are restricting your calorie intake or you eat lots of refined rather than whole grains, you may be missing out on B vitamins. To compensate for any shortfall, you may benefit from a multivitamin supplement that contains at least 100% of the RNI of the B vitamins.

Vitamin B_6 is involved in protein and amino acid metabolism. It is needed for making red blood cells and new proteins, so getting the right amount of vitamin B_6 is very important to athletes.

Pantothenic acid (vitamin B_5) is necessary for making glucose and fatty acids from other metabolites in the body. It is also used in the manufacture of steroid hormones and brain chemicals.

Obviously, a deficiency would be detrimental to health and athletic performance.

Folic acid and vitamin B_{12}

These B vitamins are both involved with red blood cell production in the bone marrow. They are also needed for cell division, and protein and DNA manufacture. Clearly, exercise increases all of these processes and therefore your requirements for folic acid and vitamin B_{12}. As vitamin B_{12} is not found naturally in any plant sources, vegans must obtain vitamin B_{12} from fortified foods such as non-dairy milk alternatives, yeast extract, nutritional yeast and certain breakfast cereals, or a supplement (*see* p. 274).

Beta-carotene

Beta-carotene is one of 600 carotenoid pigments that give fruit and vegetables their yellow, orange and red colours. They are not vitamins but act as antioxidants by protecting cells from oxidative damage (*see* p. 231). Beta-carotene enhances the antioxidant function of vitamin E, helping to regenerate it after it has disarmed free radicals. However, carotenoids function most effectively together, so it is best to take these nutrients packaged together, in a multivitamin supplement or in food.

Calcium

Calcium is an important mineral in bone formation, but it also plays an important role in muscle growth, muscle contraction and nerve transmission. While the body is able to increase or decrease the absorption of this mineral according to its needs, extra calcium is recommended for female athletes with low oestrogen levels (*see* pp. 266–7). Weight-bearing exercise, such as running and weight training, increases bone mass and calcium absorption so it is important to get enough calcium in your diet.

Iron

Iron is important for athletes. Its major function is in the formation of haemoglobin (which transports oxygen in the blood) and myoglobin (which transports oxygen in the muscle cells). Many muscle enzymes involved in energy metabolism require iron. It is also required for immune function. It is estimated that 15–35% of female athletes and 3–11% of male athletes have iron deficiency (Sim *et al.*, 2019).

Iron deficiency can reduce the amount of oxygen delivered to the muscles during exercise, as well as the amount of energy that can be generated in muscle cells. It reduces your maximal oxygen consumption (VO_2max), your endurance capacity and your performance. Symptoms of low iron status include lethargy, chronic fatigue, pallor, headaches, light-headedness, above-normal

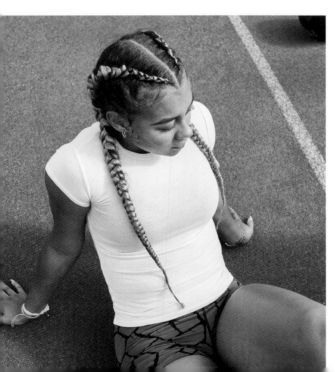

breathlessness during exercise and palpitations, frequent injuries, loss of endurance and power, loss of appetite and negative mood states. For this reason, athletes should be screened regularly for iron status (Sim *et al.*, 2019; Thomas *et al.*, 2016). Early diagnosis can help to prevent iron stores from declining further and therefore avoid training and performance interruptions.

How is iron deficiency defined in athletes?

Iron deficiency in the general population is usually diagnosed with a simple blood test that measures ferritin (a protein in the blood that stores iron), which gives a fairly accurate indication of the body's iron stores. For athletes, it is recommended that doctors also measure haemoglobin concentration (the iron-containing protein in red blood cells that carries oxygen around the body) and transferrin saturation (which tells you how much iron in the blood is bound to the protein transferrin). There are three stages of iron deficiency (Sim *et al.*, 2019):

- **Stage 1 (iron deficiency)** – Iron stores are depleted, and ferritin levels fall below 35 mcg/litre). Haemoglobin levels are normal (>115 g/litre) and transferrin saturation is normal (>16%).
- **Stage 2 (iron-deficient non-anaemia)** – Red blood cell formation starts to become impaired but not enough to cause anaemia. Ferritin levels fall further (<20 mcg/litre), transferrin saturation falls (<16%), but haemoglobin levels are normal (>115 g/litre).
- **Stage 3 (Iron deficiency anaemia)** – Haemoglobin production falls, resulting in anaemia (haemoglobin <115 g/litre; ferritin <12 mcg/litre; transferrin saturation <16%).

What are the causes of iron deficiency?

Athletes are at higher risk of developing iron deficiency than the general population. Intense exercise causes an increased inflammatory response, which increases levels of the iron-regulatory hormone hepcidin for 3–6 hours post-exercise (Peeling *et al.*, 2008). When hepcidin levels rise, iron absorption decreases. This means that any iron consumed in meals during this post-workout period may not be absorbed.

There is also potentially iron loss due to *haematuria*, due to bruising of the bladder lining caused by repeated pounding by the abdominal contents during running. Another condition, called *haemoglobinuria* (the presence of haemoglobin in the urine), can result from repetitive foot strikes associated with poor running gait or pounding on hard surfaces. This causes some destruction of red blood cells in the soles of the feet. However, iron losses via any of these routes are relatively small.

Certain athletes are more susceptible to iron deficiency. These include: 1) female athletes who menstruate, because blood losses are higher; 2) athletes with a low energy intake because iron intakes are likely to be insufficient to meet the body's requirement; 3) athletes who avoid red meat may not compensate by eating other sources of iron.

Table 6.1	THE IRON CONTENT OF VARIOUS FOODS	
Food	Portion size	mg iron
Calves' liver	Average (100 g)	12.2
Bran flakes	1 bowl (50 g)	10.0
Dried apricots (ready-to-eat)	5 (200 g)	7.0
Red lentils (boiled)	4 tbsp (160 g)	4.0
Prunes (ready-to-eat)	10 (110 g)	3.0
Baked beans	1 small tin (205 g)	2.9
Chickpeas (boiled)	4 tbsp (140 g)	2.8
Pumpkin seeds	Small handful (25 g)	2.5
Lean beef fillet (grilled)	Average (105 g)	2.4
Spinach	3 tbsp (100 g)	2.1
Wholemeal bread	2 large slices (80 g)	2.0
Wholemeal roll	1 (50 g)	1.8
Cashew nuts	30 (30 g)	1.8
Walnuts	12 halves (40 g)	1.2
Eggs	1 large (61 g)	1.2
Broccoli	2 spears (90 g)	1.0
Brown chicken meat	2 slices (100 g)	0.8

How can you treat an iron deficiency?

If you have been diagnosed with iron deficiency, there are three main strategies you can take:

1. Increase your iron intake. Iron-rich foods include meat and offal, sardines, tuna, wholegrain cereals, egg yolks, beans, lentils, green leafy vegetables, dried apricots, nuts and seeds. However, the absorption of iron from food is relatively inefficient. For example, meat-eating athletes may only absorb 5–35% of the iron in meat, whereas plant-based athletes may only absorb 2–20%) of the iron in plants. However, it is still possible to get enough iron from a plant-based diet (*see* pp. 269–72). The absorption of non-haeme iron can be increased by consuming foods rich in vitamin C (e.g. citrus fruit, berries) and citric acid (in fruit and vegetables). It may be reduced by calcium, tannins (in coffee and tea) and phytates (the main storage form of phosphorus in plants). The UK recommended intake of iron is 8.7 mg/day for men; 14.8 mg/day for women aged 19 to 50; and 8.7 mg/day for women over 50. However, athletes need more iron than the general population – perhaps as much as 30 –70% more, depending on iron losses (DellaValle, 2013).
2. Taking iron supplements in either liquid or tablet form. The standard recommended dose is 60–100 mg iron per day taken in the form of iron sulphate for 3 months, although doses depend on gender, weight and iron level. Supplements are best taken in the morning when hepicidin levels are at their lowest. This will help maximise absorption. Studies suggest that iron absorption from supplements is highest if iron is given on alternate days (Stoffel *et al.*, 2020). However, if you are not deficient then you shouldn't take supplements above the recommended intake as they may cause constipation and gastrointestinal (GI) upset.

   Athletes may be advised to take supplements before and during altitude training to maintain iron balance (Garvican-Lewis *et al.*, 2018). Altitude training places extra demands on the body's iron stores in order to manufacture new red blood cells. Low iron stores before or during training at altitude would blunt training adaptations.
3. Intravenous or intramuscular iron injections. Studies show these can increase ferritin levels two- to four-fold relatively rapidly and have the added advantage of bypassing the gut, avoiding GI issues.

Consuming iron-rich foods in the morning when hepcidin levels are low will avoid the inhibition of iron uptake caused by high levels induced by intense exercise later in the day, and may help reduce the risk of iron deficiency.

CAN VITAMIN AND MINERAL SUPPLEMENTS IMPROVE YOUR PERFORMANCE?

Unless you are deficient, vitamin and mineral supplements will not enhance your exercise performance or health. Many studies have been carried out over the years using varying doses of supplements. In the vast majority of cases, scientists have been unable to measure significant improvements in the performance of healthy athletes. Where a beneficial effect has been observed – for example, increased endurance – this has tended to be in athletes who had suboptimal vitamin or mineral status. Taking supplements simply restored the athletes' nutrient stores to 'normal' levels.

In other words, low body stores or deficient intakes can adversely affect your performance, but vitamin and mineral supplements taken in excess of your requirements will not necessarily produce a further improvement in performance. More does not mean better!

The scientific consensus is that vitamin and mineral supplements are unnecessary for those consuming a varied diet that provides enough energy to maintain your body weight (Rodriguez *et al.*, 2009).

To find out if you are deficient in any nutrient, consult a registered sports nutrition practitioner or registered dietitian (look for the initials RNutr or RD, *see* Online resources on p. 406) who will be able to analyse your diet and give you advice about whether supplements will have health benefits for you. Alternatively, you may purchase a home vitamin and mineral blood test from a private provider.

What is sports anaemia?

Athletes sometimes experience a transient decrease in haemoglobin in the early stages of a training programme or when training load increases. This is called 'dilutional' or 'sports anaemia'. It is not the same as iron-deficiency anaemia – it is simply a consequence of endurance training, and does not need any treatment. Intense exercise increases the volume of plasma in the blood, diluting the levels of haemoglobin. As a result, this decrease can sometimes incorrectly suggest there is an iron deficiency.

Check that it includes an accredited lab analysis and a review by a registered healthcare professional.

WHO MAY BENEFIT FROM TAKING SUPPLEMENTS?

Many athletes take some form of vitamin or mineral supplement, the most popular being multivitamins. A study of male triathletes found that over 60% routinely took vitamin supplements (Knez and Peake, 2010). All athletes consumed less vitamin D than the recommended daily intake but everyone consumed adequate amounts of all other nutrients. Obviously, supplements are not a substitute for poor or lazy eating habits. If you think you may be lacking in vitamins and minerals, try to adjust your diet to include more vitamin- and mineral-rich foods, or seek the advice of a registered sports nutrition practitioner or dietitian.

CAN HIGH DOSES OF SUPPLEMENTS BE HARMFUL?

Except perhaps in the case of vitamin A from liver (owing to modern animal feeding practices), it is almost impossible to overdose on vitamins and minerals from food. Problems are more likely to arise from the indiscriminate use of supplements, so always follow the guidelines on the label or the advice of a registered sports nutrition practitioner or dietitian.

Certain vitamins and minerals in supplement form taken in high doses can be harmful. As a rule of thumb, never take more than 10 times the RNI of the fat-soluble vitamins A and D, and no more than the RNI for any mineral. The Expert Group on Vitamins and Minerals in the UK have published safe upper levels for vitamins and minerals (Food Standards Agency, 2003). In particular, it warns against high doses of:

- Chromium in the form of chromium picolinate – may cause cancer, although up to 10 mg/day of other forms of chromium is unlikely to be harmful.
- Vitamin C – although excess vitamin C is excreted in the urine, levels above 1000 mg/day may result in stomach cramps, diarrhoea and nausea.
- Iron – levels above 17 mg/day may result in constipation and discomfort through an upset or bloated stomach.
- Vitamin D – large doses can cause weakness, thirst, increased urination and, if taken for a long period, result in high blood pressure and kidney stones.
- Vitamin A – large doses over a prolonged period can cause nausea, skin changes such as flakiness, liver damage and birth defects in unborn babies. Pregnant women are advised to avoid vitamin A supplements, fish liver oils and concentrated food sources of vitamin A such as liver and liver pâté.
- Vitamin B_6 – doses over 10 mg/day taken for a long period may lead to numbness, persistent pins and needles and unsteadiness (a type of neuropathy).

HOW ARE SUPPLEMENTS REGULATED?

Food supplements are not regulated like medicines, so there is not a 100% guarantee that they are safe and effective or that they contain what is stated on the label. Instead, they are regulated under food law. In the UK, vitamin and mineral supplements are regulated under the EU Food Supplements Directive (2002, amended August 2005). Manufacturers can only use nutrients and ingredients from a 'permitted' list, and then within maximum limits. Each ingredient must undergo extensive safety tests before it is allowed on the permitted list and, therefore, into a supplement. All health claims are required to be assessed and authorised by the European Food Safety Authority (EFSA) before they can be used. Manufacturers must also provide scientific proof to support a product's claims and ensure that it is clearly labelled. If you are subject to anti-doping regulations, opt for products tested by a credible third party, such as Informed Sport or NSF Certified for Sport (US). These ensure that there are no banned substances in the products.

CAN SUPPLEMENTS CAUSE IMBALANCES?

Taking single vitamins or minerals without the advice of a healthcare professional can easily lead to imbalances and deficiencies. Many interact with each other, competing for absorption, or enhancing or impairing each other's functions. For example, iron, zinc and calcium share the same absorption and transport system, so taking large doses of iron can reduce the uptake of zinc and calcium. For healthy bones, a finely tuned balance of vitamin D, calcium, phosphorus, magnesium, zinc, manganese, fluoride, chloride, copper and boron is required. Vitamin C enhances the absorption of iron, converting it from its inactive ferric form to the active ferrous form. Most of the B vitamins are involved in energy metabolism, so a short-term shortage of one may be compensated for by a larger than normal use of another.

If in doubt about supplements, it is safest to choose a multivitamin and mineral formulation rather than take individual supplements. With the exception of vitamin D, single supplements should be taken only upon the advice of a registered healthcare professional.

HOW SHOULD I CHOOSE A MULTIVITAMIN/MINERAL SUPPLEMENT?

While diet should always come first, a well-formulated multivitamin and mineral supplement acts as a nutritional safety net to ensure you obtain all the nutrients you need from your diet. Here are some basic guidelines:

- Check the supplement contains a wide range of vitamins and minerals.
- Check the percentages. In general, the amounts of each vitamin should be approximately 100% of the NRV stated on the label, but below the safe upper limit (SUL) (*see* pp. 352–61). By law, supplements can contain up to 50% more or 20% less vitamin, and 45% more and 20% less mineral than what's listed on the label.
- Avoid supplements containing more than 100% of the NRV of any mineral as these nutrients compete for absorption and can be harmful in doses higher than the NRV.
- There is no proof that so-called 'natural' or 'food state' vitamin supplements are better absorbed than synthetic vitamins. The majority have an identical chemical structure.

Vitamins as antioxidants

WHAT ARE ANTIOXIDANTS?

Antioxidants are enzymes and nutrients in the blood that 'disarm' free radicals or reactive oxygen species (ROS) (*see* below) and render them harmless. They work as ROS scavengers by donating one of their own electrons to 'neutralise' the ROS. Fortunately, your body has a number of natural defences against ROS. They include various enzymes (e.g. superoxide dismutase, glutathione, peroxidase) which have minerals such as manganese, selenium and zinc incorporated in their structure; vitamins C and E, as well as hundreds of other natural substances in plants, called phytochemicals. These include polyphenols, carotenoids (such as beta-carotene), and tannins.

WHAT ARE REACTIVE OXYGEN SPECIES?

Reactive oxygen species (ROS) are atoms or molecules with an unpaired electron and are produced all the time in our bodies as a result of normal metabolic and biochemical reactions, including energy production. They can easily generate other ROS by snatching an electron from any nearby molecule, and exposure to cigarette smoke, pollution, exhaust fumes, UV light and stress can increase their formation. ROS include superoxide anion radical, singlet oxygen, hydroxyl radical and perhydroxyl radical

In large numbers, ROS have the potential to cause damage in the body. ROS damage is thought to be responsible for heart disease, many cancers, ageing and post-exercise muscle soreness. Unchecked ROS can damage cell membranes and genetic material (DNA), destroy enzymes, disrupt red blood cell membranes, and oxidise LDL cholesterol in the bloodstream, thus also increasing the risk of atherosclerosis or the furring of arteries – the first stage of heart disease. Studies have demonstrated increased levels of ROS following exercise and these have been held partly responsible for muscle soreness, pain, discomfort, oedema (fluid retention) and tenderness post-exercise (Halliwell and Gutteridge, 1985).

Not all ROSs are damaging. Some help to kill germs, fight bacteria and heal cuts. The problem arises when too many are formed and they cannot be controlled by the body's defence system.

HOW DOES EXERCISE AFFECT ROS LEVELS?

Because exercise increases oxygen consumption, there is an increased generation of ROS. No one knows exactly how or why exercise does this, but it is thought to be connected to energy metabolism. During the final steps of ATP production (from carbohydrates or fats), electrons (the negative particles of atoms) sometimes go off course and collide with other molecules, creating ROS.

Another source is the damage done to muscle cell membranes during high-intensity eccentric exercise, such as heavy weight training or plyometric exercise, causing minor tears and injury to the muscles that results in the production of ROS.

Other factors such as increased lactic acid production, increased haemoglobin breakdown and heat generation may be involved, too. In essence, the more you exercise, the more ROS you generate.

WHAT ARE THE BEST SOURCES OF ANTIOXIDANTS?

The best source of antioxidants is the natural one: food! There are hundreds of natural substances in food called phytochemicals. These substances, which are found in plant foods, have antioxidant properties that are not present in supplements. Each appears to have a slightly different effect and to protect against different types of cancer and other degenerative diseases. For example, the phytochemicals in soya beans may prevent the development of hormone dependent cancers,

such as breast, ovarian and prostate cancer, while those in garlic can slow down tumour development. It is therefore wise to obtain as wide a range of phytochemicals from food as possible.

Table 6.2 (p.106) lists the food sources for the various antioxidants.

Summary of key points

- Vitamin and mineral requirements depend on age, body size, activity level and individual metabolism.
- DVRs should be used as a guide for the general population; they are not targets and do not take account of the needs of athletes.
- Regular and intense exercise increases the requirements for a number of vitamins and minerals. However, there are no official recommendations for athletes.
- Low intakes can adversely affect health and performance. However, high intakes exceeding requirements will not necessarily improve performance.
- Vitamins A, D and B_6 and a number of minerals may be toxic in high doses (more than 10 x RNI). Indiscriminate supplementation may lead to nutritional imbalances and deficiencies.
- Due to an erratic lifestyle or restricted food intake, many athletes consume suboptimal amounts of vitamins and minerals. Therefore a supplement containing a broad spectrum of vitamins and minerals would benefit their long-term health and performance.
- A well-formulated supplement should contain 100% of the NRV for vitamins (but below the safe upper limit) and no more than 100% of the NRV for minerals.

Table 6.2	FOOD SOURCES OF ANTIOXIDANTS	
	Antioxidant	**Source**
Vitamins	Vitamin C	Most fruit and vegetables, especially blackcurrants, strawberries, oranges, tomatoes, broccoli, green peppers, baked potatoes
	Folate	Spinach, broccoli, curly kale, green cabbage and other green leafy vegetables
	Vitamin E	Sunflower/safflower/corn oil, sunflower seeds, sesame seeds, almonds, peanuts, peanut butter, avocado, oily fish, egg yolk
Minerals	Selenium	Whole grains, vegetables, meat
	Copper	Whole grains, nuts, liver
	Manganese	Wheatgerm, bread, cereals, nuts
	Zinc	Bread, wholegrain pasta, grains, nuts, seeds, eggs
Carotenoids	Beta-carotene	Carrots, red peppers, spinach, spring greens, sweet potatoes, mango, cantaloupe melon, dried apricots
	Alpha- and gamma-carotene	Red coloured fruit, red and green coloured vegetables Tomatoes, watermelon
Flavonoids	Flavanols and polyphenols	Fruit, vegetables, tea, coffee, red wine, garlic, onions, dark chocolate
Phytochemicals	Canthaxanthin	Tomatoes, watermelon
	Coumaric acid	Green peppers, tomatoes, carrots
	Allicin saponins	Onions, garlic, leeks
	Glucosinolates	Broccoli, cabbage, cauliflower, Brussels sprouts
	Sulforaphane	Broccoli
	Lycopene	Tomatoes
	Lutein	Green vegetables
	D-limonene	Pith of citrus fruits
	Quercetin	Onions, garlic, apples, grapes
	Phenols	Grapes
	Resveratrol	Grape skins, red wine
	Ellagic acid	Grapes, strawberries, cherries

Sports
Supplements

The most effective way to develop your natural sports ability and achieve your fitness goals is through consistent and efficient training combined with optimal nutrition. Despite this, there is a huge variety of sports supplements promising greater performance gains.

It's hardly surprising that many athletes believe supplements to be an essential component for sports success and it has been estimated that 40–100% are using some form of supplement (Garthe and Maughan, 2018). For example, a study of 440 elite male and female athletes at the University of Calgary Sport Medicine Centre found that 87% used supplements regularly (Lun *et al.*, 2012). A study of Canadian varsity athletes found that 99% took supplements (Kristiansen *et al.*, 2005). A US study of collegiate varsity athletes found that 65% used some type of supplement regularly (Herbold *et al.*, 2004). The most commonly used supplements in the studies were vitamin/minerals, carbohydrate supplements, creatine and protein supplements.

The main reasons given by athletes for their supplement choices include to correct or prevent nutrient deficiencies, to provide a convenient form of energy or nutrients, to enhance athletic performance, to reduce body fat or increase muscle mass, and to promote rapid recovery (Garthe and Maughan, 2018).

Sifting through the multitude of products on offer can be an overwhelming task for athletes. It can be hard to pinpoint which ones work,

Definition of sports supplements and ergogenic aids

Sports supplements are a category of nutritional supplements whose purpose is to supplement the normal diet to improve general health and well-being or enhance sporting performance. They may include tablets, capsules, powders, drinks and bars, which claim to help with building muscle, increasing endurance, weight gain or loss, improving suppleness, rehydrating, aiding recovery or overcoming a nutrient deficiency.

Ergogenic aids are defined as any external influence created to enhance sport performance. They can include sports supplements as well as illegal drugs and methods.

especially when advertising claims sound so persuasive. Scientific research may be exaggerated or used selectively by manufacturers trying to sell a product. Testimonials from well-known athletes are also a common ploy that is used to hype products.

According to a recent consensus statement by the International Olympic Committee, the majority of sports supplements have little evidence to back them up (Maughan *et al.*, 2018). At best, they are unnecessary, and, at worst, harmful or prohibited. There are relatively few products that are supported by robust research and offer performance or health benefits. This chapter examines the evidence for some of the following sports supplements and provides an expert rating on their effectiveness and safety.

1. Antioxidant supplements
2. Arginine
3. Branched-chain amino acid supplements
4. Beta-alanine
5. Beetroot juice (nitrate)
6. Bicarbonate
7. Caffeine
8. Cannabidiol (CBD)
9. Cherry juice
10. Conjugated linoleic acid (CLA)
11. Collagen
12. Colostrum
13. Creatine
14. Energy bars
15. Energy gels
16. Ephedrine/ma huang/'fat burners'/thermogenic supplements
17. Fat burners (ephedrine-free)
18. Glutamine
19. HMB
20. Hydrogel energy drinks
21. Ketones
22. Leucine
23. Omega-3 fatty acids
24. Polyphenols
25. Probiotics
26. Protein supplements
27. Pro-hormones/steroid precursors/testosterone boosters
28. Taurine
29. Testosterone boosters
30. ZMA

Are sports supplements safe?

There is currently no specific European or national legislation governing the safety of sports supplements. As they are classified as foods, supplements are not subject to the same strict manufacturing, safety testing or labelling requirements as licensed medicines. This means that there is no guarantee that a supplement lives up to its claims.

Moreover, as many supplements are sold through the internet, it is difficult to regulate the market and there remains the risk of purchasing contaminated products. Contaminants – anabolic androgenic steroids and other prohibited stimulants – have been found in many different supplements. Inadvertent contamination may be caused by cross-contamination during manufacturing, impurities within ingredients or cross-contamination between ingredients in the supply chain.

The most common supplements associated with inadvertent doping are those claiming to modulate hormone regulation, stimulate muscle mass gain, increase fat loss, and/or boost energy. These may contain banned substances such as

Guidelines for evaluating the claims of sports supplements[*]

How valid is the claim?
- Does the claim made by the manufacturer of the product match the science of nutrition and exercise, as you know it? If it sounds too good to be true then it probably isn't valid.
- Does the amount and form of the active ingredient claimed to be present in the supplement match that used in the scientific studies on this ergogenic aid?
- Does the claim make sense for the sport for which the claim is made?

How good is the supportive evidence?
- Is the evidence presented based on testimonials or scientific studies?
- What is the quality of the science? Check the credentials of the researchers (look for university-based or independent) and the journal in which the research was published (look for a peer-reviewed journal reference). Did the manufacturer sponsor the research?
- Read the study to find out whether it was properly designed and carried out. Check that it contains phrases such as 'double-blind placebo controlled', i.e. that a 'control group' was included in the study and that a realistic amount of the ergogenic substance/placebo was used.
- The results should be clearly presented in an unbiased manner with appropriate statistical procedures. Check that the results seem feasible and the conclusions follow from the data.

Is the supplement safe and legal?
- Are there any adverse effects?
- Does the supplement contain toxic or unknown substances?
- Is the substance contraindicated in people with a particular health problem?
- Is the product illegal or banned by any athletic organisations?
- Has the product been independently batch-tested for banned substance by a certification programme, such as Informed Sport or NSF Certified for Sport (US)?

[*] Adapted from Butterfield (1996), Clark (1995).

ephedrine, androstenedione, androstenediol, dehydroepiandrosterone (DHEA), 19-norandrostenedione, 19-norandrostenediol, amphetamines and ephedra (ma huang).

The largest survey was from the International Olympic Committee-accredited laboratory in Cologne. They looked for steroids in 634 sports supplements and found 15% contained substances – including nandrolone – that would lead to a failed drugs test (Geyer *et al.*, 2004); 19% of UK samples were contaminated. In another report, Swiss researchers found different substances than those declared on the labels, including testosterone, in seven out of 17 pro-hormone supplements, i.e. 41% of the supplements (Kamber *et al.*, 2001).

An analysis of 152 sports supplements purchased through standard retail outlets within the UK found that over 10% were contaminated with steroids and/or stimulants (Judkins, 2008).

A 2012 investigation by the Medicines and Healthcare Products Regulatory Agency (MHRA) found 84 illegal products such as energy and muscle gain products containing dangerous ingredients such as steroids, stimulants and hormones (MHRA, 2012). More recently, an analysis of 66 'high risk' sports supplements (e.g. supplements claiming to change hormone levels or stimulate muscle mass gain) purchased from the internet found that 38% contained undeclared doping substances, including high levels of stimulants and anabolic steroids (Duiven *et al.*, 2021). It should be noted that this survey did not include 'low risk' supplements (e.g. protein powders), so is not applicable to all supplements.

Most of the above-mentioned surveys were carried out before independent batch-testing and certification became widespread. Since then, a large number of supplement companies have signed up to certification programmes and therefore the risk of inadvertent contamination – particularly of 'low risk' supplements – is likely to be significantly lower.

Antioxidant supplements

WHAT ARE THEY?

Antioxidant supplements may contain one or more of the following nutrients: beta-carotene, vitamin C, vitamin E, zinc, magnesium, copper, lycopene (a pigment found in tomatoes), selenium, co-enzyme Q10, catechins (found in green tea), methionine (an amino acid) and anthocyanidins (pigments found in purple or red fruit).

How can I minimise the risk of inadvertent doping?

No guarantee can be given that any particular supplement, including vitamins and minerals, ergogenic aids and herbal remedies, is free from prohibited substances as these products are not licensed and are not subject to the same strict manufacturing and labelling requirements as licensed medicines. Anti-doping rules are based on the principle of strict liability and therefore supplements are taken at an athlete's risk. While the risk of using a contaminated supplement will never be eliminated, should you decide to take a supplement you can minimise the risk of inadvertent doping by looking for voluntary certifications by companies such as Informed Sport or NSF Certified for Sport (US) on the label. This indicates that the product has been independently tested for most (though not all) banned substances. You'll find all registered products listed on the companies' websites: www.wetestyoutrust.com and www.nsfsport.com. However, it is important to realise that even when using certified products, you are still risking a positive drug test. Any product can be contaminated since there is no regulation in place to prevent this. If you are in doubt as to whether to take supplements or not, seek the advice of a qualified medical professional or UK Anti-Doping (UKAD) Accredited Advisor.

WHAT DO THEY DO?

Energy production produces free radicals, or reactive oxygen species (ROS), with levels increasing during exercise. When ROS generation exceeds the body's antioxidant capacity they can damage cell membranes and DNA and impair muscle function, hastening fatigue. The imbalance is sometimes called 'oxidative stress'. The idea behind antioxidant supplementation is to offset exercise-induced ROS damage, counteract fatigue and to speed recovery.

WHAT IS THE EVIDENCE?

Although previous studies have suggested antioxidant supplementation may be beneficial, these have been criticised due to small subject numbers and poor study design. Newer studies suggest that antioxidant supplements either have no effect on performance or can actually decrease training efficiency and prevent adaptation of muscles to training – the very opposite of what athletes want (Nikolaidis *et al.*, 2012). Although supplements reduce post-exercise oxidative stress, this isn't a good thing because oxidative stress and therefore a change in the redox state is needed to drive training adpatations. In other words, redox signalling and inflammation are desirable and are considered essential for training adaptations. Reactive oxygen species generated during intense exercise signal to the body that it needs to adapt to the stress of training by becoming stronger and more efficient. By prematurely quenching these ROS with high doses of antioxidant supplements, you could be preventing muscle adaptations.

Studies suggest that exercise itself increases the oxidative capacity of muscles by enhancing the action of antioxidant enzymes such as glutathione peroxidase, catalase and superoxide dismutase (Draeger *et al.*, 2014). Thus, taking supplements during training (i.e. when training adaptations are the goal) will provide no further benefit. A review of more than 150 studies by Australian researchers concluded that there is insufficient evidence that antioxidant supplements improve performance (Peternelj and Coombes, 2011).

A double-blind randomised controlled trial found that vitamin C (1000 mg) and E (235 mg) supplements blunted the endurance training-induced increase of mitochondrial proteins, which is important for improving muscular endurance (Paulsen *et al.*, 2013). There was no difference in aerobic capacity (VO_2max) or performance between those taking supplements or a placebo. The researchers concluded that vitamins C and E hampered cellular adaptations in the muscles and therefore provided no performance benefit.

In another study, cyclists taking antioxidant supplements experienced no performance benefit during 12 weeks of strenuous endurance training compared with those taking a placebo (Yfanti *et al.*, 2010). Similarly, another study found that vitamin C and vitamin E supplementation had no effect on muscle performance or recovery following 4 weeks of eccentric training (Theodorou *et al.*, 2011). In another, footballers who took an antioxidant supplement experienced no increase in aerobic capacity (VO_2max) after 6 weeks of training, while those taking a placebo did (Skaug *et al.*, 2014).

DO I NEED THEM?

There is little benefit to be gained from taking high dose antioxidant supplements during training. Instead of improving performance or promoting recovery, supplements may actually hamper it by disrupting the mechanisms designed to deal with exercise-derived oxidative stress. The consensus statement by the American College of Sports Medicine cautions against the use of antioxidant supplements (Rodriguez *et al.*, 2009). However, supplements may have some benefit immediately prior to competition when training adaptations are not needed.

Getting your vitamins and minerals through a varied and balanced diet remains the best approach to maintaining an optimal antioxidant status. There's good evidence to suggest that a diet rich in foods that are naturally high in antioxidants is associated with better health outcomes.

ARE THERE ANY SIDE EFFECTS?

Antioxidant supplementation may delay recovery and even result in reduced performance.

Arginine

WHAT IS IT?

L-arginine is a non-essential amino acid made naturally in the body. It is sold as l-arginine, arginine alpha keto-glutarate (A-AKG) or arginine keto iso-caproate (A-KIC). Supplements are marketed to athletes (and bodybuilders in particular) for promoting and prolonging muscle pumps.

WHAT DO THEY DO?

Arginine is an amino acid that is readily converted to nitric oxide (NO) in the body. NO is a gas that is involved in vasodilation, which is the process that increases blood flow to muscles, allowing better delivery of nutrients and oxygen. The idea behind supplementation is to increase blood flow, or the muscle 'pump', when lifting weights, and promote recovery and muscle growth.

WHAT IS THE EVIDENCE?

Little research supports these assertions directly. Most studies suggest that arginine supplements have no effect on NO production or exercise performance in elite athletes (Alvares et al., 2012 Liu *et al.*, 2009). In one study, there was no difference in NO levels, blood flow or performance in athletes taking A-AKG supplements or a placebo (Willoughby *et al.*, 2011). An analysis of several studies concludes that NO supplements may produce a small benefit for beginners, but not for more highly trained athletes and not for females (Bescos *et al.*, 2012).

DO I NEED THEM?

Arginine is unlikely to benefit your performance – it does not increase NO levels to an appreciable extent. Other NO boosters, such as beetroot juice, are likely to be more effective (*see* pp. 115–17).

ARE THERE ANY SIDE EFFECTS?

Side effects are unlikely from the doses recommended on the supplement label.

Branched-chain amino acid supplements

WHAT ARE THEY?

Branched-chain amino acids (BCAAs) include valine, leucine and isoleucine. These three essential amino acids (EAAs) make up one-third of muscle proteins.

WHAT DO THEY DO?

It is claimed that BCAA supplements 1) enhance endurance and delay fatigue by providing a fuel source to muscles when muscle glycogen is depleted, 2) reduce muscle soreness following muscle-damaging exercise and 3) increase muscle protein synthesis (MPS).

WHAT IS THE EVIDENCE?

The evidence that BCAA supplements enhance endurance performance is mixed. Early studies suggested that BCAA supplements during and after prolonged exercise are oxidised as fuel and may reduce muscle breakdown and preserve muscle in athletes (Williams, 2005). However, not all studies have shown positive results.

There is a small amount of evidence that BCAAs may reduce muscle soreness after muscle-damaging exercise but the benefits are small (Nosaka *et al.,* 2006; Shimomura *et al.,* 2006). However, a more recent study of distance runners found that supplements did not improve marathon performance, nor reduce muscle damage compared with a placebo (Areces *et al.,* 2014).

While leucine consumed along with suboptimal doses of protein has been shown to increase MPS (Churchward-Venne *et al.,* 2012), there is no evidence that BCAA supplements alone can increase MPS (Wolfe, 2017). A review of studies showed that BCAA supplementation showed no benefits for strength or muscle mass when sufficient daily protein is consumed (Plotkin *et al.,* 2021). The International Society of Sports Nutrition does not recommend the use of BCAAs to increase performance or maximise muscle protein synthesis (Kerksick *et al.,* 2018).

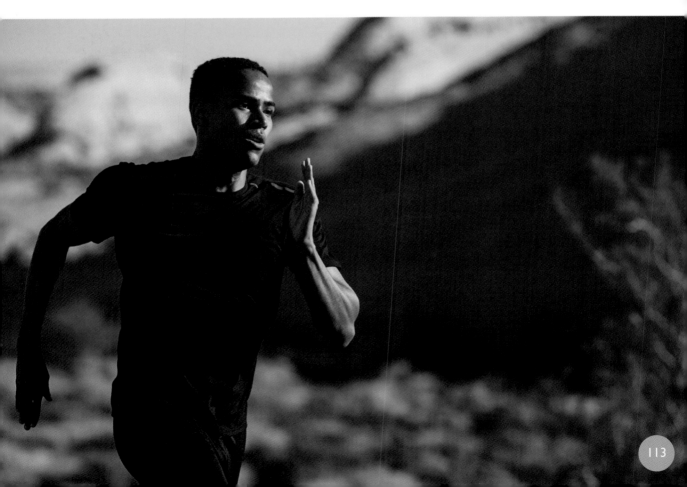

DO I NEED THEM?

There appears to be little benefit in taking BCAA supplements if sufficient calories, protein and carbohydrate are being consumed. In other words, there is no evidence that BCAAs are better than protein-containing foods for stimulating MPS.

ARE THERE ANY SIDE EFFECTS?

BCAAs are relatively safe because they are normally found in protein in the diet. Excessive intake may reduce the absorption of other amino acids.

Beta-alanine

WHAT IS IT?

Beta-alanine is an amino acid that is used to make carnosine (a dipeptide formed from beta-alanine and histidine). Carnosine is an important intracellular buffer in muscles – it buffers the acidity (hydrogen ions) produced during high-intensity exercise. Supplements are available in powder or capsule form.

WHAT DOES IT DO?

Beta-alanine supplements increases muscle carnosine levels. One study found that taking 5–6 g/day increases muscle carnosine content by 60% after 4 weeks and 80% after 10 weeks (Harris et al., 2006). This raises the buffering capacity of the muscles, increasing the ability of muscles to tolerate high-intensity exercise for longer. Normally, a build-up of acidity results in fatigue. Supplementation may therefore increase power output and performance in anaerobic exercise, and decrease perceived exertion.

WHAT IS THE EVIDENCE?

Beta-alanine is one of the five performance-enhancing supplements supported by the International Olympic Committee for use in sports (Maughan et al., 2018). A large number of studies have shown that supplementation increases the body's capacity for high-intensity exercise efforts. One of the first was carried out at Ghent University, Belgium, and showed that beta-alanine supplements reduced fatigue when performing a set of knee extensions (Derave et al., 2007). Another study at the College of New Jersey found that beta-alanine supplements resulted in increased training volume and reduced subjective feelings of fatigue in football players (Hoffman et al., 2008).

Australian researchers found that runners who took beta-alanine supplements for 28 days achieved significantly faster 800 m race times compared with those who took a placebo (Ducker et al., 2013). Another study measured significant improvements in power output and time-trial performance in cyclists after 4 weeks of beta-alanine supplementation (Howe et al., 2013). Similarly, a study by Belgian researchers found that beta-alanine supplementation for 8 weeks significantly enhanced sprint performance at the end of a simulated endurance cycle race (Van Thienen et al., 2009).

More recently, a systematic review of 40 studies concluded that beta-alanine supplementation leads to improved performance in short-duration, high-intensity activities lasting between 30 seconds and 10 minutes (Saunders et al., 2017). Similar findings were shown in previous reviews, which also indicated an average performance improvement of 2 –3% in recreational athletes and 0.5–1% in elite athletes (Quesnele et al., 2014; Hobson et al., 2012).

DO I NEED IT?

If your sport or activity involves sustained high-intensity efforts lasting between 30 seconds and 10 minutes, or you play team sports such as rugby, football and tennis that involve repeated sprints then beta-alanine may be of benefit. It may also be advantageous in races such as 100–400 m swimming, 4-km cycling, 800–1500 m running and 2000 m rowing, and for resistance training. The optimum dose is 65 mg/kg BW, equivalent to 4.5 g for a 70 kg athlete. It is most effective when taken in divided doses (0.8–1.6 mg every 3–4 hours) over 10–12 weeks. Once supplementation stops, muscle carnosine gradually return to baseline levels so a maintenance dose of 1.2 g/day is recommended if you want to sustain the benefits (Maughan *et al.*, 2018; Stegen *et al.*, 2014). However, the research to date has involved relatively small numbers of athletes, so recommendations may change as further research is carried out.

ARE THERE ANY SIDE EFFECTS?

There have been reports of parathesia (skin tingling) shortly after taking a dose, although this appears to be harmless, and is associated mainly with higher doses. Smaller doses, sustained-release formulations or supplements taken with food are less likely to cause side effects. Importantly, the long-term effects of beta-alanine supplements are not known.

Beetroot juice (nitrate)

WHAT IS IT?

Beetroot juice (and beetroot) is a rich source of nitrate. Nitrate is also found in other vegetables, such as spinach, rocket, lettuce, kale, chard, pak choi, cabbage, endive, leeks and broccoli. Nitrate may also be taken in the form of sodium nitrate supplements.

WHAT DOES IT DO?

Beetroot juice increases the amount of nitrate in the blood. Nitrate is converted into nitrite (by oral bacteria acting on saliva) and then into nitric oxide (NO) in the body. NO can also be made in the body from the amino acid arginine. It plays an important role in vasodilation and regulating blood pressure. However, its performance-enhancing effects are thought to be due to its effects on muscle cells. It improves muscle contractile and/or mitochondrial efficiency, lowering the oxygen cost of exercise.

WHAT IS THE EVIDENCE?

A meta-analysis of 80 studies showed that nitrate supplementation in the form of beetroot juice enhances endurance performance by approximately 3% (Senefeld *et al.*, 2020). This echoes the findings of a previous review of 17 studies by UK and Australian researchers, which concluded that nitrate significantly improved endurance, as measured by time to exhaustion (Hoon *et al.*, 2013 (a)). Although time to exhaustion isn't a direct measure of performance, this finding could translate into a 1–2% reduction in race times.

Beetroot juice also reduces resting blood pressure (Siervo *et al.*, 2013) and the oxygen cost of exercise, meaning that athletes can sustain a given exercise intensity for longer or exercise at a higher intensity for the same oxygen uptake. For example, researchers at the University of Exeter, found that drinking 500 ml beetroot juice a day for a week enabled volunteers to run 15% longer before becoming exhausted (Lansley *et* al., 2011(a)). This was due to the higher levels of nitrate measured in the blood, which enabled a higher power output for the same oxygen uptake. A further study by the same researchers found that cyclists given 500 ml beetroot juice 2½ hours before a time-trial race improved their performance by 2.8% in a 4 km race and 2.7% in a 16.1 km race (Lansley et al., 2011(b)). Maastricht University researchers found that 170 ml beetroot juice concentrate over 6 days improved 10 km time-trial performance and power output in cyclists (Cermak et al., 2012). However, whole beetroot works equally well. Athletes who consumed 200 g cooked beetroot an hour before exercise were able to run faster in the latter stages of a 5 km run (Murphy et al., 2012). These results suggest that the nitrates in beetroot juice reduce oxygen uptake, improve exercise economy and allow athletes to exercise longer. This may give you the edge in events lasting 4–30 minutes or during intense intermittent exercise and team sports.

More recently, studies have suggested that beetroot juice also has the potential to improve performance in high-intensity intermittent sports (e.g. repeated sprints). Exeter University researchers found that consuming 70 ml (1 shot) of concentrated beetroot juice for 5 days improved 20 m sprint and high-intensity intermittent running performance in competitive team sport players (Thompson et al., 2016). Another study showed that soccer players were able to run 3.4% longer distances in a repeated sprint test when they were supplemented with beetroot juice for 6 days beforehand compared to a placebo (Nyakayiru et al., 2017).

Beetroot juice may also improve performance in resistance training. In one study, consuming 70 ml concentrated beetroot juice 2 hours before exercise was shown to improve training quality and volume in bench press performance (Williams et al., 2020).

However, the majority of studies showing a positive effect involved non-elite (untrained or recreational) athletes, not elite athletes. Whether beetroot juice also benefits performance in highly trained or elite athletes is unclear. Australian researchers found that beetroot juice supplementation did not improve performance in elite cyclists (Lane et al., 2013(c)). Even when combined with caffeine, beetroot juice (2 x 70 ml shots) made no difference to their performance in a 60-minute simulated time-trial. Another study with elite cyclists found little difference in time-trial performance following beetroot juice supplementation (Hoon et al., 2014). So, to date, beetroot juice appears to be a more effective ergogenic aid for non-elite (with a VO_2max <65 ml/kg/min) than elite athletes (VO_2max >65 ml/kg/min) (Senefeld et al., 2020). However, 65 ml/kg/min is a high threshold, which captures the vast majority of people.

Additionally, beetroot juice may not benefit female athletes in the same way as it does male athletes (Senefeld et al., 2020). The reasons are not clear but it may simply be due to the fact that females are under-represented in studies of beetroot juice supplementation (and more generally in sports science). To date, women have made up just 10% of sample sizes.

DO I NEED IT?

Beetroot may help improve your performance time in endurance activities lasting between 4 and 30 minutes, as well as in anaerobic and high-intensity activities involving single or multiple sprints. You can expect a performance increase of approximately 3%, which represents a significant advantage in many events. The optimal dose is likely to be 400–600 mg (5.6–8.4 mmol) nitrate, equivalent to one or two 70 ml concentrated beetroot 'shots' or 1 litre of regular beetroot juice or 400 g cooked beetroot (Wylie *et al.*, 2013; Senefeld *et al.*, 2020), the former format being likely to be the most practical option.

The optimal timing appears to be 2–3 hours pre-exercise as nitrate and nitrite levels in the blood peak 2–3 hours after consumption and then gradually fall over 12 hours. Alternatively, you may prefer 'nitrate loading' for 3–7 days prior to a competition to ensure blood levels of NO remain high (Cermak *et al.*, 2012). In practice, a combination of both strategies may be used, i.e. load for a few days followed by an acute dose 2–3 hours before the event.

Avoid using antibacterial mouthwash as this removes the beneficial bacteria in the mouth that convert some of the nitrate to nitrite and thus reduces the benefits of beetroot juice.

ARE THERE ANY SIDE EFFECTS?

No side effects of beetroot have been reported to date apart from a harmless, temporary pink colouration of urine and stools. There have been questions as to whether beetroot juice could theoretically increase cancer risk (dietary nitrates can be converted to nitrite in the body and then go on to react with amino acids to produce carcinogenic compounds called nitrosamines). However, research has shown that these harmful effects are associated with nitrates and nitrites from processed meat, not from vegetables (Gilchrist *et al.*, 2010; Hord *et al.*, 2009).

Bicarbonate

WHAT IS IT?

Sodium bicarbonate is a 'pH buffer', an extracellular anion that helps maintain pH gradients between the cells and blood. It is also a raising agent and a main ingredient of baking powder.

WHAT DOES IT DO?

Bicarbonate is already found in the blood, but consuming supplements ('bicarbonate loading') will increase the concentration further. Bicarbonate increases the pH of the blood, making it more alkaline. During high-intensity (anaerobic) exercise, hydrogen ions are produced, which gradually accumulate and result in fatigue ('the burn'!). However, by raising the pH of the blood, hydrogen ions can pass more easily from the muscle cells to the blood, where they can be removed (buffered), which allows you to continue exercising at a high intensity a little longer. It also means lactate is removed faster so you can recover faster.

WHAT IS THE EVIDENCE?

Research has shown improvement in high-intensity events lasting around 60 seconds, with benefits decreasing up to 10 minutes (Carr *et al.*, 2011). The average improvement is 1.7% with a bicarbonate dose of 0.3 g/kg BW. A study with elite cyclists found that bicarbonate supplementation significantly improved 4-minute cycling performance compared with a placebo (Driller *et al.*, 2012).

However, not all studies have shown beneficial effects of bicarbonate. For example, an Australian study with 8 swimmers found that bicarbonate loading did not result in faster times in 200 m freestyle (approximately 2 minutes' duration) compared with taking a placebo (Joyce *et al.*, 2012). Another study with New Zealand rugby players found that bicarbonate loading produced no difference in performance in rugby-specific skills (Cameron *et al.*, 2010). The discrepancies in findings may be explained by the type of exercise examined by the studies, which may not have been high enough in intensity for bicarbonate loading to have had an effect.

DO I NEED IT?

You may benefit from bicarbonate if you are competing in high-intensity events lasting 1–10 minutes – for example, sprint and middle-distance swimming, running and rowing events – or in events that involve multiple sprints, e.g. tennis, football, rugby. However, the side effects may cancel out any potential improvement.

The most common dose for bicarbonate loading is 0.2–0.3 g/kg. This equates to 14–21 g for a 70 kg person. It should be consumed gradually with at least 500 ml water 60–90 minutes before the start of exercise to minimise GI symptoms.

ARE THERE ANY SIDE EFFECTS?

Typical side effects include gastrointestinal upset, nausea, stomach pain, diarrhoea and vomiting. Bicarbonate loading may also cause water retention, which may be a disadvantage in many events. These side effects could negate any possible performance advantage. Symptoms may be reduced by taking the loading dose in divided doses over a 2–2½ hour period before the event, along with a small carbohydrate-rich meal and plenty of water.If you will be competing in several events over a few days, you could try taking 0.5 g/kg/day over the course of

1–3 days and then stop 12–24 hours before the event. Alternatively, you can take enteric-coated capsules, which have been formulated to bypass the stomach and therefore reduce the risk of gastrointestinal effects. Theoretically, the benefits will persist but with less risk of side effects.

Caffeine

WHAT IS IT?

Caffeine is a stimulant and has a pharmacological action on the body so is classed as a drug rather than a nutrient. It was once classed as a banned substance but was removed from the World Anti-Doping Agency (WADA) Prohibited List in 2004. This change was based on the recognition that caffeine enhances performance at doses that are indistinguishable from everyday caffeine use, and that the previous practice of monitoring caffeine use via urinary caffeine concentrations is not reliable.

It is found in everyday drinks and foods such as coffee, tea and cola, herbs such as guarana, and chocolate. It may also be added to energy drinks and sports drinks and gels. Table 7.1 lists the caffeine content of popular drinks and foods. The amounts used in research range from 1–15 mg/kg BW, which is equivalent to 70–1050 mg for a 70 kg athlete. Studies normally use caffeine pills rather than drinks.

WHAT DOES IT DO?

Caffeine acts on the central and peripheral nervous system, blocking a sleep-inducing brain chemical called adenosine, thus increasing alertness and concentration, reducing the perception of effort and allowing exercise to be maintained at a higher intensity for a longer period. It also increases endorphin (a 'feel-good' hormone) release and improves neuromuscular function.

It was once believed that caffeine enhances endurance performance because it promotes an increase in the utilisation of fat as an exercise fuel and 'spares' the use of glycogen. In fact, studies now show that the effect of caffeine on 'glycogen sparing' during submaximal exercise is short-lived and inconsistent – not all athletes respond in this way. Therefore, it is unlikely to explain the enhancement of exercise capacity and performance seen in many studies.

WHAT IS THE EVIDENCE?

A large number of studies show that caffeine can enhance performance by 2–4% in numerous different sports (Guest *et al.*, 2021; Maughan *et al.*, 2018; Goldstein *et al.*, 2010; Dodd, 1993; Graham and Spriet, 1991; Spriet, 1995). For example, a meta-analysis of 46 studies showed that anhydrous caffeine (i.e. in pill or powder form) has a small but significant effect on endurance performance when taken in doses of 3–6 mg/kg BW (Southward *et al.*, 2018). Overall, it improved average power output by 3% and time-trial performance by 2.2%. Similarly, a previous review of 21 time-trial studies found that caffeine improved endurance performance by an average of 3.2% (Ganio *et al.*, 2009). The optimal dose is not clear, though – one study showed no difference in cycling time-trial performance between 3 mg and 6 mg caffeine/kg BW (Desbrow *et al.*, 2012). Others suggest that <3 mg/kg BW also has an ergogenic effect when consumed with carbohydrate (Spriet, 2014(a)). For example, cyclists completed a time-trial significantly faster after consuming either 1.5 or 3 mg caffeine/kg BW compared to a placebo (Talanian and Spriet,

Table 7.1	THE CAFFEINE CONTENT OF POPULAR DRINKS AND FOODS	
Product	**Caffeine content, mg/cup**
Instant coffee (1 cup, 236 ml)	57 mg
Espresso (1 shot, 44 ml)	77 mg
Cappuccino (1 cup, 236 ml)	75 mg
Latte (1 cup, 236 ml)	75 mg
Brewed (237 ml)	96 mg
Tea (1 cup, 236 ml)	42 mg
Green tea (1 cup, 236 ml)	18 mg
Red Bull energy drink (1 can, 250 ml)	80 mg
Coca Cola (1 can, 330 ml)	32 mg
Energy gel (1 sachet)	25–75 mg
Dark chocolate (1 square, 10 g)	8 mg

Source: www.caffeineinformer.com

2016). Similarly, in a study at the University of Texas, cyclists who consumed 160 mg caffeine in the form of an energy drink completed a 1-hour time-trial 3 minutes 4 seconds faster than those who took a placebo (Ivy *et al.*, 2009).

Caffeine has also been shown to improve performance during anaerobic activities of 1–2 minutes' duration and for repeated sprints. For example, one study showed that rugby players who consumed 300 mg caffeine before exercise achieved greater performance gains in repeated sprints and tackles compared with those taking a placebo (Wellington *et al.*, 2017). Another study with footballers found that consuming a caffeinated drink 1 hour before training and then at 15-minute intervals improved sprinting performance and reduced the perception of fatigue (Gant *et al.*, 2010).

Two meta-analyses have shown that caffeine may also improve muscle strength and power by 2–7% (Grgic and Pickering, 2019; Grgic *et al.*, 2018).

Individual responses to caffeine vary, with some people experiencing greater performance-enhancing effects than others. This is thought to be due to genetic variation, which can predispose people to be 'fast' or 'slow' caffeine metabolisers (Guest *et al.*, 2018). Fast metabolisers break down caffeine quicker and experience a greater performance-enhancing effect than slow metabolisers.

DO I NEED IT?

Caffeine is likely to benefit performance in many types of endurance and short-term high-intensity activities. For anhydrous caffeine (i.e. pill or powder form), the optimal pre-exercise dose is

Does caffeine promote hypohydration?

Although caffeine is a diuretic, a daily intake of less than 4 mg/kg (equivalent to four cups of coffee) provides similar hydrating qualities to water (Killer *et al.*, 2014). At this level, caffeine is considered safe and unlikely to have any detrimental effect on performance or health (Armstrong, 2002). Taking caffeine regularly (e.g. drinking coffee) builds up your caffeine tolerance so you experience smaller diuretic effects.

According to a study from Ohio State University, caffeine taken immediately before exercise does not promote hypohydration (Wemple, 1997) (see p. 147). Six cyclists consumed a sports drink with or without caffeine over a 3-hour cycle ride. Researchers found that there was no difference in performance or urine volume during exercise. Only at rest was there an increase in urine output.

In another study, when 18 healthy men consumed 1.75 litres of three different fluids at rest, the caffeine-containing drink did not change their hydration status (Grandjean, 2000).

Researchers at Maastricht University found that cyclists were able to rehydrate after a long cycle equally well with water or a caffeine-containing cola drink (Brouns, 1998). Urine output was the same after both drinks. However, large doses of caffeine – over 600 mg, enough to cause a marked ergogenic effect – may result in a larger fluid loss. A study at the University of Connecticut, found that both caffeine-containing cola and caffeine-free cola maintained hydration in athletes (during the non-exercise periods) over 3 successive days of training (Fiala *et al.*, 2004). The athletes drank water during training sessions but rehydrated with either caffeinated or caffeine-free drinks. A further study by the same researchers confirmed that moderate caffeine intakes (up to 452 mg caffeine/kg BW/day) did not increase urine output compared with a placebo and concluded that caffeine does not cause a fluid electrolyte imbalance in the body (Armstrong *et al.*, 2005).

3–6 mg/kg BW, equivalent to 210–420 mg for a 70 kg athlete (Maughan *et al.*, 2018). However, lower doses of caffeine (<3 mg/kg BW) will also have an ergogenic effect when consumed with carbohydrate (e.g. in the form of gels or energy drinks) before or during exercise.

Performance benefits occur soon after consumption – it appears in the bloods within 5–15 minutes and peaks between 40 and 80 minutes – so you may opt to consume it approximately 60 minutes before exercise, spread throughout exercise, or late in exercise as fatigue is beginning to occur (Guest *et al.*, 2021). However, the optimal timing will depend on the form of caffeine. For example, caffeine in chewing gum is absorbed faster than anhydrous caffeine. Coffee will have a similar ergogenic effect to anhydrous caffeine (Higgins *et al.*, 2015; Hodgson *et al.*, 2013(a)). Bear in mind, though, the caffeine content in coffee can vary greatly depending on the preparation method, brand and variety.

As individual responses vary, you should experiment in training – not during competition – to find the dose and protocol that suits you.

It was once thought that cutting down on caffeine for several days before competition results in a more marked ergogenic effect. However, studies show that there is no difference in the performance response to caffeine between non-users and users of caffeine, and that withdrawing from caffeine does not increase the improvement in performance.

ARE THERE ANY SIDE EFFECTS?
The effects of an acute intake of caffeine follow a U-shaped curve. Low–moderate doses produce positive effects and a sense of well-being, but higher doses of caffeine (6–9 mg/kg BW) can

have negative effects. It may increase the heart rate, impair fine motor control and technique, and cause anxiety or over-arousal, trembling and sleeplessness. Some people are more susceptible to these than others. If you are sensitive to caffeine, it is best to avoid it.

Scientific research shows, on balance, no link between long-term caffeine use and health problems such as hypertension and bone mineral loss. The connection between raised cholesterol levels and heavy coffee consumption is now known to be caused by certain fats in coffee, which are more pronounced in boiled coffee than in instant or filter coffee.

Cannabidiol (CBD)

WHAT IS IT?
CBD is one of around 120 cannabinoids produced by the cannabis plant. There are two strains of cannabis plant: 1) hemp (which has a low concentration of tetrahydrocannabinol (THC), the illegal psychoactive compound of marijuana) and 2) marijuana (which has a high THC concentration). CBD is produced from hemp and does not have psychotropic effects. It is available in the form of oils, capsules, sprays, tinctures and gummies.

WHAT DOES IT DO?
CBD is purported to relieve pain, reduce inflammation and improve sleep quality, making it an attractive supplement for many athletes. Exactly how it exerts these effects has yet to be elucidated. It is plausible that CBD reduces inflammation by binding receptors in immune tissues, thus reducing the immune response to high-intensity exercise. In terms of improving sleep quality, it

has been proposed that CBD inhibits adenosine re-uptake in the brain.

WHAT IS THE EVIDENCE?

Despite the attractive claims and relatively widespread use, there is currently no robust evidence to support the claims for CBD in athletes (Kasper *et al.*, 2020; Close *et al.*, 2019). The evidence to date is mainly anecdotal or based on studies with animals in laboratories.

DO I NEED IT?

CBD cannot be recommended to athletes owing to a lack of evidence and safety data for it. Although it is not currently listed on the World Anti-Doping Agency's Prohibited List, you should be aware that CBD carries a high risk of inadvertent doping as it may be contaminated with THC or other prohibited cannabinoids. One analysis of CBD products sold online found that 25% contained less CBD than labelled and 21% contained THC at levels higher than is currently permitted by the FDA (Bonn-Miller *et al.*, 2017). Unfortunately, there is currently no reliable independent testing or certified products available, so it is not possible to know whether a product is safe to take. UK Anti-Doping cautions against its use. Despite this, one study found that its use is relatively widespread among rugby players, with 26% reporting currently or previously using CBD to provide pain relief or improve sleep quality (Kasper *et al.*, 2020).

ARE THERE ANY SIDE EFFECTS?

There are reports of liver toxicity at high doses.

Cherry juice

WHAT IS IT?

Montmorency cherry juice is available as a concentrate, or in freeze-dried powdered form as capsules.

WHAT DOES IT DO?

Montmorency cherry juice is a rich source of flavonoids and anthocyanins, which have potent antioxidant and anti-inflammatory effects. It is thought that these compounds can help alleviate delayed onset muscle soreness (DOMS) and reduce inflammation that occurs after muscle-damaging exercise and quicken the recovery process.

WHAT IS THE EVIDENCE?

A number of studies suggest that Montmorency cherry juice may promote muscle recovery following intense exercise. Researchers at London South Bank University gave 10 athletes 30 ml of Montmorency cherry juice concentrate twice daily for 7 days prior to and 2 days after an intense strength training regimen (Bowtell *et al.*, 2011). The researchers found that the athletes' muscle recovery was significantly faster after consuming cherry juice compared to a placebo. It is thought that the antioxidant flavonoid compounds in the cherry juice may have reduced the oxidative damage to muscles, which normally occurs when muscles are worked to their maximum, thereby allowing the muscles to recover more quickly.

A study in runners carried out at Northumbria University, found that consuming Montmorency cherry juice for 5 days before and 2 days after a marathon improved muscle recovery and reduced inflammation (Howatson *et al.*, 2010). And another study by the same research group demonstrated that cyclists who consumed 30 ml Montmorency cherry juice concentrate for 5 days had less muscle damage and exercise-induced inflammation following a 109-minute cycling trial (Bell *et al.*, 2015). More recently, a study with recreational female athletes found that supplementing with Montmorency cherry juice for 4 days before and after muscle-damaging exercise reduced DOMS and accelerated recovery (Brown *et al.*, 2019). However, not all studies have shown positive results. Studies with professional soccer players (Abbot *et al.*, 2020) and with rugby league players (Morehen *et al.*, 2020) found that cherry juice concentrate had no effect on muscle recovery or soreness after a match compared with a placebo.

DO I NEED IT?

Consuming 30 ml Montmorency cherry juice concentrate for 4–5 days prior to and 2 days after a strenuous event (or a workout involving eccentric exercise) may reduce exercise-induced inflammation, muscle soreness and pain and accelerate recovery. Although not all studies have shown beneficial effects, on balance the supplement speeds functional recovery and, unlike high-dose antioxidant supplements (such as vitamins C and E), it does not interfere with the inflammation that is necessary for chronic training adaptations (*see* pp. 110–12). It therefore appears to be a more effective option than antioxidant supplements, which can interfere with post-training recovery. However, the benefits are mainly seen in athletes who consume diets low in polyphenols, which suggests that getting your polyphenols from a varied diet rich in fruit and vegetables (rather than from supplements) is likely to be best approach.

ARE THERE ANY SIDE EFFECTS?

No side effects have been found.

Conjugated linoleic acid (CLA)

WHAT IS IT?

CLA is an unsaturated fatty acid (in fact, it is a mixture of linoleic acid isomers) found naturally in small amounts in full-fat milk, meat and cheese. Supplements are made from sunflower and safflower oils.

WHAT DOES IT DO?

It is marketed as a fat-loss supplement. It is thought that CLA works by stimulating the enzyme hormone sensitive lipase (which releases fat from fat cells) and suppressing the hormone lipoprotein lipase (which transports fat into fat cells).

WHAT IS THE EVIDENCE?

Most of the research evidence for CLA is based on animal studies, which suggested that it promotes fat loss, increases muscle mass and reduces muscle breakdown. For this reason, CLA has been marketed as a supplement for weight loss. But there have been relatively few studies with humans and these have produced mixed results. Some have found that CLA supplements reduce fat levels and increase strength while others found no change in body composition. In studies that found positive results, CLA was used in conjunction with other supplements, making it difficult to assess its true effect (Falcone *et al.*, 2015). A randomised controlled study involving 28 overweight women found that CLA supplementation in conjunction with an 8-week aerobic exercise programme had no effect on body composition compared with a placebo (Ribeiro *et al.*, 2016). Similarly, researchers at the University of Memphis found no significant difference in body composition, fat loss or strength following 28 days of resistance training between volunteers taking CLA supplements and those taking a placebo (Kreider *et al.*, 2002). A review of studies by Brazilian researchers found that there is very little evidence that CLA reduces body fat in humans (Lehnen *et al.*, 2015).

DO I NEED IT?
It is unlikely that CLA supplements help reduce your body fat or increase muscle mass.

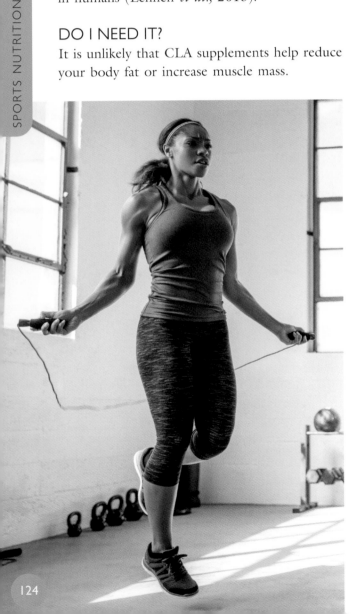

ARE THERE ANY SIDE EFFECTS?
No side effects have been reported to date.

Collagen
WHAT IS IT?
Collagen is the main protein in tendons, bones, ligaments and cartilage, where it provides strength and structure (stiffness). It is made in the body from the amino acids proline, glycine and hydroxyproline. Collagen supplements in the form of gelatine or collagen hydrolysate (collagen that has been broken down into smaller peptides to make it more readily absorbed by the body) are widely available and marketed to athletes.

WHAT DOES IT DO?
It is claimed that collagen supplementation increases the availability of collagen-forming amino acids, increases collagen synthesis in the tissues, and thus prevents or accelerate recovery from musculoskeletal injuries.

WHAT IS THE EVIDENCE?
A joint US-Australian study found that volunteers who took 15 g of vitamin C-enriched gelatine (a food form of collagen) 1 hour before performing 6 minutes of high-intensity exercise (skipping) three times a day for 3 days, had higher levels of collagen-forming amino acids and markers linked to collagen synthesis in their blood during the recovery period (Shaw *et al.*, 2017). The gelatine supplement also improved the mechanics of engineered lab-grown ligaments. However, whether this translates to injury prevention or tissue repair has not been proven.

A further study comparing the effects of various collagen supplements found that vitamin-C enriched gelatine and hydrolysed collagen both raised levels of collagen markers (Lis and Baar, 2019). However, results were very variable, so no firm conclusions can be drawn.

DO I NEED IT?

Research on the benefits of collagen supplements is at an early stage and there is no concrete evidence that they reduce the risk of tendon and ligament injuries nor that they promote faster recovery from injury. There have been no studies to date comparing collagen supplements with other proteins, so it could just be that consuming extra protein may help injury recovery (*see* p. 247).

Colostrum

WHAT IS IT?

Colostrum supplements are derived from bovine colostrum, the milk produced in the first few days after the birth of a calf. It has a high concentration of immune and growth compounds, such as immunoglobulins and antimicrobial proteins.

WHAT DOES IT DO?

It is claimed that bovine colostrum supplements enhance immunity and improve performance, recovery and body composition.

WHAT IS THE EVIDENCE?

It is unclear whether supplements help reduce the suppression of the immune system associated with prolonged intense exercise. Some studies found a reduction in self-reported upper respiratory tract infections (Brinkworth and Buckley, 2003), but others have found no effect (Crooks *et al.*, 2006). University of

Queensland researchers measured an increase in immunoglobulins but no significant difference in incidence of upper respiratory tract infection (URTI) among a group of cyclists during high-intensity training (Shing *et al.*, 2007). A review of studies concluded that daily supplementation with bovine colostrum helps maintain intestinal barrier integrity and immune function and reduces the chances of URTI or URTI symptoms in athletes undertaking heavy training (Davison, 2012). Another review of studies concluded that colostrum supplements may benefit performance and recovery during periods of high-intensity training as a result of increased plasma IGF-1, improved intramuscular buffering capacity, increases in lean body mass and increases in salivary IgA (Shing *et al.*, 2009).

There is inconclusive evidence that colostrum supplements improve performance, strength and power. One study at the University of South Australia suggests that supplements improve anaerobic power after 8 weeks (Buckley *et al.*, 2003), but another study by the same researchers found that supplements had no effect on body composition after 8 weeks of weight training (Brinkworth, 2004).

DO I NEED IT?

While supplements may help boost your immunity during periods of strenuous training, it is not certain whether they will reduce your risk of upper respiratory tract infection. It is unlikely that supplements have any benefit on your athletic performance.

ARE THERE ANY SIDE EFFECTS?

There are no known side effects.

Creatine

WHAT IS IT?

Creatine is a protein that is made naturally in the body from three amino acids (arginine, glycine and methionine), but can also be found in meat and fish or taken in higher doses as a supplement. It is most commonly available as creatine monohydrate, but it is often an ingredient in 'all-in-one' meal replacement drinks and supplement 'stacks'.

WHAT DOES IT DO?

Creatine combines with phosphorus to form phosphocreatine (PC) in your muscle cells. This is an energy-rich compound that fuels your muscles during high-intensity activities, such as lifting weights or sprinting. Creatine supplementation raises PC levels typically around 2% (Hultman *et al.*, 1996). This enables you to sustain all-out effort longer than usual and recover faster between sets, leading to greater training adaptations. Creatine supplements also help promote protein manufacture and muscle hypertrophy (by drawing water into the cells), increasing lean body mass; reduce muscle acidity (it buffers excess hydrogen ions), thus allowing more lactic acid to be produced before fatigue sets in; and reduce muscle protein breakdown following intense exercise, resulting in greater strength and improved ability to do repeated sets. Additionally, creatine may enhance post-exercise recovery, injury prevention, thermoregulation, rehabilitation and recovery from concussion.

WHAT IS THE EVIDENCE?

Hundreds of studies have measured the effects of creatine supplements on anaerobic performance

How does creatine work?

The observed gains in weight are due partly to an increase in cell volume and partly to muscle synthesis. Creatine causes water to move across cell membranes. When muscle cell creatine concentration goes up, water is drawn into the cell, an effect that boosts the thickness of muscle fibres by around 15%. The water content of muscle fibres stretches the cells' outer sheaths – a mechanical force that can trigger anabolic reactions. This may stimulate protein synthesis and result in increased lean tissue (Haussinger *et al.*, 1996).

Creatine may have a direct effect on protein synthesis. In studies at the University of Memphis, athletes taking creatine gained more body mass than those taking the placebo, yet both groups ended up with the same body water content (Kreider *et al.*, 1996; Clark, 1997).

and the majority have proven it to be an effective aid for increasing strength and muscle mass as well as enhancing performance in high-intensity activities (Gualano *et al.*, 2012). The greatest improvements are found in high power output efforts repeated for a number of bouts.

The International Society of Sports Nutrition (ISSN) describes creatine as 'the most effective ergogenic nutritional supplement currently available to athletes in terms of increasing high-intensity exercise capacity and lean body mass during training' (Kreider *et al.*, 2017). A review of 22 studies concluded that creatine supplementation increases maximum strength (i.e. 1 rep maximum)

What is the best form of creatine?

Creatine monohydrate is the most extensively studied and widely available form of creatine. It is a white powder that dissolves readily in water and is virtually tasteless. It is the most concentrated form available commercially and the least expensive. Creatine monohydrate comprises a molecule of creatine with a molecule of water attached to it so it is more stable.

Although other forms of creatine such as creatine serum, creatine citrate and creatine phosphate are available, there is no evidence that they are better absorbed, produce higher levels of phosphocreatine in the muscle cells or result in greater increases in performance or muscle mass (Jäger et al., 2011).

Will I lose strength when I stop taking creatine supplements?

When you stop taking supplements, elevated muscle creatine stores will drop very slowly to normal levels over a period of 4 weeks (Greenhaff, 1997). During supplementation, your body's own synthesis of creatine is depressed but this is reversible. In other words, you automatically step up creatine manufacture once you stop supplementation. Certainly, fears that your body permanently shuts down normal creatine manufacture are unfounded. You may experience weight loss and there are anecdotal reports about athletes experiencing small reductions in strength and power, although not back to pre-supplementation levels.

It has been proposed that creatine is best taken in cycles, such as 3–5 months followed by a 1-month break.

by an average 8% as well as endurance strength, i.e. maximum reps at a submaximal load, by 14% (Cooper et al., 2012; Rawson and Volek, 2003). Another review found that 70% of creatine studies showed a positive effect on performance, and 30% showed no effect (Kreider, 2003(b)).

Creatine supplementation results in lean mass and total mass gains of typically 1–3% lean body weight (approx. 0.8–3 kg) after a 5-day loading dose, compared with controls – although not all studies show positive results (Buford et al., 2007). The observed gains in weight are due partly to an increase in cell fluid volume (i.e. water weight) and partly to muscle synthesis.

Creatine appears to enhance performance in both men and women. Researchers at McMaster University, Ontario, gave 12 male and 12 female volunteers either creatine supplements or a placebo before a high-intensity sprint cycling test (Tarnopolsky and MacLennan, 2000). Creatine improved performance equally in both sexes.

Researchers at the Australian Institute of Sport found that creatine improved sprint times and agility run times in football players (Cox et al., 2002). A study in former Yugoslavia found that creatine supplementation improved sprint power, dribbling and vertical jump performance in young football players, but had no effect on endurance (Ostojic, 2004).

If creatine improves the quality of resistance training over time, this would increase adaptation and lead to faster gains in mass, strength and power. The vast majority of studies indeed show that short-term creatine supplementation increases body mass.

There is less evidence for the use of creatine with aerobic-based sports – only a few laboratory studies have shown an improvement in performance. This is probably due to the fact that the PC energy system is less important during endurance activities. However, it can increase performance in endurance events that include high-intensity efforts, such as road cycling. One study at Louisiana State University suggests creatine supplements may be able to boost athletes' lactate threshold and therefore prove beneficial for certain aerobic-based sports (Nelson *et al.*, 1997).

DO I NEED IT?

If you train with weights or do any sport that includes repeated high-intensity movements, such as sprints, jumps or throws (as in, say, rugby and football) for bouts of up to 30 seconds, creatine supplements may help increase your performance, strength and muscle mass. It may also enhance endurance activities that include high-intensity bouts of 30–150 seconds. Sports events that may benefit from creatine supplementation include track sprints (60–200 m), swim sprints (50 m), pursuit cycling, basketball, hockey, track events (400, 800 m), swim events (100–200 m), combat sports, rowing, canoeing, interval training in endurance athletes, bodybuilding, American Football, rugby, powerlifting, track/field events and weightlifting (Kreider *et al.*, 2017).

In some people (approx. two out of every 10), muscle creatine concentrations increase only very slightly. It may be partly due to differences in muscle fibre types. Fast-twitch (FT) fibres tend to build up higher concentrations of creatine than slow-twitch (ST) fibres. This means that athletes with a naturally low FT fibre composition may experience smaller gains from creatine supplements. Taking creatine with carbohydrate may help solve the problem as carbohydrate raises insulin, which, in turn, helps creatine uptake by muscle cells.

HOW MUCH CREATINE?

The quickest method of increasing muscle creatine stores is to consume 0.3 g/kg BW/day of creatine monohydrate for 5–7 days, followed by 3–5 g/day thereafter to maintain elevated stores. A popular creatine-loading protocol is 4 x 5–7 g doses per day over a period of 5 days, i.e. 20–25 g daily.

Other protocols involve smaller doses of creatine monohydrate (e.g. 3–5 g/day) for a 3–4 week period (Hultman *et al.*, 1996) or 6 daily doses of 0.5–1 g (i.e. 6 x 1 g doses) with food to increase the absorption rate (Harris, 1998). According to a Canadian study, relatively low doses of creatine supplementation can significantly improve weight training performance to the same extent as higher doses (Burke *et al.*, 2000).

Studies have shown that insulin helps shunt creatine faster into the muscle cells (Green *et al.*, 1996; Steenge *et al.*, 1998). Taking creatine along with carbohydrate – which stimulates insulin release – will increase the uptake of creatine by the muscle cells and raise levels of PC. The exact amount of carbohydrate needed to produce an insulin spike is debatable but estimates range from 35 g to around 100 g.

Creatine uptake is also greater immediately after exercise, so adding creatine to the post-exercise meal will help to boost muscle creatine levels.

ARE THERE ANY SIDE EFFECTS?

Creatine appears to be safe in both the short and long term. The only side effect is weight gain. This is due partly to extra water in the muscle cells and partly to increased muscle tissue. While this is desirable for bodybuilders and people who work out with weights, it could be disadvantageous in sports where there is a critical ratio of body weight and speed (e.g. running) or in weight-category sports. In swimmers, a heavier body weight may cause more drag and reduce swim efficiency. It's a matter of weighing up the potential advantage of increased maximal power and/or lean mass against the possible disadvantage of increased weight.

There have been anecdotal reports about muscle cramping, gastrointestinal discomfort, hypohydration, muscle injury, and kidney and muscle damage. However, there is no clinical data to support these statements (Lugares *et al.,* 2013; Williams *et al.,* 1999; Robinson *et al.,* 2000; Mihic *et al.,* 2000; Kreider, 2000; Greenwood *et al.,* 2003; Mayhew *et al.,* 2002; Poortmans and Francaux, 1999).

Energy bars

WHAT ARE THEY?

Energy bars consist mainly of sugar and maltodextrin, and provide around 250 calories and 25–35 g of carbohydrate/bar. Some may also have added vitamins and minerals, cereals or soya flour to boost the nutritional content.

WHAT DO THEY DO?

Energy bars provide a convenient way of consuming carbohydrate before, during or after intense exercise lasting more than 1 hour.

WHAT IS THE EVIDENCE?

An Australian study compared an energy bar (plus water) with a sports drink during exercise; it was found that both boosted blood sugar levels and endurance equally (Mason *et al.,* 1993).

In a study at the University of Texas, cyclists were given either a sports drink (containing 10% carbohydrate), an energy bar with water, or a placebo (Yaspelkis *et al.,* 1993). Those who consumed some form of carbohydrate managed to keep going 21 minutes 30 seconds longer before reaching exhaustion than those taking a placebo. The reason? The extra carbohydrate helped fuel the cyclists' muscles, reducing the dependency on glycogen. After 3 hours in the saddle, the cyclists sipping the sports drink or eating food had 35% more glycogen than those who had no carbohydrate.

DO I NEED THEM?

Any form of high-GI carbohydrate will help improve your endurance during high-intensity exercise lasting longer than 1 hour. Whether you consume carbohydrate in the form of an energy bar, drink or any other form during exercise is down to personal preference. The main benefit of energy bars is their convenience: they are easy to carry and eat! Make sure that you have your bar with enough water to replace fluids lost in sweat as well as to digest the bar. They are an acquired taste and texture, and you may need to experiment with different flavours and brands.

ARE THERE ANY SIDE EFFECTS?

If you don't consume enough water, they may cause gastrointestinal discomfort. Some products may adhere to your teeth, so ensure you rinse with water.

Energy gels

WHAT ARE THEY?

Energy gels come in small squeezy sachets and have a jelly-like texture. They consist of simple sugars (such as fructose and glucose) and maltodextrin (a carbohydrate derived from corn starch, consisting of 4–20 glucose units). They may also contain sodium, potassium and caffeine. Most brands contain between 18 and 25 g of carbohydrate per sachet.

WHAT DO THEY DO?

Gels provide a concentrated source of calories and carbohydrate that can be rapidly digested and absorbed, and are designed to be consumed during endurance exercise.

WHAT IS THE EVIDENCE?

Studies show that consuming 30–60 g of carbohydrate per hour during prolonged exercise delays fatigue and improves endurance. This translates into 1–2 sachets per hour, depending on the brand. A 2007 study from Napier University, Edinburgh, showed that gels have a similar effect on blood sugar levels and performance as sports drinks (Patterson and Gray, 2007). Soccer players who consumed an energy gel (with water) immediately before and during high-intensity interval training increased their endurance by 45% compared with a placebo.

DO I NEED THEM?

Energy gels provide a convenient way of consuming carbohydrate during intense endurance exercise lasting longer than 1 hour. Some brands are highly concentrated in carbohydrate (hypertonic) so you will need to consume plenty of water with them to avoid gastrointestinal problems, such as bloating, discomfort and nausea. However, there are isotonic brands available, which are designed to be consumed without water. On the downside, some people dislike their texture, sweetness and intensity of flavour – it's really down to personal preference – and they don't do away with the need for carrying a water bottle with you.

ARE THERE ANY SIDE EFFECTS?

Some formulations are very concentrated in sugar, which drags water from your bloodstream into your stomach, increasing the risk of stomach discomfort.

Ephedrine/ma huang/ 'fat burners'/thermogenic supplements (prohibited by WADA)

WHAT ARE THEY?

The main ingredient in 'fat burners' or thermogenics is ephedrine, a synthetic version of the Chinese herb ephedra or ma huang. Ephedrine is, in fact, a drug rather than a nutritional supplement and is prohibited by WADA. It is also used at low concentrations in cold and flu remedies (pseudoephedrine).

WHAT DOES IT DO?

Ephedrine is chemically similar to amphetamines, which act on the brain and the central nervous system. Athletes may use it – albeit illegally –

because it increases arousal, physical activity and the potential for neuromuscular performance. It is often combined with caffeine, which enhances the effects of ephedrine.

WHAT IS THE EVIDENCE?

Ephedrine is a stimulant. However, research studies generally show it has little effect on strength and endurance. This is probably because relatively low doses were used. What is more likely is that these products have a 'speed-like' effect; they make you feel more awake and alert, more motivated to train hard and more confident.

There is some evidence that ephedrine helps fat loss: partly due to an increase in thermogenesis (heat production), partly because it suppresses your appetite and partly because it makes you more active.

DO I NEED IT?

It is an addictive drug and I would strongly recommend avoiding any fat-burner containing ephedrine or ma huang because of the significant health risks. It is banned by WADA, whether in cold remedies or in supplements. Exercise and good nutrition are the safest methods for burning fat.

ARE THERE ANY SIDE EFFECTS?

Ephedrine is judged to be safe in doses containing around 18–25 mg; that's the amount used in decongestants and cold remedies. Taking too much can have serious side effects. These include increased heart rate, increased blood pressure, palpitations, anxiety, nervousness, insomnia, nausea, vomiting and dizziness. Very high doses (around 3000 mg) cause heart attacks and can even be fatal. Caffeine–ephedrine stacks produce adverse effects at even lower doses. A case of a sportsman who suffered an extensive stroke after taking high doses of 'energy pills' (caffeine–ephedrine) has been reported in the *Journal of Neurology, Neurosurgery and Psychiatry* (Vahedi, 2000).

In 2002, the American Medical Association called for a ban on ephedrine due to concerns over its side effects. Since 1997 the FDA in the US has documented at least 70 deaths and more than 1400 'adverse effects' involving supplements containing ephedrine. These included heart attacks, strokes and seizures. Ephedrine's risks far outweigh its potential benefits. It is addictive and people can develop a tolerance to it (you need to keep taking more and more to get the same effects).

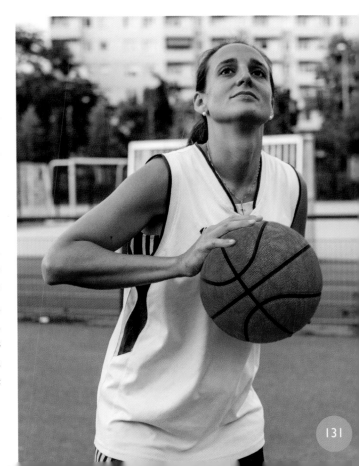

Fat burners (ephedrine-free)

WHAT ARE THEY?

Certain fat-burning and weight loss supplements claim to mimic the effects of ephedrine, boost the metabolism and enhance fat loss but without harmful side effects. The main ingredients in these products include *citrus aurantium* (synephrine or bitter orange extract); green tea extract and *Coleus forskohlii* extract (a herb, similar to mint).

WHAT DO THEY DO?

Citrus aurantium is a weak stimulant, chemically similar to ephedrine and caffeine. It contains a compound called synephrine which, according to manufacturers, reduces appetite, increases the metabolic rate and promotes fat burning. However, despite the hype, there is no sound scientific evidence to back up the weight loss claims.

The active constituents in green tea are a family of polyphenols called catechins (the main type is epigallocatechin gallate, EGCG) and flavanols, which possess potent antioxidant activity. The theory behind *Coleus forskohlii* as a dietary supplement is that its content of forskolin can be used to stimulate adenyl cyclase activity, which will increase cAMP (cyclic adenosine monophosphate) levels in the fat cell, which will in turn activate another enzyme (hormone sensitive lipase) to start breaking down fat stores.

WHAT IS THE EVIDENCE?

Despite the hype, there is no sound scientific evidence to back up the weight loss claims of fat burners. The only ingredient that may have some value is green tea extract, although the research is inconclusive (Hodgson *et al.*, 2013(b); Dulloo *et al.*, 1999).

DO I NEED THEM?

The research on ephedrine-free fat burners is not robust and any fat-burning boost they provide would be relatively small or none. The doses used in some brands may be too small to provide a measurable effect. A reduced calorie intake and exercise are likely to produce better weight loss results in the long term. While synephrine is not currently banned by WADA, it may be converted into norepinephrine (octopamine) in the body, which is prohibited during competition, and therefore is best avoided. The only positive data is for green tea, but you would need to drink at least six cups daily (equivalent to 100–300 mg EGCG) to achieve a significant fat-burning effect.

ARE THERE ANY SIDE EFFECTS?

While the herbal alternatives to ephedrine are generally safer, you may get side effects with high doses. *Citrus aurantium* can increase blood pressure as much, if not more, than ephedrine. High doses of forskolin may cause heart disturbances.

Glutamine

WHAT IS IT?

Glutamine is a non-essential amino acid. It can be made in the muscle cells from other amino acids (glutamic acid, valine and isoleucine) and is the most abundant free amino acid in muscle cells. It is essential for cell growth and a critical source of energy for immune cells called lymphocytes. Many protein and meal replacement supplements contain glutamine.

WHAT DOES IT DO?

Glutamine is needed for cell growth, as well as serving as a fuel for the immune system. During periods of heavy training or stress, blood levels of glutamine fall, weakening your immune system and putting you at risk of infection. Muscle levels of glutamine also fall, which results in a loss of muscle tissue, despite continued training. Supplementation during intense training periods is thought to help offset the drop in glutamine, boost immunity, reduce the risk of overtraining syndrome and prevent upper respiratory tract infections.

Manufacturers claim that glutamine has a protein-sparing effect during intense training. This is based on the theory that glutamine helps draw water into the muscle cells, increasing the cell volume. This inhibits enzymes from breaking down muscle proteins and also counteracts the effects of stress hormones (such as cortisol), which are increased after intense exercise.

WHAT IS THE EVIDENCE?

The evidence for glutamine is divided. Some studies have suggested that supplements may reduce the risk of infection and promote muscle growth (Parry-Billings *et al.*, 1992; Rowbottom *et al.*, 1996). Researchers at Oxford University have shown that glutamine supplements taken immediately after running and again 2 hours later appeared to lower the risk of infection and boost immune cell activity in marathon runners (Castell and Newsholme, 1997). Only 19% of those taking glutamine became ill during the week following the run while 51% of those taking a placebo became ill. However, not all studies have managed to replicate these findings. A more recent review of studies concluded that while many athletes take glutamine supplements to protect against exercise-related impairment of the immune system, supplements do not prevent post-exercise changes in immune function or reduce the risk of infection (Gleeson, 2008).

Glutamine does not improve performance, body composition or muscle breakdown (Haub, 1998). According to a Canadian study, glutamine produces no increase in strength or muscle mass compared with a placebo (Candow *et al.*, 2001). After 6 weeks of weight training, those taking glutamine achieved the same gains in strength and muscle mass as those taking a placebo.

DO I NEED IT?

The case for glutamine is not clear. It is unlikely to prevent immune-suppression or improve body composition or performance.

ARE THERE ANY SIDE EFFECTS?

No side effects have been found so far.

HMB

WHAT IS IT?

HMB (beta-hydroxy beta-methylbutyrate) is made in the body from the BCAA leucine. You can also obtain it from foods such as grapefruit, alfalfa and catfish.

WHAT DOES IT DO?

No one knows exactly how HMB works, but it is thought to be involved in cellular repair. HMB is a precursor to an important component of cell membranes that helps with growth and repair of muscle tissue. HMB supplements claim to protect muscles from excessive breakdown during exercise, accelerate repair and build muscle.

WHAT IS THE EVIDENCE?

A meta-analysis of studies by Canadian researchers found no robust evidence to support the claims for HMB supplementation (Jakubowki *et al.*, 2020).

They concluded that HMB does not increase muscle mass, size or strength, and has no effect on fat loss. It appears to have little effect in experienced athletes (Kreider *et al.*, 2000). One study at the Australian Institute of Sport failed to find strength or mass improvements in 22 athletes taking 3 g per day for 6 weeks (Slater *et al.*, 2001). Researchers at the University of Queensland in Australia found no beneficial effect on reducing muscle damage or muscle soreness following resistance exercise (Paddon-Jones *et al.*, 2001).

These findings are in contrast to those of a previous review published by the International Society of Sports Nutrition, which concluded that HMB promotes recovery, reduces exercise-induced muscle breakdown and damage, promotes muscle repair, and increases muscle mass (Wilson *et al.*, 2013). However, this review relates to older studies, which used flawed methodology.

DO I NEED IT?

Overall, there is little evidence to support the use of HMB to improve body composition.

Consuming sufficient calories, protein, carbohydrate and fat in conjunction with consistent resistance training is likely to produce better results. No long-term studies have been carried out to date and, in any case, it is unlikely to benefit more experienced athletes.

ARE THERE ANY SIDE EFFECTS?

No side effects have yet been found.

Hydrogel energy drinks

WHAT ARE THEY?

Hydrogel energy drinks contain carbohydrates (maltodextrin and fructose) mixed with two gelling agents: alginate (which is extracted from algae) and pectin (which is found in fruit). They are available in powdered form that can be mixed with water to produce a drink with a concentration of approximately 150 g carbohydrate/litre.

WHAT DO THEY DO?

Hydrogel drinks purport to increase the rate of stomach emptying during exercise, enhance carbohydrate absorption, reduce the incidence and severity of GI symptoms (e.g. nausea, bloating and diarrhoea) and allow carbohydrate delivery in concentrations that greatly exceed what can typically be tolerated using commercially available sports drinks (Sutehall *et al.*, 2020).

Manufacturers claim that the alginate and pectin in the drinks encapsulates the carbohydrate in the drink once it enters the acid environment of the stomach, forming a hydrogel. This prevents carbohydrate triggering the glucose receptors in the stomach wall, which would normally slow stomach emptying and cause discomfort during intense exercise. By emptying from the stomach more rapidly, hydrogel drinks can be absorbed from the intestines more rapidly than other drinks containing an equivalent concentration of carbohydrate.

WHAT IS THE EVIDENCE?

A study at Monash University, Australia compared the effects of a hydrogel drink and a sports drink containing the same amount of carbohydrate in nine runners during 3 hours of running (McCubbin *et al.*, 2020). They found no difference in blood glucose levels, carbohydrate oxidation, GI symptoms or performance between the two drinks, suggesting that the hydrogel drink conferred no benefit. Similarly, University of Loughborough researchers showed no significant difference in performance or GI symptoms in cyclists consuming 68 g carbohydrate/hour either from hydrogel drinks or sports drinks (Mears *et al.*, 2020). Another UK study compared a hydrogel drink with a sports drink during cycling under hot, humid conditions and, again, showed no difference in performance, GI symptoms or gut barrier function (Flood *et al.*, 2020).

DO I NEED THEM?

While the theory behind hydrogel drinks sounds compelling, there is no evidence to back the claims made by manufacturers. To date, no study has shown any performance benefit or improvement in GI symptoms from consuming hydrogel drinks over and above a carbohydrate sports drink. Therefore, there is no valid reason to use hydrogels instead of sports drinks containing multiple carbohydrates. However, research until now has been carried out on non-elite athletes undertaking moderate-intensity exercise. Future research is required to find out whether hydrogel drinks may benefit elite athletes undertaking high-intensity prolonged events.

ARE THERE ANY SIDE EFFECTS?

No side effects have been documented.

Ketones

WHAT ARE THEY?

Ketones include D-β-hydroxybutyrate, acetone and acetoacetate, which are made in the liver from fatty acids. They can be used as an energy source by muscles and organs during periods of starvation or when glycogen levels are low, such as during a ketogenic (very low-carbohydrate, high-fat) diet or prolonged exercise. Supplements are available in the form of ketone esters (which are chemically similar to the ketones your body makes) and ketone salts (which are not).

WHAT DO THEY DO?

Ketone esters raise blood ketone levels more effectively than ketone salts. They are purported to enhance endurance performance by encouraging the muscles to burn fat instead of carbohydrate, thus sparing muscle glycogen. Manufacturers also claim that they aid glycogen resynthesis after endurance exercise.

WHAT IS THE EVIDENCE?

To date, only one study has shown positive effects of ketone esters. It revealed that ketone esters enabled cyclists to ride an average of 2% further in a 30-minute time-trial carried out in a laboratory (Cox *et al.*, 2016). However, subsequent studies under conditions simulating real-life competition have not found any beneficial effect on performance. A 2017 study carried out by Australian researchers showed that performance was, in fact, impaired in high-performance cyclists completing a time-trial lasting approximately 50 minutes (Leckey *et al.*, 2017). Similarly, a study by Irish researchers found no benefit of ketone esters on 10 km running performance (Evans *et al.*, 2019). More recently, Belgian researchers showed that ketone ester supplementation during a simulated cycling race did not cause glycogen sparing nor did it affect all-out performance in the final stage of the race (Poffé *et al.*, 2020). There is no evidence to support the claims for ketone salts.

DO I NEED THEM?

While the claims for ketone ester supplements are compelling, there is no evidence to date that they enhance endurance under real-life conditions. In fact, they have no discernable advantages over carbohydrate supplements and drinks. As ketone esters are expensive and are associated with potential side effects (*see* below), you would be wise to save your money until more robust evidence is found. There is no evidence to support the claims for ketone salts.

ARE THERE ANY SIDE EFFECTS?

Side effects include gut discomfort and higher perception of effort. Ketone ester drinks also have a strong, unpleasant taste.

Leucine

WHAT IS IT?

Leucine is an essential amino acid, and the most abundant of the three branched-chain amino acids (BCAAs) in muscles (the other two are isoleucine and valine).

WHAT DOES IT DO?

Leucine is an important trigger for protein synthesis. It acts as a signal to the muscle cells to make new muscle proteins, activating a compound called mammalian target of rapamycin complex 1 (mTORC1), a molecular switch that turns on the machinery that manufactures muscle proteins.

WHAT IS THE EVIDENCE?

Research suggests that leucine can stimulate protein synthesis (when consumed after exercise) and reduce protein breakdown (when consumed before exercise). In a study at Maastricht University, athletes who consumed a leucine/carbohydrate/protein drink after resis-

tance training had less muscle protein breakdown and greater muscle protein synthesis than those who consumed a supplement without leucine (Koopman *et al.*, 2005). Similarly, another study found that consuming a leucine-enriched protein drink during endurance exercise resulted in less muscle breakdown and greater muscle synthesis (Pasiakos *et al.*, 2011). A study with canoeists found that 6 weeks of leucine supplementation improved endurance performance and upper body power (Crowe *et al.*, 2006). However, there is no benefit to taking extra leucine if you consume protein (as food or drink) before or after exercise. Researchers found that consuming more than 1.8 g leucine does not produce any additional benefit (Pasiakos and McClung, 2011).

DO I NEED IT?

Getting sufficient leucine is particularly important for those wanting to build strength and muscle mass. However, it isn't necessary to get

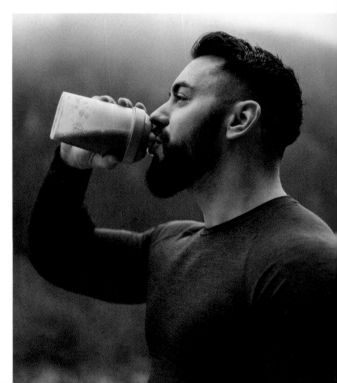

leucine in the form of supplements. It is found widely in foods, the best sources being eggs, dairy products, meat, fish and poultry. It is also found in high concentrations in whey protein. You'll need around 3 g leucine to get maximum muscle-building benefits; that's the amount found in approximately 20 g of protein from an animal protein source (*see* p. 66).

ARE THERE ANY SIDE EFFECTS?

There are no reported side effects.

Omega-3 fatty acids

WHAT ARE THEY?

Omega-3 fatty acids include alpha-linolenic acid (ALA), eicosapentaenoic acid (EPA) and docosahexaenoic acid (DHA). Supplements may be derived from the tissues of oily, cold-water fish such as tuna, cod (liver) and salmon. Vegan and vegetarian supplements contain omega-3s derived from algae.

WHAT DO THEY DO?

The main health benefit linked with omega-3s is improved cardiovascular health (*see* p. 88).

Omega-3 fatty acids form part of the structure of cell membranes and have potent anti-inflammatory properties. It is purported that supplementation may reduce inflammation in the body, including post-exercise muscle soreness, and improve muscle adaptation and recovery.

WHAT IS THE EVIDENCE?

Omega-3 supplementation in conjunction with exercise may have a number of benefits. These include improved endurance, muscle adaptation, energy metabolism, muscle recovery and injury prevention (Philpott *et al.*, 2019; Lewis *et al.*, 2020). They may also reduce the oxygen cost of exercise, although the benefits in terms of endurance have not been proven (Kawabata *et al.*, 2014; Watt *et al.*, 2002; Hingley *et al.*, 2017).

In contrast, studies have failed to show that omega-3 supplements enhance muscle growth following resistance training. Researchers at the University of Stirling found that supplements (in conjunction with protein supplementation) made no significant difference to MPS following an 8-week resistance training programme (McGlory *et al.*, 2016).

There is growing evidence that omega-3 supplements may promote muscle recovery. One study found that women who consumed 3 g/day of DHA for 7 days experienced less muscle soreness and stiffness following eccentric exercise compared with a placebo (Corder *et al.*, 2016). A study with soccer players showed that omega-3 supplementation reduced muscle damage and muscle soreness in the 72 hours following muscle-damaging exercise (Philpott *et al.*, 2018).

Omega-3s also appear to play a key role in immune function. Researchers found 3 g fish oil supplementation for 60 days before a marathon prevented a drop in immune function induced by the race, although the researchers did not measure whether this led to a reduced incidence of colds or infection (Santos *et al.*, 2013).

DO I NEED THEM?

Omega-3 supplements appear to have a number of benefits for athletes, including reduced muscle damage after eccentric exercise, enhanced muscle recovery and reduced muscle soreness. If you don't eat oily fish regularly, supplements are a good option for ensuring adequate omega-3 intake. The UK government recommends a minimum intake of 450 mg EPA and DHA per day, which can also be met with two portions of fish per week (including one oily). The Academy of Nutrition and Dietetics and Dietitians of Canada recommends 500 mg EPA + DPA per day; the European Food Safety Authority recommends 250 mg EPA + DPA per day (European Food Safety Authority, 2009).

ARE THERE ANY SIDE EFFECTS?
Very high doses (more than 3 g/day) may increase the risk of bleeding. This is due to the ability of omega-3s to break down blood clots.

Polyphenols
WHAT ARE THEY?
Polyphenols are plant chemicals that give fruits and vegetables their distinctive tastes and colours (as well as helping them fight off disease). A number of polyphenol supplements are marketed to athletes, including curcumin (from turmeric), resveratrol (from grapes), cocoa flavanols, quercetin (from apples and onions), green tea extracts, blueberry, pomegranate and blackcurrant extracts, and Montmorency cherry juice concentrate (*see* pp. 122–3).

WHAT DO THEY DO?
Polyphenols act as powerful vasodilators and may therefore improve performance by increasing peripheral blood flow and oxygen delivery to the muscles during exercise (Kay *et al.*, 2012). They also have potent antioxidant properties and anti-inflammatory effects.

Polyphenols also provide 'food' for the gut microbiota, thereby promoting the growth of beneficial bacteria (e.g. *Akkermansia*, *Lactobacilli* and *Bifidobacteria*). These bacteria break down polyphenols to produce compounds that indirectly enhance performance and recovery (*see* p. 232) (Sorrenti *et al.*, 2020).

WHAT IS THE EVIDENCE?
Supplements providing around 300 mg polyphenols taken either shortly before or for several days before exercise have been shown to enhance exercise capacity and performance during endurance and repeated sprint exercise (Bowtell and Kelly, 2019). For example, one study showed that trained cyclists experienced modest improvements in end-sprint performance 1½ hours after consuming Montmorency cherry concentrate (Keane *et al.*, 2018). Another study showed that 7 days of blackcurrant supplementation improved 16.1 km cycling time-trial performance by an average of 2.4% (Cook *et al.*, 2015). These benefits have been attributed to the potent antioxidant properties of polyphenols as well as their ability to dilate blood vessels and increase oxygen delivery.

There is also evidence that supplements providing >1000 mg polyphenols for three or more days prior to and following exercise can accelerate recovery following exercise-induced muscle damage (Bowtell and Kelly, 2019). This has been demonstrated with Montmorency cherry juice concentrate (*see* pp. 122–3), and pomegranate juice (250 ml consumed twice a day for 7 days prior to and after exercise) (Trombold *et al.*, 2011). Similarly, blueberry supplementation in the form of a smoothie consumed 5 and 10 hours prior to and then for 2 days after eccentric exercise accelerated recovery in recreationally active women (McLeay *et al.*, 2012). These benefits are thought to be due to the ability of polyphenols to suppress inflammation (Mizumura and Taguchi, 2016).

DO I NEED IT?

To date, only a few studies have been carried out with polyphenols, so it is difficult to make firm recommendations. However, the results are positive and suggest that supplementing with around 300 mg polyphenols 1 hour before high-intensity exercise may be ergogenic. There is a larger body of evidence to support the use of polyphenols for recovery after intensive exercise. This suggests that supplementing with >1000 mg polyphenols per day for 3 or more days prior to and following exercise may help reduce muscle soreness and reduce recovery times. You can also get this amount from 450 g blueberries, 120 g blackcurrants or 300 g Montmorency cherries. The benefits are likely to be greater after events that induce muscle damage, such as heavy resistance training and for competitions that involve successive matches or rounds with short recovery periods.

ARE THERE ANY SIDE EFFECTS?

No side effects have been reported to date.

Probiotics

WHAT ARE THEY?

Probiotics are potentially beneficial bacteria. They are defined as live microorganisms that, when taken in adequate amounts, confer a health benefit to the host. They occur naturally in some fermented foods, including yoghurt, cheese, sauerkraut, kefir, tempeh, kombucha and sourdough bread. They can also be taken as a supplement in the form of capsules, tablets, powders and liquids. The main commercially used species are *Lactobacillus acidophilus* and *Bifidobacterium bifidum* cultures.

WHAT DO THEY DO?

Probiotic supplements work by increasing the number of beneficial bacteria in the large intestine and crowding out potentially harmful bacteria. They also help digest the components of food that can't be digested by enzymes in the small intestine, such as fibre and resistant starch. They produce beneficial substances such as short chain fatty acids that fuel our gut cells, helping strengthen the gut barrier that prevents disease-causing microorganisms getting into the bloodstream. They also produce substances that kill harmful bacteria, called bacteriocins, and help prime the immune system so our immune cells are able to attack pathogens.

Hard training, psychological stress, disturbed sleep and environmental extremes can all put a significant strain on an athlete's immune system, increasing the risk of catching infections such as upper respiratory tract infections (URI). Taking probiotics may therefore help strengthen the immune system and increase resilience to gastrointestinal and upper respiratory tract infections.

WHAT'S THE EVIDENCE?

A position statement by the International Society of Sports Nutrition concluded that probiotic supplementation may benefit immune function, gastrointestinal function, nutrient absorption, recovery and performance (Jäger *et al.*, 2019). Studies examining probiotic supplementation in athletes indicate that it reduces the incidence, severity and/or duration of URI in athletes, and may also reduce gastrointestinal illness often associated with longer bouts of training (Jäger *et al.*, 2019; Pyne *et al.*, 2015; King *et al.*, 2014; Hao *et al.*, 2015; Gleeson, 2008).

For example, a study carried out by researchers at the Australian Institute of Sport found that probiotic supplementation can dramatically cut the risk and duration of URIs in elite long-distance runners (Cox *et al.*, 2008). Those taking probiotic supplements experienced symptoms for 30 days during 4 months of intensive training compared with 72 days in the placebo group, and the severity of symptoms was less. This was attributed to higher levels of interferon (immune cells that fight viruses). In a follow-up study with competitive cyclists, 11 weeks of probiotic supplementation reduced the severity and duration of lower respiratory illness by 30% compared with a placebo (West *et al.*, 2011). There was also a reduction in the severity of gastrointestinal symptoms and athletes used cold and flu medication less frequently.

A review of 12 randomised controlled trials concluded that probiotics may reduce the incidence of URIs by 47% and the duration of illness by nearly 2 days (Hao *et al.*, 2015).

Research suggests that probiotics may also help alleviate gut problems during marathon running (Pugh *et al.*, 2019). Those who took a probiotic supplement for 28 days before a marathon experienced fewer and less severe gut symptoms in the latter stages of racing compared with those who did not take supplements. However, there was no difference in performance between groups. Those runners supplementing with probiotics also demonstrated less of a performance decrement (as evidenced by maintaining running speed) towards the end of the race.

DO I NEED THEM?

While probiotics can be useful in some situations – such as after finishing a course of antibiotics or during periods of increased URI risk such as in the weeks before and during international travel and major competition – they shouldn't replace a balanced diet rich in fruits, vegetables and fermented foods. If taking them before a major competition, start at least 14 days beforehand to allow enough time for the probiotics to colonise your gut. Probiotics are most effective in tablet or capsule form and should contain 1 billion to 10 billion viable organisms in order to survive the journey through the digestive tract. Probiotics found in food, especially liquid or semi-solid ones such as milk or yoghurt, usually need refrigeration to keep them safe.

ARE THERE ANY SIDE EFFECTS?

No adverse health effects have been reported.

Protein supplements

WHAT ARE THEY?

Protein supplements can be divided into three main categories: 1) protein powders (which you mix with milk or water into a shake); 2) ready-to-drink shakes; and 3) high-protein bars. They may contain whey protein, casein, egg, soya or other non-dairy sources (e.g. pea, brown rice and hemp protein) or a mixture of these.

WHAT DO THEY DO?

They provide a concentrated source of protein to supplement your usual food intake. Whey protein is derived from milk and contains high levels of the essential amino acids, which are readily digested, absorbed and retained by the

Whey vs. casein supplements

Most of the research on whey vs. casein shows there is no difference in muscle mass and strength gains between those taking whey or casein proteins (Dangin et al., 2001; Kreider, 2003(a); Brown et al., 2004), although some studies have suggested that whey produces greater gains in strength and muscle mass compared with casein (Cribb et al., 2006).

Whey protein, the most popular protein ingredient, is derived from milk using either a process called micro-filtration (the whey proteins are physically extracted by a microscopic filter) or by ion-exchange (the whey proteins are extracted by taking advantage of their electrical charges). It has a higher biological value (BV) than milk (and other protein sources) and is digested and absorbed relatively rapidly, making it useful for promoting post-exercise recovery. It has a higher concentration of essential amino acids (around 50%) than whole milk, about half of which are BCAAs (23–25%), which may help minimise muscle protein breakdown during and immediately after high-intensity exercise. Research at McGill University in Canada suggests that the amino acids in whey protein also stimulate glutathione production in the body (Bounous and Gold, 1991). Glutathione is a powerful antioxidant and also helps support the immune system. This is particularly useful during periods of intense training, when the immune system is suppressed. Whey protein may also help to stimulate muscle growth by increasing insulin-like growth factor-1 (IGF-1) production – a powerful anabolic hormone made in the liver that enhances protein manufacture in muscles.

Casein, also derived from milk, comprises larger protein molecules, which are digested and absorbed more slowly than whey. It also has a high BV and a high content of the amino acid glutamine (around 20%) – a high glutamine intake may help spare muscle mass during intense exercise and prevent exercise-induced suppression of the immune system. As casein is a 'slow-acting' protein, it may be beneficial taken before sleep for promoting overnight recovery.

A study at Maastricht University found that protein synthesis was 22% higher in resistance-trained males who consumed 40 g of protein in the form of a casein drink before sleep (Res et al., 2012). Casein produced a sustained rise in amino acids throughout the night and increased whole body protein synthesis compared with a placebo.

body for muscle repair. Whey protein may also help enhance immune function. Casein, also derived from milk, provides a slower-digested protein, as well as high levels of amino acids. Soya protein is less widely used in supplements but is a good option for vegans and people with high cholesterol levels – 25 g of soya protein daily (as part of a diet low in saturated fat) can help reduce cholesterol levels. Other non-dairy proteins such as pea, brown rice and hemp are often combined so they provide the full range of essential amino acids.

WHAT IS THE EVIDENCE?

Studies have shown that consuming either a casein or whey supplement immediately after resistance training raises blood levels of amino acids and promotes muscle protein synthesis (Tipton *et al.*, 2004). Male volunteers who consumed a whey protein supplement (1.2 g/kg BW/day) during 6 weeks of resistance training achieved greater muscle mass and strength gains compared with those who took a placebo (Candow *et al.*, 2006), but others have reported no or minimal effects (Campbell *et al.*, 1995; Haub *et al.*, 2002).

In one study, those consuming 20 g of whey supplement before and after resistance exercise had greater increases in muscle mass and muscle strength over 10 weeks compared with those consuming a placebo (Willoughby *et al.*, 2007). Another study found that when athletes consumed a whey supplement immediately before and after a training session they could perform more reps and lift heavier weights 24 hours and 48 hours after the workout compared with those taking a placebo (Hoffman *et al.*, 2008). Compared with casein or soya protein, whey supplements may be a better option in the immediate post-exercise period as whey is absorbed quicker, but there is no evidence that it results in greater muscle growth over 24 hours (Tang *et al.*, 2009). On the plus side, whey may also help support immunity. Researchers found that those who consumed whey supplements following a 40 km cycling time-trial experienced a smaller drop in glutathione levels, which is linked with lowered immunity (Middleton and Bell, 2004).

However, in studies where athletes were already consuming adequate amounts of protein in their diet, taking additional protein in the form of supplements before and after their workouts made no difference to muscle synthesis or strength (Weisgarber *et al.*, 2012). A meta-analysis of 49 studies concluded that protein supplements may augment muscle and strength gains but the benefits are relatively very small (Morton *et al.*, 2018). Resistance training alone resulted in an average muscle mass gain of 1.1 kg over 13 weeks; protein supplementation (average 35 g/day) increased those gains by a mere 0.3 kg. In other words, resistance training has a far greater effect on strength and muscle mass than protein supplementation. Protein supplementation has only a minor benefit. What's more, gains were only seen with up to protein intakes of 1.6 g/kg BW/day – anything above this produced no further gains in muscle mass or strength. The timing, post-exercise dose and source of protein had little if any effect.

DO I NEED THEM?

It is undisputed that resistance training increases muscle protein turnover and therefore the daily protein requirement. But it remains to be proven whether supplements are necessary to increase muscle mass and strength or whether you can get sufficient protein from food.

Supplementation may help you meet your daily protein requirements, but provided these are met it makes little difference where you obtain your protein from. It is highly likely that consuming adequate amounts of any high-quality protein source (*see* p. 160 – 'High quality') immediately after resistance training will promote similar gains in MPS (Tipton *et al.*, 2004). Whole foods are generally a better option than supplements. Not only do they supply protein, but the interaction of the other nutrients contained within the food matrix may actually increase the use of protein for muscle repair. The International Association of Athletic Federations (IAAF) recommends whole-food sources of protein rather than supplements (Burke *et al.*, 2019).

If you are already consuming sufficient protein in your diet (1.2–2.0 g/kg BW/day) and getting around 20–25 g protein per meal then additional protein from supplements is unlikely to produce further gains in muscle mass, strength or performance.

However, protein supplements may benefit you if you have particularly high protein requirements (e.g. for athletes weighing 100 kg or more), you are on a calorie-restricted diet or you cannot consume enough protein from food alone (e.g. a vegetarian or vegan diet). Estimate your daily protein intake from food and compare that with your protein requirement.

Perhaps the main benefit of protein supplements and the best-argued case for taking them is their convenience. Whether in the form of drinks, bars, flapjacks, cookies or gels, they are portable, easy to consume on the go and provide a defined quantity of protein.

ARE THERE ANY SIDE EFFECTS?

An excessive intake of protein, whether from food or supplements, is not harmful but offers no health or performance advantage. Concerns about excess protein harming the liver and kidneys or causing calcium loss from the bones have been disproved.

Pro-hormones/steroid precursors/testosterone boosters

WHAT ARE THEY?

Pro-hormone supplements include dehydro-epiandrosterone (DHEA), androstenedione ('andro') and norandrostenedione, weak androgenic steroid compounds. They are produced naturally in the body and converted into testosterone. Supplements are marketed to bodybuilders and other athletes for increased strength and muscle mass.

WHAT DO THEY DO?

Manufacturers claim the supplements will increase testosterone levels in the body and produce similar muscle-building effects to anabolic steroids, but without the side effects.

WHAT IS THE EVIDENCE?

Current research does not support supplement manufacturers' claims. Studies show that andro supplements and DHEA have no significant testosterone-raising effects, and no effect on muscle mass or strength (King *et al.*, 1999; Broeder *et al.*, 2000; Powers, 2002). A study at Iowa State University found that 8 weeks of supplementation with andro, DHEA, saw palmetto, *Tribulus terrestris* and chrysin, combined with a weight training programme, failed to raise testosterone levels or increase muscle strength or mass – despite of increased levels of androstenedione – compared with a placebo (Brown *et al.*, 2000).

DO I NEED THEM?

It is unlikely that pro-hormones work and they may produce unwanted side effects (*see* below). They are on the World Anti-Doping Agency's prohibited list (WADA, 2014). All athletic associations, including the International Olympic Committee (IOC), ban pro-hormones. Pro-hormones are highly controversial supplements and, despite the rigorous marketing, there is no research to prove the testosterone-building claims.

ARE THERE ANY SIDE EFFECTS?

Studies have found that pro-hormones increase oestrogen (which can lead to gynecomastia, male breast development) and decrease HDL (high density lipoproteins or good cholesterol) levels (King *et al.,* 1999). Reduced HDL carries a greater heart disease risk. Other side effects include acne, enlarged prostate and water retention.

Some supplements include anti-oestrogen substances, such as chrysin (dihydroxyflavone), to counteract the side effects, but there is no evidence that they work either (Brown *et al.,* 2000).

Taurine

WHAT IS IT?

Taurine is a non-essential amino acid produced naturally in the body. It is also found in meat, fish, eggs and milk. It is the second most abundant amino acid in muscle tissue. Taurine is sold as a single supplement, but more commonly as an ingredient in certain protein drinks, creatine-based products and sports drinks. It is marketed to athletes for increasing muscle mass and reducing muscle tissue breakdown during intense exercise.

WHAT DOES IT DO?

Taurine has multiple roles in the body, including brain and nervous system function, blood pressure regulation, fat digestion, absorption of fat-soluble vitamins and control of blood cholesterol levels. It is used as a supplement because it is thought to decrease muscle breakdown during

exercise. The theory behind taurine is that it may act in a similar way to insulin, transporting amino acids and sugar from the bloodstream into muscle cells. This would cause an increase in cell volume, triggering protein synthesis and decreasing protein breakdown.

WHAT IS THE EVIDENCE?

Intense exercise depletes taurine levels in the body, but there is no sound research to support the claims for taurine supplements. In a randomised double-blind crossover trial, US researchers found no difference in either strength or muscular endurance in athletes following consumption of 500 ml sugar-free Red Bull energy drink (containing taurine and caffeine) compared with a drink containing caffeine (without taurine) or a placebo (without caffeine or taurine) (Eckerson *et al.,* 2013).

DO I NEED IT?

As you can obtain taurine from food (animal protein sources), there appears to be no convincing reason to recommend taking the supplements for athletic performance or muscle gain.

ARE THERE ANY SIDE EFFECTS?

Taurine is harmless in the amounts found in protein and creatine supplements. Very high doses of single supplements may cause toxicity.

Testosterone boosters

WHAT ARE THEY?

These include *Tribulus terrestris* (a flowering plant), horny goat weed (a leafy plant), and zinc. They are marketed as natural alternatives to anabolic steroids.

WHAT DO THEY DO?

Manufacturers claim that the phytochemicals in the plants increase testosterone production and therefore increase muscle mass and strength as well as boosting libido.

WHAT IS THE EVIDENCE?

There is no evidence supporting the claims for *Tribulus terrestris* or horny goat weed. A 4-week study of 21 healthy young men failed to find any measurable differences in testosterone levels between those taking a *Tribulus terrestris* supplement and a placebo group (Neychev and Mitev, 2005). Similarly, a study of 22 Australian elite rugby players found no difference in testosterone levels or any improvement in strength or body composition after 5 weeks of supplementation with *Tribulus terrestris* compared with a placebo (Rogerson *et al.*, 2007).

Despite the manufacturers' claims, there have been no studies on horny goat weed and testosterone levels in humans – only studies with rats!

Zinc supplements do not raise testosterone levels unless you have a deficiency, i.e. abnormally low testosterone levels. By correcting the deficiency, you may notice a short-term improvement in strength and muscle mass.

ARE THERE ANY SIDE EFFECTS?

Tribulus supplements are unlikely to produce side effects. However, they are contraindicated for people with breast or prostate cancer.

DO I NEED THEM?

Despite the claims, testosterone boosters do not increase testosterone, improve muscle mass or enhance athletic performance. Although some manufacturers claim *Tribulus terrestris* will not lead to a positive drug test, others have suggested it may increase the urinary testosterone epitestosterone (T:E) ratio, which may place athletes at risk of a positive drug test. So you should avoid anything containing this supplement if you compete in a drug-tested sport.

ZMA

WHAT IS IT?

ZMA (zinc monomethionine aspartate and magnesium aspartate) is a supplement that combines zinc, magnesium, vitamin B_6 and aspartate in a specific formula. It is marketed to bodybuilders and strength athletes as a testosterone booster.

WHAT DOES IT DO?

Manufacturers claim that ZMA can boost testosterone production, strength, muscle mass and recovery after exercise. Zinc is needed for growth, cell reproduction and testosterone production. In theory, a deficiency may reduce the body's anabolic hormone levels and adversely affect muscle mass and strength. Magnesium helps reduce levels of the stress hormone cortisol (high levels are produced during periods of intense training), which would otherwise promote muscle breakdown. A magnesium deficiency may increase catabolism. ZMA supplements may therefore help increase anabolic hormone levels and keep high levels of cortisol at bay by correcting a zinc and magnesium deficiency.

WHAT IS THE EVIDENCE?

Both zinc and magnesium deficiencies can impair performance (Nielson and Lukaski, 2006). It is feasible that ZMA supplementation corrects underlying zinc and/or magnesium deficiencies, thus 'normalising' various body processes and improving testosterone levels. This is supported by one study, which found ZMA increased testosterone and strength in a group of football players (Brilla and Conte, 2000). However, this was a small study with a high drop-out rate, and has not been replicated since.

A more rigorous randomised, double-blind study with 42 experienced weight-trainers found that supplementation with ZMA for 8 weeks failed to increase testosterone levels, strength, muscle mass, anaerobic capacity or muscular endurance compared with a placebo (Wilborn *et al.*, 2004).

DO I NEED IT?

Unless you are deficient in zinc or magnesium, taking ZMA won't help you gain muscle mass or get stronger. You can obtain zinc from whole grains, including wholemeal bread, nuts, beans and lentils. Magnesium is found in whole grains, vegetables, fruit and milk.

ARE THERE ANY SIDE EFFECTS?

Do not exceed the safe upper limit (SUL) of 25 mg daily for zinc; 400 mg daily for magnesium. High levels of zinc – more than 50 mg – can interfere with the absorption of iron and other minerals, leading to iron deficiency. Check the zinc content of any other supplement you may be taking.

Summary of key points

	Endurance/ recovery	Muscle mass/ strength	Weight loss	General health
Strong evidence	• Caffeine • Carbohydrate • drinks, bars and gels • Beta-alanine • Beetroot juice • Bicarbonate	• Creatine • Protein	• Calorie-reduced diet • Exercise	• Probiotics • Vitamin D
Moderate or emerging evidence	• Cherry juice • Glutamine	• Leucine • HMB • BCAAs		• Multivitamins • Fish oil/ omega-3s
Lack of evidence or prohibited by WADA	• Antioxidants • Vitamin C • Vitamin E • Arginine • Taurine	• Pro-hormones • ZMA • Colostrum • Testosterone boosters • *Tribulus terrestris* • Horny goat weed	• CLA • Fat burners • Ephedrine • Synephrine • Ma huang	• Colostrum

//Hydration

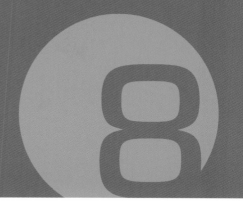

Exercise is thirsty work.

Whenever you exercise you lose water, not only through sweating but also as water vapour in the air that you breathe out. During exercise in warm and hot conditions, your body's fluid losses can be very high and, if the fluid is not replaced quickly, hypohydration (a state of reduced body water) will follow. This, if large enough, will have an adverse effect on your physical and mental performance, yet it can be avoided, or at least minimised, by appropriate drinking strategies during exercise.

This chapter explains the effects of hypohydration on performance and how to reduce the risk of both hypohydration and overhydration, which can lead to hyponatraemia. It provides guidance on fluid intake before, during and after exercise, discusses planned drinking vs drinking to thirst strategies, and summarises the science behind the formulation of sports drinks. Do they offer an advantage over plain water and can they improve performance? Finally, this chapter looks at the effects of alcohol on performance and health.

WHY DO I SWEAT?

First, let us consider what happens to your body when you exercise. When you start exercising, your muscles produce extra heat. In fact, about 75% of the energy you put into exercise is converted into heat, which is then lost. This is why exercise makes you feel warmer. Extra heat has to be dissipated to keep your core body temperature within safe limits – around 37–39°C. If your temperature rises too high, normal body functions are upset and eventually heat stroke can result.

The most effective method of heat dispersal during exercise is sweating, which acts as a cooling mechanism allowing evaporation to occur. Water from your body is carried to your skin via your blood capillaries and as it evaporates you lose heat. For every litre of sweat that evaporates, you will lose around 600 kcal of heat energy from your body. You can lose some heat through convection, conduction and radiation, but the amounts are relatively small compared with sweating.

HOW MUCH WATER DO I LOSE?

Water makes up 50–70% of your body weight, depending on your body composition (lean body mass has a much higher water content than fat tissue). On average you lose between 1 and 3 litres a day through the urine, faeces, respiration and sweat and this needs to be replaced through your food and drink intake to maintain water balance. The amount of sweat that you produce and, therefore, the amount of water that you lose, depends on:

- exercise intensity
- exercise duration
- the temperature and humidity of your surroundings
- body size
- amount and type of clothing

In general, the higher the intensity and duration of your activity, and the hotter and more humid the environment, the more water you will lose. During exercise, an average person could lose anywhere between 0.5 and 2.5 litres/hour. In more extreme conditions of heat and humidity, sweat rates may be as high as 3–4 litres/hour.

Some people sweat more profusely than others, even when they are doing the same exercise in the same surroundings. This depends partly on body weight and size (a smaller body produces less sweat), your fitness level (the fitter and better acclimatised to warm conditions you are, the more readily you sweat due to better thermoregulation), and individual factors (some people simply sweat more than others!). In general, women tend to produce less sweat than men, due to their smaller body size and their greater economy in fluid loss.

WHAT ARE THE RISKS OF HYPOHYDRATION?

Hypohydration during exercise develops when your fluid intake is insufficient to keep pace with your sweat losses. When this happens, blood volume decreases (hypovolemia) and osmolality increases (meaning you have a higher-than-normal concentration of particles in your blood)

Definition of terms

- *Euhydration* refers to a normal state of hydration.
- *Hyperhydration* refers to a state of increased body water.
- *Dehydration* refers to the process of losing body water.
- *Hypohydration* refers to a state of reduced body water, typically a body water deficit of >2% of body weight (BW).

because it provides the fluid for sweat and sweat is hypotonic (i.e. less concentrated) relative to plasma. This places extra strain on the heart, lungs and circulatory system. It means the heart has to work harder to pump blood round your body and blood pressure rises. The strain on your body's systems means that exercise feels much harder, you will fatigue earlier and your performance will drop. Hypohydration also leads to a rise in core body temperature (hyperthermia), increased glycogen use, mental fatigue, a drop in concentration and low mood (Sawka and Coyle, 1999). Ultimately, hypohydration will impair aerobic performance when exercise is performed in warm and hot conditions (Sawka *et al.*, 2015). Maximal aerobic capacity may fall by 10–20% during endurance exercise lasting more than 90 minutes (Armstrong *et al.*, 1985). In one study with cyclists, time-trial performance was 13% slower when cyclists were 3.1% hypohydrated by the end of the trial (Logan-Sprenger *et al.*, 2015). If allowed to progress, hypohydration can have more serious health and performance consequences (ACSM, 2007; Montain and Coyle, 1992; Noakes, 1993).

Ironically, the more hypohydrated you become, the less able your body is to sweat. This is because hypohydration results in a smaller blood volume (due to excessive loss of fluid), and so a compromise has to be made between maintaining the blood flow to muscles and maintaining the blood flow to the surface of the skin to carry away heat. Usually the blood flow to the skin is reduced, causing your core body temperature to rise.

Clearly, these symptoms will have an impact on performance. Although there is considerable difference between individuals, the scientific consensus is that fluid deficits greater than 2% BW will affect your aerobic and cognitive performance, in warm and hot conditions (Sawka *et al.*, 2015; Thomas *et al.*, 2016; Sawka *et al.*, 2007; Cheuvront *et al.*, 2003; Sawka, 1992; Below *et al.*, 1995; McConnell *et al.*, 1997). However, it has less impact on performance in cool conditions, and little effect on strength, power and sprint exercise. A drop in the performance of anaerobic activities, sport-specific skills and aerobic performance in cool weather usually occurs once you have lost 3–5% of BW (Sawka *et al.*, 2007; Shirreffs and Sawka, 2011).

IS THERE A HYPOHYDRATION THRESHOLD?

The current consensus is that performance is impaired when hypohydration exceeds 2% BW (James *et al.*, 2019(b)). However, the threshold at which hypohydration affects performance has been hotly debated in recent years, with several studies suggesting that fluid losses greater than 2% BW can be well tolerated by elite athlete in real-world settings. For example, one meta-analysis of five studies concluded that elite cyclists were able to tolerate hypohydration up to 4% BW loss in outdoor conditions (Goulet, 2011). Similarly, a study of elite Ethiopian distance runners found that they consumed comparatively little fluid (1.75 litres per day) and did not drink anything before or during training (Beis *et al.*, 2011). A 2006 study of Ironman triathletes in Australia

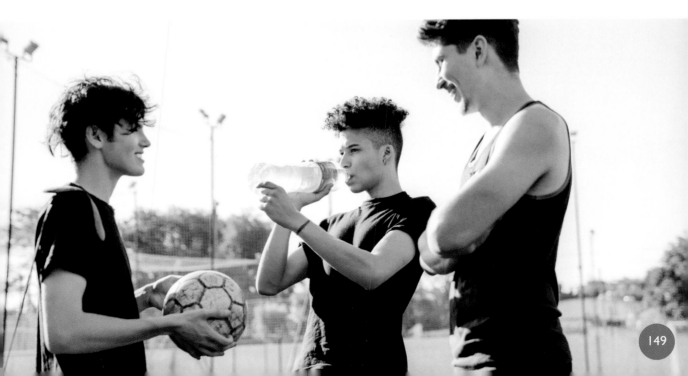

found that performance could be sustained and core temperature maintained despite fluid losses of up to 3% of BW (Laursen *et al.*, 2006). Another study with marathon runners measured a 3% BW loss, suggesting that athletes can race well even with significant levels of hypohydration present at the end (Zouhal *et al.*, 2011).

These findings may be partly explained by individual differences in tolerance but also by the fact that, in outdoor settings, surrounding temperatures are generally lower and air flow is greater than in lab settings, resulting in a natural cooling effect and less strain on athletes' cardiovascular systems.

These studies did not distinguish between thirst and hypohydration, so it is possible that the uncomfortable sensation of thirst impairs performance, rather than a shortage of fluid in the body. More recent studies using a contemporary method of 'blinding' subjects to their hydration status by delivering fluid directly to the stomach via a gastric feeding tube found that hypohydration of 3% BW caused a drop in performance regardless of whether subjects thought they were hypohydrated or not (Funnell *et al.*, 2019). Cyclists who were blinded or unaware of their hydration status experienced a similar drop in performance as those who were aware of their hydration status (11% vs.10%).

In summary, the threshold at which a performance drop occurs will vary from one individual to the next and may be anywhere from 1.5 to 19.2% fluid loss (James *et al.*, 2017; Funnell *et al.*, 2019). Some athletes may experience a drop in performance at low levels of hypohydration while other may be able to tolerate much higher fluid losses. In practice, this is likely down to how familiar you are with experiencing hypohydration during exercise. It is possible to attenuate the negative effects of hypohydration by repeated exposure to hypohydration. For many athletes, this often happens unintentionally as they regularly under-consume fluid during training.

CAN I MINIMISE MY FLUID LOSS?

You cannot prevent your body from losing fluid. After all, this is a natural and desirable way to regulate body temperature. On the other hand, you can prevent your body from becoming hypohydrated by offsetting fluid losses as far as possible. The best way to do this is to make sure you are hydrated before you start exercising, and to drink adequate fluids during and after exercise.

HOW DO YOU KNOW IF YOU ARE HYPOHYDRATED?

Many people, both athletes and non-athletes, suffer mild hypohydration without realising it. Hypohydration is cumulative, which means you can easily dehydrate over successive days of training or competition if you fail to rehydrate fully between workouts or races.

The most simple method to assess hydration status is to look at urine colour and compare against a urine colour chart. From a practical point of view, you should be producing a dilute, pale-coloured urine. Concentrated, dark-coloured urine of a small volume indicates you are hypohydrated and is a signal that you should drink more before you exercise. Indeed, many coaches and trainers advise their players or athletes to monitor their urine output and colour because this is a surprisingly accurate way of assessing hydration status. University of Connecticut researchers found that urine colour correlated very accurately with hydration status – as good as measurements of specific gravity and osmolality of the urine (Armstrong *et al.*, 1998). Urine described as 'very pale yellow' or 'pale yellow' indicates you are within 1% of optimal hydration.

Hydration status may also be assessed by tracking early morning body weight since daily changes in body weight generally reflect changes in body water. It is assumed that a loss of 1 g BW is equivalent to 1 ml water. If body weight changes by more than 1% or 0.5–1 kg, this suggests that you may be hypohydrated.

Urine specific gravity (a measure of the concentration of dissolved particles e.g. electrolytes, urea, phosphates, proteins and glucose, compared with water density) and urinary osmolality (concentration of particles) can also be measured. If you are properly hydrated, urinary osmolality should be between 300 and 900 mOsmol/kg. Higher values indicate that you are hypohydrated (Thomas *et al.*, 2016). Urine specific gravity should be <1.025, with higher values indicating hypohydration (Kenefick and Cheuvront, 2012)

HOW DO SWEATSUITS AFFECT FLUID LOSS?

Many athletes in weight-category sports use sweatsuits, plastic, neoprene and other clothing to 'make weight' for competition. By preventing sweat evaporation, the clothing prevents heat loss. This will cause the body temperature to rise more and more. In an attempt to expel this excess heat, your body will continue to produce more sweat, thus losing increasing amounts of

Can you 'fluid load' before exercise?

'Loading up' or 'pre-hydrating' with fluid before an event seems advantageous for those competing in ultra-endurance events, activities during which there is little opportunity to drink, or in hot humid conditions. Unfortunately, you cannot achieve hyperhydration by consuming large volumes of water or sports drinks before the event. The body simply excretes surplus fluid and you will end up paying frequent visits to the toilet or bushes. However, there is a method of hyperhydration that involves the consumption of 1.2–1.5 glycerol/kg BW along with 7.5 g salt and 500 ml fluid spread out over 2 hours before exercise. Glycerol is a hyperhydrating agent, or a 'plasma expander', which, through its strong osmotic activity, drags water into the extra-cellular fluid. This results in an increase in total body fluid. In theory, you will be able to maintain blood volume longer, increase sweating and reduce the rise in core body temperature that occurs during exercise. Studies at the Australian Institute of Sport found that by doing this, athletes retained an extra 600 ml of fluid and improved performance in a time-trial by 2.4% (Hitchins *et al.*, 1999). A study at the University of Glasgow found that hyperhydrating with a combination of creatine and glycerol resulted in increased total body water but did not improve performance in a 16 km time-trial compared with normal hydration (Easton *et al.*, 2007). Until recently, glycerol was a banned substance for competitive athletes by the World Anti-Doping Agency (WADA). In January 2018, it was officially removed from the banned list.

fluid. You will become hypohydrated, with the undesirable consequences this entails.

This is definitely not a good idea! While the aim is to restore the fluid deficit between weigh-in and the start of competition, in practice this is often difficult to achieve in a short time period. If you compete in a hypohydrated state, as mentioned above, your ability to exercise will be impaired – you will suffer fatigue much sooner and will have to slow down or stop altogether. Obviously, this is not a good state in which to train or compete.

Losing weight through exercise in sweatsuits is not only potentially dangerous, but has no effect whatsoever on fat loss. Any weight loss will simply be fluid, which will be regained immediately when you next eat or drink. The exercise may seem harder because you will be sweating more, but this will not affect the body's rate of fat breakdown. If anything, you are likely to lose *less* fat, because you cannot exercise as hard or for as long when you wear a sweatsuit.

How much should I drink?

1. Before exercise

Your main priority is to ensure you are hydrated before exercise. It is clear that if you begin a training session or competition in a hypohydrated state, your performance will suffer and you will be at a competitive disadvantage (Shirreffs and Sawka, 2011).

Obviously, prevention is better than cure. Make sure you are hydrated before you begin exercising, especially in hot and humid weather. The easiest way to check your hydration status is by monitoring body mass first thing in the morning and the colour and volume of your urine. It should be pale yellow, not completely clear. The American College of Sports Medicine (ACSM) recommends drinking 5–10 ml of fluid/kg BW slowly in the 2–4 hours before exercise to promote hydration and allow enough time for excretion of excess water (Thomas *et al.*, 2016; Sawka *et al.*, 2007). That's equivalent to 300–600 ml for a 60 kg person, or 350–700 ml for a 70 kg person. If this does not result in urine production within 2 hours or if your urine is dark coloured, you should continue drinking. But don't force yourself to drink so much that you gain weight. The 2010 International Olympic Committee (IOC) Consensus Conference on Nutrition and Sport cautions against over-drinking before and during exercise, because of the risk of water intoxication (hyponatraemia).

2. During exercise

Previous advice from the American College of Sports Medicine (ACSM, 1996) to drink 'as much as possible' or 'to replace the weight lost during exercise' is no longer valid. In its latest position stand, the ACSM makes no *specific* recommendations about how much to drink because sweat rates and sweat composition vary considerably from one person to the next, depending on exercise intensity, duration, fitness, heat acclimatisation, altitude, heat and humidity (Sawka *et al.*, 2007). Instead, it advises drinking enough fluid during exercise so that hypohydration is limited to less than 2% of BW. However, the Statement of the Third International Exercise-Associated Hyponatremia Consensus Development Conference recommends a drink to thirst strategy (Hew-Butler *et al.*, 2015).

A CONTROVERSY: DRINKING TO THIRST OR TO A PLAN?

While there is scientific agreement that hypohydration impairs performance, there is long-standing controversy about drinking guidelines during exercise, with some scientists argue that fluid intake during exercise should be planned while others argue that simply drinking to thirst is optimal. This has produced two schools of thought related to guidelines for fluid intake, namely 'planned drinking' and 'drinking to thirst'.

Drinking to thirst

It seems too simple to be true but, according to this school of thinking, drinking to thirst will protect you from the risks of both hypo- and hyperhydration during exercise. Indeed, a number of studies with runners and cyclists suggest that drinking to thirst is just as effective as planned drinking in terms of averting hypohydration and performance impairment (Hoffman *et al.*, 2016; Berkulo *et al.*, 2016; Noakes, 2007; Noakes, 2010; Noakes, 2012; Daries *et al.*, 2000).

Drinking to thirst may be appropriate during activities when anticipated sweat losses are likely to be <2% BW, for example when you are exercising for less than 90 minutes; exercising in cool conditions; or during lower-intensity exercise such as ultra-running. A study with recreational runners showed that sweat losses are likely to be <2% BW for distances up to 21 km (Kenefick and Cheuvront, 2012). Provided you have easy access to fluids, drinking to thirst would be a practical strategy.

Planned drinking

Planned drinking refers to drinking pre-determined amounts of fluid in order to minimise

Fluid calculator

Here's a rough guide to calculating your sweat rate and calculating how much to drink during exercise.

1. Weigh yourself before your workout.
2. Exercise for 1 hour, recording how much fluid you drink.
3. Weigh yourself immediately after your exercise session.
4. Calculate the difference between your pre- and post-workout weight. You can assume that almost all of your weight loss is sweat (although this is not strictly accurate as some will also come from water loss in expired breath, and from the breakdown of carbohydrate and fat). So a weight loss of 1 kg represents a fluid loss of about 1 litre.
5. Add to this value the volume of fluid consumed. This is your hourly sweat rate.
6. Divide your hourly sweat rate by 4 to give you a guideline for how much to drink every 15 minutes under those particular environmental conditions.
7. Repeat the test for different environmental conditions.

fluid losses. According to this school of thinking, athletes tend to under-consume fluids during exercise when sweat losses are high and prolonged, leading to excessive hypohydration and impaired performance (Cheuvront *et al.*, 2007). Therefore, a planned drinking strategy that replaces fluid according to sweat losses (as calculated from body weight losses) is needed in order to prevent hypohydration and hypo-natraemia. One study of recreational runners showed that sweat losses are likely to be >2% BW for distances over 21 km, more so among faster runners than slower runners, and more so in hot weather (Kenefick and Cheuvront, 2012). In other words, fluid replacement becomes more critical as exercise duration, pace and surrounding temperature increase, so a planned drinking strategy would be more appropriate than a drink to thirst strategy.

You can work out how much fluid you lose through sweating by weighing yourself before and after a typical workout, then aim to drink sufficient to ensure a weight loss of no more than about 2% BW (see p. 153 'Fluid calculator'). For example, this would be equivalent to a 1.4 kg loss for a 70 kg athlete. For most recreational athletes, an intake of 400–800 ml/hour prevents hypohydration as well as overhydration, with the upper level being in warmer environments for faster and heavier athletes, and the lower level in cooler conditions for slower athletes (Sawka et al., 2007; Thomas et al., 2016).

In conclusion, planned drinking may be more appropriate during activities of longer duration (>90 minutes), particularly in the heat, as well as high-intensity activities with high sweat rates, and events when carbohydrate intake of more than 60 g/hour is required. Experimenting in training with a planned fluid intake will help you develop a personalised drinking strategy for competition. There may be circumstances where it is not possible to consume sufficient fluid to replace your sweat losses (e.g. during hot, humid conditions; lack of provisions of fluid during an event). To help minimise performance impairment, you can practise training under competition conditions to familiarise yourself with changes in hydration you may experience.

IS IT POSSIBLE TO DRINK TOO MUCH DURING EXERCISE?

Sometimes athletes consume more fluid than they are losing through sweating and overhydrate. Over-drinking can result in hyponatraemia, a condition where the concentration of sodium in your blood falls to an abnormally low level (<130 mmol/litre). It is rare compared to hypohydration but can occur during endurance events, such as marathons and ultra-distance races when athletes

Does drink temperature make a difference?

From a practical point of view, the ACSM recommend cool drinks (0.5 °C) to help reduce core temperature (Thomas et al., 2016). You will also be inclined to drink more if the drink is palatable and in a container that makes it easy to drink. Studies have shown that, during exercise, athletes voluntarily drink more of a flavoured sweetened drink than water, be it a sports drink, diluted fruit juice or fruit squash (Passe et al., 2004; Wilk and Bar-Or, 1996; Minehan, 2002). Drinks bottles with sports caps are probably the most popular containers. It is also important to make drinks readily accessible: for example, for swim training, have drinks bottles at the poolside; for games played on a pitch or court (soccer, hockey, rugby, netball, tennis), have the bottles available adjacent to the pitch or court.

drink too much water (Noakes, 2000; Speedy *et al.,* 1999; Barr and Costill, 1989). When this happens, the body's water content increases and cells begin to swell. Symptoms include headache, nausea, bloating, water retention, disorientation and confusion. In extreme cases, it can result in lapses in consciousness, cerebral oedema, seizures, coma or death due to swelling of the brain. However, some of these symptoms are also associated with hypohydration so it's important not to confuse the two conditions and to be aware of how much you are drinking.

A study of 1089 triathletes who participated in the Ironman European Championships between 2005 and 2013 found that 115 (10.6%) had documented hyponatraemia: 95 had mild hyponatremia (8.7%), 17 severe hyponatraemia (1.6%), and 3 critical hyponatraemia (0.3%) (Danz *et al.,* 2016).

Smaller individuals could be at greater risk for overhydrating because they tend to have lower sweating rates and may overestimate their water deficit and over-drink. Slower runners who take longer to complete the race are also are at higher risk because they have more time to drink.

You can minimise your risk of hyponatraemia by ensuring you do not drink more fluid than you lose through sweating, and only to the point at which you are at most maintaining, not gaining, weight. Monitor your weight during training: if you gain weight during your workout or event, you are drinking too much. During endurance events, such as a marathon or triathlon, do not feel compelled to drink at every fluid station. Drink less if you begin to have a queasy, sloshy feeling in your stomach.

What causes cramps during exercise?

It is widely believed that cramps are due to hypohydration or lack of electrolytes. However, there is little evidence to support these theories. One study of 209 Ironman athletes found no significant difference in the levels of hypohydration or sodium loss between those who developed cramp and those who didn't, thus challenging the prevailing electrolyte depletion hypothesis of cramps (Schwellnus *et al.,* 2011).

Instead, it is thought that cramps are due to a disturbance in the nerves that control the muscles. A neural switch gets stuck in the 'on' position, causing a prolonged and painful contraction. This is called the 'altered neuromuscular control hypothesis'. It has been shown to occur more frequently during high-intensity exercise or at the beginning of unaccustomed workouts (Minetto *et al.,* 2013). Researchers also believe that there is an element of genetic susceptibility, that some people are simply more prone to cramp than others. The remedy is to reduce your exercise intensity, stretch and try to relax the affected muscle(s). Correcting any muscle imbalances and developing a more efficient technique for your sport may also help avoid cramp.

3. After exercise

Both water and sodium need to be replaced to restore normal fluid balance after exercise (Shirreffs *et al.,* 1996). This can be achieved by water plus accompanying food (if there is no urgency for recovery) or a sports drink containing sodium (Shirreffs and Sawka, 2011). You need to consume a drink volume greater than your sweat loss since sweating continues for a while after exercise. Researchers recommend you should consume about 1.25–1.5 times the volume of fluid lost during exercise (Sawka *et al.*, 2007; IAAF, 2007; Shirreffs *et al.*, 2004). The simplest way to work out how much you need to drink is to calculate your fluid losses during exercise, then multiply by 1.25 and 1.5. For example, if your fluid loss is 500 ml, you will need to consume 625–750 ml in the post-exercise period to restore fluid balance. You should not drink the whole amount straight away, as a rapid increase in blood volume promotes urination and increases the risk of hyponatraemia. Consume as much as you feel comfortable with, then drink the remainder in divided doses until you are fully hydrated.

Sports drinks that contain sodium are more effective than water for restoring fluid balance after exercise, particularly when fluid losses are high or for those athletes who train twice a day and need to recover rapidly. The problem with drinking water is that it causes a drop in blood osmolality (i.e. it dilutes the blood), reducing your thirst and increasing urine output, and so you may stop drinking before you are rehydrated (Maughan *et al.*, 1996; Gonzalez-Alonzo *et al.*, 1992). A rise in osmolality plays an important role in driving the thirst mechanism. A low osmolality (e.g. low sodium concentration) in the blood signals to the brain a low thirst sensation. Conversely, a high osmolality (e.g. sodium concentration) in the blood signals greater thirst and thus drives you to drink. Hence, the popular strategy of putting salted peanuts and crisps at the bar to encourage customers to buy more drink to quench their thirst! Similarly, sports drinks, increase the urge to drink and decrease urine production.

However, research at Loughborough University suggests that skimmed milk may be an even better option for promoting post-exercise rehydration (Shirreffs *et al.*, 2007). Volunteers who drank skimmed milk after exercise were able to restore fully their fluid losses throughout the 5-hour recovery period, but were unable to do so after drinking either water or a sports drink, returning to net negative fluid balance after 1 hour. More recently, a study at Griffith University, Australia, showed that milk, soya milk alternative and a milk-based supplement all rehydrated athletes more effectively than a sports drink following a workout that induced 2% hypohydration (Desbrow *et al.*, 2014a).

A UK study comparing the hydrating properties of 13 different drinks found that skimmed and whole milk, orange juice and an oral rehydration solution all resulted in better fluid retention after 2 hours, compared with water (Maughan *et al.*, 2016). Contrary to popular belief, lager, coffee and tea did not have a significant diuretic effect and hydrated the body as well as water.

HOW MUCH SHOULD I DRINK ON NON-EXERCISING DAYS?

The current European Food Safety Authority (EFSA) Dietary Reference Value for water intakes is 2.5 litres/day for men and 2.0 litres/day for women (EFSA, 2010). However, this is simply a guideline and the amount you need to drink depends on your fluid losses incurred through sweating, breathing and urine production. Most people can rely on their sense of thirst as a good indicator of when they should drink.

Table 8.1	SUMMARY OF RECOMMENDATIONS FOR CARBOHYDRATE INTAKE DURING EXERCISE	
Exercise duration	Recommended amount of carbohydrate	Type of carbohydrate
<45 minutes	None	None
45–75 minutes	Very small amounts (mouth rinse)	Any
1–2 hours	Up to 30 g/h	Any
2–3 hours	Up to 60 g/h	Glucose, maltodextrin
3 hours	Up to 90 g/h	Multiple transportable carbohydrates (glucose + fructose or maltodextrin + fructose in 2:1 ratio)

Source: adapted from Burke *et al.*, 2011.

In a non-exercising state, it does not matter where you get your fluid from – coffee, tea, fruit juice, soup, squash and milk all count towards the total intake.

What should I drink?

During low- or moderate-intensity activities such as 'easy pace' swimming, cycling, jogging or walking carried out for less than 45 minutes, fluid losses are likely to be relatively small and can be replaced fast enough with water. There is little benefit to be gained from consuming sports drinks compared with water during these types of activities.

For higher-intensity exercise lasting between 45 and 75 minutes, you may either consume an isotonic drink containing 40–80 g carbohydrate/ litre (depending on your exercise intensity) or, if you are prone to gastrointestinal problems during exercise, try 'mouth rinsing' (swilling the drink in your mouth then it spitting out, *see* pp. 43–44).

Both strategies may improve performance but through different mechanisms.

During endurance exercise lasting longer than 60–90 minutes where muscle glycogen stores are a limiting factor, consuming carbohydrate as well as fluid will help maintain blood glucose concentration, delay fatigue and increase endurance. In other words, consuming an isotonic drink containing 40–80 g carbohydrate/litre will help avoid early glycogen depletion and low blood sugar, as well as hypohydration, as all three can result in fatigue (*see* pp. 30–31).

How much carbohydrate should you consume?

For high-intensity exercise lasting 1–2½ hours, the consensus recommendation is an intake of 30–60 g carbohydrate/hour, depending on exercise intensity (Thomas *et al.*, 2016; IOC, 2011; Burke *et al.*, 2011; Rodriguez *et al.*, 2009; Coggan and Coyle, 1991). This will help to maintain blood sugar concentration, delay fatigue and increase endurance (*see* pp. 43–46). This range corresponds to the maximum rate at which glucose can be absorbed in the small intestines (*see* p. 46). Most ready-to-drink sports drinks contain 40–80 g carbohydrate/litre, so drinking 500 ml per hour would provide 20–40 g/h.

During hot and humid conditions, you may be losing more than 1 litre of sweat per hour. Therefore, you should increase your drink volume (although still be guided by your thirst), if possible, and use a more dilute drink (around 20–40 g/litre). More concentrated fluids take longer to absorb (ACSM, 1996).

For high-intensity exercise lasting more than 2½ hours, an intake up to 90 g carbohydrate/h is recommended (Burke *et al.*, 2011). However, this can only be achieved by consuming drinks that provide a mixture of glucose (or malto-dextrin) and fructose ('multiple transportable carbohydrates'). Studies have found that drinks containing a mixture of glucose (or maltodextrin) and fructose in a 2:1 ratio allows the body to absorb carbohydrate faster and therefore supply the muscles with more carbohydrate than glucose-only drinks (Jeukendrup, 2014; Thomas *et al.*, 2016; IOC, 2011; Jeukendrup, 2008) (*see* p. 46). Ready-to-drink and powdered energy drinks are now widely available (*see* p. 160).

During high-intensity exercise in cool condi-tions when your sweat rate is low, sports drinks containing maltodextrin may be a better option than those based on glucose because they provide more fuel for a smaller volume.

The key to choosing the right drink during exercise is to experiment in training to find one that suits you best. Once you have a rough idea of which drinks suit you, aim to do a few work-outs using the same schedule you plan to use in the event. Simulate event conditions as far as possible, using the same drinks and practise taking them at the same frequency as the one you'll use during the race.

Why do I feel nauseous when I drink during exercise?

If you feel nauseous or experience other gastrointestinal symptoms when you drink during exercise, this may either indicate that you are hypohydrated or be related to the fact you are exercising at a very high intensity for a prolonged period. In the former case, you need to be aware that even a fairly small degree of hypohydration (around 2% of body weight) slows down stomach emptying and upsets the normal rhythmical movement of your gut. This can result in bloating, nausea and vomiting. Avoid this by ensuring you start exercise hydrated and then continue drinking little and often during your workout. In the latter case, it is the nature of the activity (i.e. high-intensity prolonged exercise) that affects gut motility, causing discomfort and nausea. If you are prone to such symptoms during training or competition or if you struggle to consume large volumes of fluid during long workouts or events then you should train your gut to tolerate progressively greater amounts of fluid. Start with small amounts and increase gradually over time. With practice, the stomach will learn to accommodate larger volumes of fluid and empty faster so you feel more comfortable.

What does 'osmolality' mean?

Osmolality is a measure of the number of dissolved particles in a fluid. A drink with a high osmolality means that it contains more particles per litre than one with a low osmolality. These particles may include sugars, maltodextrin, sodium or other electrolytes. The osmolality of the drink determines which way the fluid will move across a membrane (e.g. the gut wall). For example, if a drink with a relatively high osmolality is consumed then water moves from the bloodstream and gut cells into the gut. This is called *net secretion*. If a drink with a relatively low osmolality is consumed then water is absorbed from the gut (i.e. the drink) to the gut cells and bloodstream. Thus there is *net water absorption*.

WHY DO SOME PEOPLE GET GUT PROBLEMS FROM SPORTS DRINKS?

There are lots of anecdotal reports suggesting sports drinks can cause stomach discomfort or heaviness during exercise. This is likely due to the higher osmolality (*see* above) and carbohydrate concentration of the drink compared to water. It is known that more concentrated drinks empty more slowly from the stomach and are absorbed more slowly from the intestines, which would explain the increased gastrointestinal (GI) discomfort that some athletes experience. Indeed, a study at the Gatorade Sports Science Institute, Illinois, found that athletes experienced greater stomach discomfort during circuit training after drinking an 8% sports drink compared with a 6% drink (Shi *et al.*, 2004). Many people find

that diluting sports drinks helps alleviate these problems, but there's a balance to be struck between obtaining enough carbohydrate to fuel your exercise and avoiding GI discomfort. If the drink is too dilute, you may not consume enough carbohydrate to achieve peak performance. It has been claimed that hydrogel drinks overcome the problem of stomach discomfort (*see* pp.134–5). The hydrogel supposedly encapsulates the carbohydrates in the drink, effectively hiding them from the sensors in the stomach. This, in turn, allows you to consume drinks with a relatively high concentration of carbohydrate without causing GI problems. However, studies to date have failed to show any reduction in GI symptoms or performance. The bottom line is: work out from trial and error the concentration of sports drink that suits you best.

The science of sports drinks

WHAT TYPES OF SPORTS DRINKS ARE AVAILABLE?

Sports drinks can be divided into two main categories: fluid replacement drinks and energy drinks:

1. Fluid replacement drinks are dilute solutions of electrolytes and sugars. The sugars most commonly added are glucose, sucrose, fructose and maltodextrin. They can be subdivided into low-cal or 'lite' drinks, typically containing <20 g sugars/litre; and isotonic drinks, typically containing 40–80 g sugars/litre. The main aim of these drinks is to replace fluid faster than plain water, although the sugars will also help maintain blood sugar levels, spare glycogen and provide fuel. These drinks may be either hypotonic or isotonic (*see* p. 160).

2. Energy drinks provide a higher concentration of carbohydrate than fluid replacement drinks, typically 60–90 g/litre. The carbohydrate is usually in the form of maltodextrin and fructose. They provide larger amounts of carbohydrate per 100 ml but at an equal or lower osmolality than the same concentration of glucose. They will, of course, provide fluid as well. The combination of glucose and fructose increases carbohydrate absorption and oxidation during exercise. Ready-to-drink brands are generally isotonic. Powders that you make up into a drink may be made hypotonic or isotonic (*see* below).

WHAT IS THE DIFFERENCE BETWEEN HYPOTONIC, ISOTONIC AND HYPERTONIC DRINKS?

The concentration, or 'tonicity' of a drink affects the rate at which water, carbohydrate and electrolytes are absorbed into your bloodstream. The three main categories of sports drinks are:

1. Hypotonic drinks, often marketed as a 'lite' sports drinks, have a relatively low osmolality, which means they contain fewer particles (carbohydrate and electrolytes) per 100 ml than the body's own fluids. As they are more dilute, they are absorbed faster than water. Typically, a hypotonic drink contains less than 20 g carbohydrate/litre.

2. Isotonic drinks have the same osmolality as the body's fluids, which means it contains about the same number of particles (carbohydrate and electrolytes) per 100 ml and is therefore absorbed as fast as or faster than water. They include both fluid replacement sports drinks and energy drinks and typically contain 40–80 g carbohydrate/litre and 60–90 g carbohydrate/litre respectively. In theory, isotonic drinks provide the ideal compromise between rehydration and refuelling.

3. Hypertonic drinks include cola, ready-to-drink soft drinks and fruit juice. They have a higher osmolality than body fluids, as they contain more particles (carbohydrate and electrolytes) per 100 ml. This means they are absorbed more slowly than plain water. A hypertonic drink typically contains more than 80 g carbohydrate/litre.

WHEN SHOULD I OPT FOR A SPORTS DRINK INSTEAD OF WATER?

Opting for an isotonic sports drink would benefit your performance during any moderate or high-intensity event lasting longer than about 60–90 minutes. Numerous studies have shown that sports drinks containing about 40–80 g carbohydrate/litre promote both hydration and increased blood sugar levels, and enhance performance during intense and/or prolonged exercise (Coggan and Coyle, 1991; Coyle, 2004; Jeukendrup, 2004). If you are exercising longer than 2 hours or doing any event where sodium sweat losses are high (more then 3–4 g sodium in sweat), you should opt for a sports drink that also contains sodium (Coyle, 2004).

One of the first of such studies showed that cyclists completed a time-trial 3 minutes faster following consumption of a sports drink (60 g carbohydrate/litre), compared with water or a more dilute sports drink (25 g/litre) (Davis *et al.*, 1988).

In a study at Loughborough University, seven endurance runners drank similar volumes of either water, or two different sports drinks (55 g or 69 g carbohydrate/litre) before and during a 42 km treadmill run (Tsintzas *et al.*, 1995). Those who

Sports drinks and tooth enamel

Research at Birmingham University has found that sports drinks can dissolve tooth enamel and the hard dentine underneath, resulting in tooth erosion (Venables *et al.*, 2005). Their high acidity levels means that they can erode up to 30 times more tooth enamel than water. A 2007 study comparing the 'buffering capacity' of various drinks found that popular sports drinks and energy drinks have a greater potential to cause tooth erosion than cola (Owens, 2007). Drinking them during exercise makes the effects worse because exercise reduces saliva needed to combat the drink's acidity. Similar erosive problems can occur when drinking soft drinks and fruit juice. In a survey of 302 athletes from 25 different sports competing at the 2012 Olympics, 55% had evidence of caries, 45% had dental erosion and 18% said that their oral health had a negative impact on their training and performance (Needleman *et al.*, 2014). More recently, a survey of 352 athletes from 11 sports reported higher rates of tooth decay and dental erosion compared with the general population, which the researchers attributed to their consumption of sports drinks, energy gels and bars during training and competition (Gallagher *et al.*, 2018).

The best advice is to use a drinks bottle with a flip straw or nozzle that can be directed away from the teeth to reduce overall exposure to the acids and sugars, alternate with water during exercise, and to avoid sipping on them constantly or swishing around your mouth. Researchers are hoping to produce a sports drink that is less harmful to the teeth.

drank the sports drinks produced running times on average 3.9 minutes and 2.4 minutes faster, respectively, compared with water.

At the University of Texas at Austin, eight cyclists performed a time-trial lasting approximately 10 minutes after completing 50 minutes of high-intensity cycling. Those who drank a sports drink (60 g carbohydrate/litre) reduced the time taken to cycle the final trial by 6% compared with those who drank water (Below *et al.*, 1995).

WHAT ARE ELECTROLYTES?

Electrolytes are mineral salts dissolved in fluid, and carry an electrical charge. They include sodium, chloride, potassium and magnesium, and help to regulate the fluid balance between different body compartments (for example, the amount of fluid inside and outside a muscle cell) and the volume of fluid in the bloodstream. The water movement is controlled by the concentration of electrolytes on either side of the cell membrane. For example, an increase in the concentration of sodium outside a cell will cause water to move to it from inside the cell. Similarly, a drop in sodium concentration will cause water to move from the outside to the inside of the cell. Potassium draws water across a membrane, so a high potassium concentration inside cells increases the cell's water content.

WHY DO SPORTS DRINKS CONTAIN SODIUM?

Sodium in sports drinks increases the urge to drink, improves palatability and promotes fluid retention. The increase in sodium concentration and decrease in blood volume that accompany exercise increase your natural thirst sensation, making you want to drink. If you drink plain water it effectively dilutes the sodium, thus reducing your urge to drink before you are fully hydrated. Therefore, consuming a small amount of sodium (0.23–0.69 g/litre) in a sports drink will encourage you to drink more fluid (Sawka *et al.*, 2007).

Sodium is only necessary when you are exercising longer than 2 hours or doing any event where sodium sweat losses are high (more then 3–4 g sodium in sweat) (Coyle, 2004). Electrolyte replacement is only beneficial when sweat losses are high and prolonged, and you lose around 3–4 g sodium (Coyle, 2004).

If you're exercising for less than 2 hours and/or sweat losses are not excessive, sodium will not benefit performance (Shirreffs and Sawka, 2011). It was originally thought that sodium in sport drinks speeds water absorption in the intestines. However, research at the University of Iowa has since disproved this (Gisolphi *et al.*, 1995). Researchers discovered that after you have consumed any kind of drink, sodium passes from the blood plasma into the intestine, where it then stimulates water absorption. In other words, the body sorts out the sodium concentration of the liquid in your intestines all by itself, so the addition of sodium to sports drinks is unnecessary.

WHY DO SPORTS DRINKS CONTAIN CARBOHYDRATE (SUGARS)?

Carbohydrate in sports drinks serves two purposes: 1) they promote water absorption (Gisolphi *et al.*, 1992) and 2) they provide an additional source of energy (Coggan and Coyle, 1987; Febbraio *et al.*, 2000; Bosch *et al.*, 1994).

Relatively dilute solutions of carbohydrate (hypotonic or isotonic) stimulate water absorption from the small intestine into the bloodstream. A carbohydrate concentration usually in the range 40–80 g/litre is used in isotonic sports drinks to accelerate water absorption. More concentrated drinks (hypertonic), above 80 g/litre, tend to slow down the stomach emptying and therefore reduce the speed of fluid replacement (Murray *et al.*, 1999).

WHAT IS MALTODEXTRIN?

Between a sugar (1–2 units) and a starch (several 100,000 units), although closer to the former, is maltodextrin (glucose polymers). These are chains of between 4 and 20 glucose molecules produced from boiling corn starch under controlled commercial conditions.

The advantage of using maltodextrin instead of glucose or sucrose in a drink is that a higher concentration of carbohydrate can be achieved (usually between 100 and 200 g/litre) at a lower osmolality. That's because each molecule contains several glucose units yet still exerts the same osmotic pressure as just one molecule of glucose. So an isotonic or hypotonic drink can be produced with a carbohydrate content greater than 80 g/litre.

Also, maltodextrin is less sweet than simple sugars, so you can achieve a fairly concentrated drink that does not taste too sickly. In fact, most maltodextrin drinks and gels are fairly tasteless unless they have added artificial flavours or sweeteners.

WHAT ARE 'MULTIPLE TRANSPORTABLE CARBOHYDRATES'?

This term refers to a mixture of carbohydrates (e.g. glucose and fructose; maltodextrin and fructose) in sports drinks. These carbohydrates are

Table 8.2	DIY SPORTS DRINKS	
Hypotonic		**Isotonic**
• 20–40 g sucrose • I litre warm water • I–1.5 g (¼ tsp) salt (optional) • Sugar-free/low-calorie squash for flavouring (optional)		• 40–80 g sucrose • I litre warm water • I–1.5 g (¼ tsp) salt (optional) • Sugar-free/low-calorie squash for flavouring (optional)
• 100 ml fruit squash • 900 ml water • I–1.5 g (¼ tsp) salt (optional)		• 200 ml fruit squash • 800 ml water • I–1.5 g (¼ tsp) salt (optional)
• 250 ml fruit juice • 750 ml water • I–1.5 g (¼ tsp) salt (optional)		• 500 ml fruit juice • 500 ml water • I–1.5 g (¼ tsp) salt (optional)

absorbed from the intestine by different transporters, and using a mixture rather than a single type of carbohydrate in a sports drink overcomes the usual limitation of gut uptake of glucose (*see* pp 43–6). Studies show that drinks containing multiple transportable carbohydrates increases the absorption, muscle uptake and oxidation of carbohydrate during exercise compared with glucose-only drinks (Jeukendrup, 2010; IOC, 2011; Jeukendrup, 2008).

SHOULD I CHOOSE STILL OR CARBONATED SPORTS DRINKS?

Experiments at East Carolina University and Ball State University found that carbonated and still sports drinks produced equal hydration in the body (Hickey *et al.*, 1994). However, the carbonated drinks tended to produce a higher incidence of mild heartburn and stomach discomfort. In practice, many athletes find that carbonated drinks make them feel full and 'gassy', which may well limit the amount they drink.

CAN I MAKE MY OWN SPORTS DRINKS?

You can make your own sports drink from sugar, water and, if appropriate, salt. Mix the ingredients together in a bottle or jug and allow to cool in the fridge. Table 8.2 includes some recipes for making your own sports drink.

Other non-alcoholic drinks

CAN ORDINARY SOFT DRINKS AND FRUIT JUICE IMPROVE PERFORMANCE?

Ordinary soft drinks (typically between 90 and 200 g carbohydrate/litre) and fruit juices (typically between 110 and 130 g carbohydrate/litre) are hypertonic; in other words, they are more concentrated than body fluids, so are not ideal as fluid replacers during exercise. They empty more slowly from the stomach than plain water because they must first be diluted with water from the body, thus causing a temporary net reduction in body fluid.

If you dilute one part fruit juice with one part water, you will get an isotonic drink, ideal for rehydrating and refuelling during or after exercise (see Table 8.2).

CAN 'LITE' SPORTS DRINKS IMPROVE PERFORMANCE?

These types of drinks are hypotonic, containing around 20 g sugar/litre along with artificial sweeteners, flavourings and electrolytes. Their sodium content means they may promote fluid retention and stimulate thirst more than plain water, and the flavours make the drinks palatable – but they don't deliver much carbohydrate energy. They would therefore not be advantageous for intense workouts lasting longer than 1 hour and, even for shorter workouts, offer few advantages over plain water, apart from improving palatability and encouraging you to drink more.

ARE 'DIET' DRINKS SUITABLE DURING EXERCISE?

'Diet' or low-calorie drinks contain artificial sweeteners in place of sugars and have a very low sodium concentration. They will help replace fluid at approximately the same speed as plain water but offer no performance advantage. Artificial sweeteners have no known advantage or disadvantage on performance. Choose these types of drink only if you dislike the taste of water, and under the same circumstances that you would normally choose water, i.e. for low- to moderat-intensity exercise lasting less than 1 hour.

CAN ENERGY DRINKS WITH CAFFEINE IMPROVE MY PERFORMANCE?

Energy drinks containing caffeine have been shown to improve various aspects of aerobic and anaerobic performance in many studies (Guest et al., 2021). A review and meta-analysis of 34 studies concluded that caffeinated energy drinks improved endurance performance, muscular strength and endurance, jumping and sport-specific actions (Souzo et al., 2017). In a study at the University of Saskatchewan, Canada, consuming a caffeinated energy drink (2 mg caffeine/kg BW) 1 hour before exercise significantly increased bench press muscle endurance (Forbes et al., 2007).

The exact mechanism is not clear, but it is thought that the performance benefits are due partly to carbohydrate and partly to caffeine and the amino acid taurine (see p. 144) in the drinks. The optimal dose of caffeine is 3–6 mg/kg BW, equivalent to 210–420 mg for a 70 kg person. However, lower doses, around 2 mg/kg BW have also been shown to be effective. Energy drinks typically contain 80 mg caffeine/250 ml, about the same as in a cup of coffee. Performance benefits occur soon after consumption, so caffeine may be consumed 10–60 minutes before exercise, spread throughout exercise, or late in exercise as fatigue is beginning to occur (Campbell et al., 2013). As individual responses vary, you should experiment during training to find the dose and protocol that suits you. The effects of caffeine on performance is covered earlier (see pp. 118–21).

Alcohol

HOW DOES ALCOHOL AFFECT PERFORMANCE AND RECOVERY?

Alcohol features prominently in post-training and post-event celebrations in many sports. However, misuse of alcohol can interfere with performance goals in a number of ways. Alcoholic drinks not only add extra calories to your daily intake but when you consume alcohol it suppresses fat oxidation and increases the likelihood of gaining unwanted body fat. Consuming alcohol before exercise may appear to make you more alert and confident but, even in small amounts it will have a negative effect on coordination, reaction time, balance and judgement; increase injury risk, and may impair strength, power, muscular endurance, speed and endurance (ACSM, 1982).

However, athletes are more likely to consume alcohol after exercise. Studies have shown that high intakes can increase the risk of alcohol-related illness and reduce hormonal and immune function. It can also reduce muscle protein synthesis and muscle adaptation, which is likely to inhibit recovery and adaptation to exercise (Parr et al., 2014). Subjects who consumed alcohol either with protein or carbohydrate had a lower rate of MPS than those who did not consume alcohol. It is thought that alcohol suppresses the anabolic response in muscle, which would clearly impair recovery and adaptation to training and subsequent performance. However, this study was designed to mimic binge drinking and thus the alcohol intake was high (12 units). A smaller alcohol intake, e.g. a pint of beer, may not have the same effect. Alcohol has also been shown to reduce the rate of glycogen resynthesis after exercise, although this is only really apparent when it displaces carbohydrate (Burke et al., 2003). However, if you wish to consume alcohol after exercise, researchers suggest limiting your intake to 0.5 g/kg BW, equivalent to 4 units of alcohol or 2 pints of beer (see Table 8.3) (Barnes, 2014). This level of consumption is unlikely to impact recovery.

CAN I DRINK ALCOHOL ON NON-TRAINING DAYS?

There is no reason why you cannot enjoy alcohol in moderation on non-training days. The UK government recommends 14 units a week as a safe upper limit (Department of Health, 2016) (see Table 8.3 for the number of units in various drinks). Ideally, this should be spread evenly over 3 days or more and you should try to have alcohol-free days. There is some evidence that a moderate intake of alcohol brings a small reduction in heart disease risk, but it is now thought that these benefits are outweighed by the increased risk of other diseases such as cancer (GBD 2016 Alcohol Collaborators, 2016).

Table 8.3	UNITS OF ALCOHOL IN VARIOUS DRINKS
Type of drink	**Number of alcohol units**
Single shot (25 ml) spirits	1
1 pint standard strength (ABV 3.6%) beer/lager/cider	2
1 bottle (330 ml) beer/lager/cider (ABV 5%)	1.7
1 pint higher-strength beer/lager/cider (ABV 5.2%)	3
1 standard glass (175 ml) red, white or rosé wine	2.1
1 large glass (250 ml) red, white or rosé wine	3
1 (275 ml) Alcopop (ABV 5.5%)	1.5

Source: www.nhs.uk

WHAT EXACTLY HAPPENS TO ALCOHOL IN THE BODY?

When you drink alcohol, about 20% is absorbed into the bloodstream through the stomach and the remainder through the small intestine. Most of this alcohol is then broken down in the liver (it cannot be stored, as it is toxic) into a substance called acetyl CoA and then, ultimately, into ATP (adenosine triphosphate or energy). Obviously, while this is occurring, less glycogen and fat are used to produce ATP in other parts of the body.

However, the liver can carry out this job only at a fixed rate of approximately 1 unit alcohol/hour. If you drink more alcohol than this, it is dealt with by a different enzyme system in the liver (the microsomal ethanol oxidising system, MEO) to make it less toxic to the body. The more alcohol you drink on a regular basis, the more MEO enzymes are produced, which is why you can develop an increased tolerance to alcohol – you need to drink more to experience the same physiological effects.

Initially, alcohol reduces inhibitions, increases self-confidence and makes you feel more at ease. However, it is actually a depressant rather than a stimulant, reducing your psychomotor (coordination) skills. It is potentially toxic to all of the cells and organs in your body and, if it builds up to high concentrations, it can cause damage to the liver, stomach and brain.

Too much alcohol causes hangovers – headache, thirst, nausea, vomiting and heartburn. These symptoms are due partly to hypohydration and a swelling of the blood vessels in the head. Congeners, substances found mainly in darker alcoholic drinks such as rum and red wine, are also responsible for many of the hangover symptoms.

Prevention is better than cure, so make sure you follow the government guidelines. The best way to deal with a hangover is to drink plenty of water or, better still, a sports drink. Do not attempt to train or compete with a hangover!

Summary of key points

- Fluid losses during exercise depend on exercise duration and intensity, temperature and humidity, body size and fitness level.
- Hypohydration causes cardiovascular stress and increases core body temperature.
- Hypohydration >2% BW impairs aerobic exercise and cognitive performance, particularly in warm and hot conditions.
- A drop in the performance of anaerobic activities, sport-specific skills and aerobic performance in cool weather usually occurs with hypohydration 3–5% BW.
- Hydration status may be assessed by monitoring urine output and colour, body weight, urine specific gravity or urine osmolality.
- A fluid intake of 5–10 ml/kg BW in the 2–4 hours before exercise is recommended before exercise to ensure normal hydration.
- Aim to drink enough fluid during exercise so that hypohydration is limited to less than 2% BW.
- Drinking to thirst may be appropriate during activities when anticipated sweat losses are likely to be <2% BW, for example, when you are exercising for less than 90 minutes; exercising in cool conditions; or during lower-intensity exercise such as ultra-running.
- Planned drinking may be more appropriate during activities of longer duration (>90 minutes), particularly in the heat, as well as

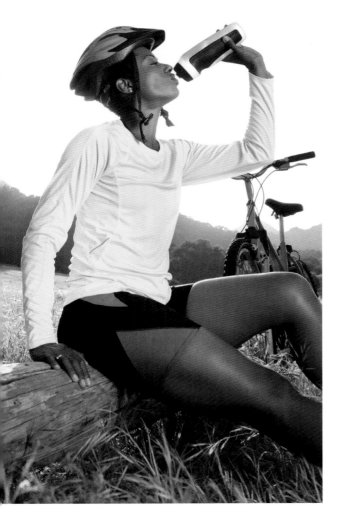

high-intensity activities with high sweat rates, and events when carbohydrate intake of more than 60 g/hour is required.

- Over-drinking can result in hyponatraemia (<130 mmol sodium/litre plasma). Symptoms include headache, nausea, bloating, water retention, disorientation and confusion. To avoid the risk of hyponatraemia during exercise, drink only to the point at which you are maintaining, not gaining, weight.

- After exercise, it is recommended to consume 1.25–1.5 times the volume of fluid lost during exercise.
- During low- or moderate-intensity activities <45 minutes, water is an effective fluid replacement drink.
- During higher-intensity exercise >60–90 minutes, a sports drink containing 40–80 g carbohydrate/litre will promote fluid replacement as well as provide fuel.
- For exercise 1–2½ h duration, a carbohydrate intake of 30–60 g/hour is recommended to maintain blood sugar concentration, delay fatigue and increase endurance. For high-intensity exercise >2½ h, an intake up to 90 g carbohydrate/h is recommended in the form of multiple transportable carbohydrates.
- Hypotonic (<40 g/litre) and isotonic (40–80 g/litre) sports drinks are appropriate when rapid fluid replacement is the main priority.
- Energy drinks based on maltodextrin (60–90 g/litre) are appropriate when fuel replacement is a major priority or fluid losses are small.
- The main purpose of sodium in a sports drink is to increase the urge to drink, promote fluid retention and increase palatability.
- The main purpose of carbohydrate in a sports drink is to promote water absorption and provide a source of energy.
- Energy drinks containing caffeine have been shown to improve various aspects of aerobic and anaerobic performance.
- Alcohol before exercise has a negative effect on strength, endurance, coordination, power and speed, and increases injury risk.
- Alcohol after exercise can reduce muscle protein synthesis and muscle adaptation, which is likely to inhibit recovery.

Body
// Composition

9

As athletes in almost every sport strive to get leaner and competitive standards get higher, the relationship between body composition, health and performance becomes increasingly important. However, the optimal body composition for fitness or sports performance is not necessarily a desirable one from a health point of view. This chapter covers the different methods for measuring body fat percentage and body fat distribution, and considers their relevance to performance. It highlights the dangers of attaining very low body fat levels, and gives realistic guidance on recommended body fat ranges.

DOES BODY FAT AFFECT PERFORMANCE?

Carrying around excess body weight in the form of fat is a distinct disadvantage in almost every sport. It can adversely affect strength, speed and endurance. Surplus fat is basically surplus baggage. Carrying around this extra weight is not only unnecessary, but also costly in terms of energy expenditure. There are three main categories of sports where high levels of body fat can have a detrimental effect on performance:

1. *Gravitational sports*, such as distance running, road and mountain bike cycling, triathlon, climbing, cross-country skiing, ski jumping, and jumping in athletics, where excess body fat impairs performance because moving the body against gravity is an essential part of these sports. For example, in distance running and road cycling, surplus fat can reduce speed and increase fatigue. It is like carrying a couple of heavy shopping bags with you; they make it harder for you to get up speed, slow you down and cause you to tire quickly. It is best to leave your shopping bags at home, or at least to lighten the load. In explosive sports (e.g. sprinting/ jumping), where you must transfer or lift the weight of your whole body very quickly, extra fat again is non-functional weight, slowing you down, reducing your power and decreasing your mechanical efficiency. Muscle is useful weight, whereas excess fat is not.

2. *Weight-category sports*, such as weightlifting, boxing, wrestling, martial arts, lightweight rowing and jockey, where greater emphasis is put on body weight, particularly during the competitive season. The person with the greatest percentage of muscle and the smallest percentage of fat has the advantage.

3. *Aesthetic sports*, such as bodybuilding, figure skating, artistic and rhythmic gymnastics, diving, dance and synchronised swimming, where success depends on body shape and composition as well as physical skill.

In virtually every sport, it is the leanest body that wins. Reducing your body fat while maintaining lean mass and health will result in improved performance.

CAN HIGH LEVELS OF BODY FAT BE AN ADVANTAGE IN CERTAIN SPORTS?

Until recently, it was believed that extra weight – even in the form of fat – was an advantage for certain sports in which momentum is important (e.g. discus, hammer throwing, judo, wrestling).

A heavy body can generate more momentum to throw an object or knock over an opponent, but there is no advantage of this weight being fat. It would be better if it were in the form of muscle. Muscle is stronger and more powerful than fat – although, admittedly, it is harder to acquire! If two athletes both weighed 100 kg, but one comprised 90 kg lean (10 kg fat) mass, and the other 70 kg lean (30 kg fat) mass, the leaner one would obviously have the advantage. Perhaps the only sport where fat could be considered a necessary advantage is sumo wrestling – it would be almost impossible to acquire a very large body mass without fat gain.

HOW CAN I TELL IF I AM CARRYING TOO MUCH FAT?

Looking in the mirror is the quickest and simplest way to see if you are carrying excess body fat by everyday standards, but this will not give the accurate information that you need for your sport. Many people also tend to perceive themselves as fatter or thinner than they really are. It is useful, therefore, to employ some sort of measurement system so that you can work towards a definite goal.

Standing on a set of scales, reading your weight and comparing it to standard weight and height charts is simple. However, it has several drawbacks. Weights and heights given in charts are based on average weights of a sample population. They are only *average* weights for *average* people, not ideal weights, and give no indication of body composition or health risk.

To get a general picture of your health risk, you can calculate your Body Mass Index (BMI) from your weight and height measurements.

WHAT IS THE BODY MASS INDEX?

Doctors and researchers often use a measurement called the Body Mass Index (BMI) to classify different grades of body weight and to assess health risk. It is sometimes referred to as the Quetelet Index after the Belgian statistician Adolphe Quetelet, who observed that for people of normal weight there is more or less a constant ratio between weight and the square of height. The BMI assumes that there is no single ideal weight for a person of a certain height, and that there is a healthy weight range for any given height.

The BMI is calculated by dividing a person's weight (in kg) by the square of his or her height (in m). For example, if your weight is 60 kg and height 1.7 m, your BMI is 21.

$$\frac{60}{1.7 \times 1.7} = 21$$

A quick online BMI calculator can be found on www.nhs.uk/live-well/healthy-weight/bmi-calculator

HOW USEFUL IS BMI?

Researchers and doctors use BMI measurements to assess a person's risk of acquiring certain health-related conditions, such as heart disease. Studies have shown that people with a BMI of between 18.5 and 25 have the lowest risk of developing diseases that are linked to obesity, e.g. cardiovascular disease, gall bladder disease, hypertension (high blood pressure) and type 2 diabetes. People with a BMI of between 25 and 29.9 are at increased risk, while those with a BMI above 30 are at a greater risk. It is important to note that BMI is a proxy of excess fat, and it is not the excess weight but the likelihood of excess fat that is linked to disease risk.

It is not true that the lower a person's BMI the better, however (*see* Table 9.1). A very low BMI is also not desirable; a BMI below 20 is associated with a higher risk of health problems, such as respiratory disease, certain cancers and metabolic complications.

Table 9.1	BMI CATEGORIES	
Category	**BMI**	
Underweight	<18.5	
Ideal	18.5–24.9	
Overweight	25–29.9	
Obese	30–39.9	
Very obese	40+	

Both those with a BMI below 18.5 and those above 30 have an increased risk of premature death (*see* Fig. 9.1).

WHAT ARE THE LIMITATIONS OF BMI?

BMI does not give information about body composition, i.e. how much weight is fat and how much lean tissue. It simply gives an indication of the health risk for *average* people – not *sportspeople*!

When you stand on the scales, you weigh everything – bone, muscle and water, as well as fat. Therefore, you do not know how much body fat you have. Muscle is denser then fat, so individuals who are athletic and/or have a muscular build may be categorised as overweight even though their body fat is low. For example, bodybuilders and rugby players with a high percentage of lean body mass and a low percentage body fat would be erroneously categorised as overweight or obese. Body fat can be underestimated in individuals who have little muscle or who are very overweight. For example, people who lose muscle as they get older may fall into the 'healthy' weight category even though they may be carrying excess fat.

Also, BMI doesn't take into account *where* fat is stored in your body. This is important because it affects your health risk as well as your body shape.

IS DISTRIBUTION OF BODY FAT IMPORTANT?

Scientists believe that the distribution of your body fat is more important than the total amount of fat. This gives a more accurate assessment of your risk of metabolic disorders such as heart disease, type 2 diabetes, high blood pressure and gall bladder disease. Fat stored mostly around the

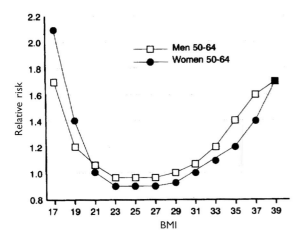

Figure 9.1 Relative risk of death according to BMI

abdomen (central obesity) gives rise to an 'apple' or 'barrel' shape, and this carries a much bigger health risk than fat stored mostly around the hips and thighs (peripheral or gynecoid obesity) in a pear shape. For most people, visceral fat is the most variable store and is one of the first places where excess fat is laid down. When the store gets too large, it begins to send out inflammatory and clot-producing compounds. It also increases the likelihood of fat spilling over into other tissues, such as the liver and pancreas, creating insulin resistance, impairing the regulation of glucose and blood lipids and increasing the risk of cardio-vascular disease. This means that a man with a 'beer belly' but slim limbs may be at greater risk of heart disease and diabetes than a pear-shaped person with the same BMI but less visceral fat.

The way we distribute fat on our body is determined partly by our genetic make-up and partly by our natural hormonal balance. Men, for example, tend to have higher levels of testos-terone, which favours fat deposition around the abdomen, between the shoulder blades and close

to the internal organs. Women have higher levels of oestrogen, which favours fat deposition around the hips, thighs, breasts and triceps. After the menopause, however, when oestrogen levels fall, fat tends to transfer from the hips and thighs to the abdomen, giving women more of an apple shape and pushing up their chances of heart disease (Davis *et al.*, 2012) (*see* p. 279).

Excess fat in the abdomen is a health risk. This is partly to do with the close proximity of the intra-abdominal fat to the liver. Fatty acids from the adipose tissue are delivered into the portal vein that goes directly to the liver. The liver thus receives a continuous supply of fat-rich blood and this stimulates increased cholesterol synthesis. A high blood cholesterol level is a major risk factor for heart disease.

HOW CAN I MEASURE MY BODY FAT DISTRIBUTION?

You can assess your body fat distribution by two methods:

1. *Waist circumference* Scientists at the Royal Infirmary, Glasgow, have found that waist circumference measurement correlates well with intra-abdominal fat and total body fat percentage (Lean *et al.*, 1995) and is more accurate than body weight or BMI in predict-ing type 2 diabetes (Wang *et al.*, 2005). A waist circumference of 94 cm (37 in) or more in men or 80 cm (31.5 in) or more in women indicates excess abdominal fat.

2. *Waist-to-height ratio* This is a more accurate method than BMI for assessing health risk (Ashwell *et al.*, 2011). Divide your waist measurement by your height. It should be no more than half your height. If your waist

measures more than half your height then your health risks are higher and your life expectancy lower. For example, if you are 1.72 m (5ft 8 in/68 in) tall, your waist size should be 86 cm (34 in) or less.

WHAT DOES BODY COMPOSITION MEAN?

Body composition can be defined as the proportion of fat mass (FM) and fat-free mass (FFM) in the body. FFM includes muscles, organs, bones and blood. FM includes fat that is stored as an energy source and fat in the central nervous system, bone marrow and the fat surrounding your organs, known as essential fat. The proportion of these various components in the body is called body composition. This is more important than total body weight. Body composition is typically expressed as a 'two compartment model', meaning that it assesses FM and FFM.

For example, two people may weigh the same, but have a different body composition. Athletes usually have a smaller percentage of body fat and a higher percentage of lean weight than less physically active people. Lean body tissue is functional (or useful) weight, whereas fat is non-functional in terms of sports performance.

HOW CAN I MEASURE BODY COMPOSITION?

Clearly, height and weight measurements are not useful for assessing your body composition. To give you a more accurate idea of how much fat and FFM you have, there are a number of techniques for measuring body composition, which vary in accuracy, reliability and cost. The only method that is 100% accurate is cadaver analysis. Clearly this is impractical, so indirect methods must be used. These are based on assumptions of body compartments so will provide only an estimate of body composition.

Underwater weighing (hydrodensitometry)

For a long time, this method was judged to be the most accurate. Its accuracy rate averages 97–98%. However, there are other methods, such as dual-energy X-ray absorptiometry and magnetic resonance imaging, which produce similar, if not more accurate, results.

Underwater weighing works on the Archimedes' principle, which states that when an object is submerged under water it creates a buoyant counter force equal to the weight of water that it has displaced. Since bone and muscle are more dense than water, a person with a higher percentage of lean mass will weigh more in water, indicating a lower percentage of fat. Since fat is less dense than water, a person with a high fat percentage will weigh less in water than on land.

In this test, the person sits on a swing-seat and is then submerged into a water tank. After expelling as much air as possible from the lungs, the person's weight is recorded. This figure is then compared with the person's weight on dry land, using standard equations on a computer, and FFM and FM calculated.

The disadvantage of this method is that the specialised equipment is expensive and bulky and found only at research institutions or laboratories, i.e. it is not readily available to the public. The person also needs to be water-confident.

Air displacement plethysmography (ADP or BOD POD)

A newer method is the ADP, which is similar to the principle behind underwater weighing but

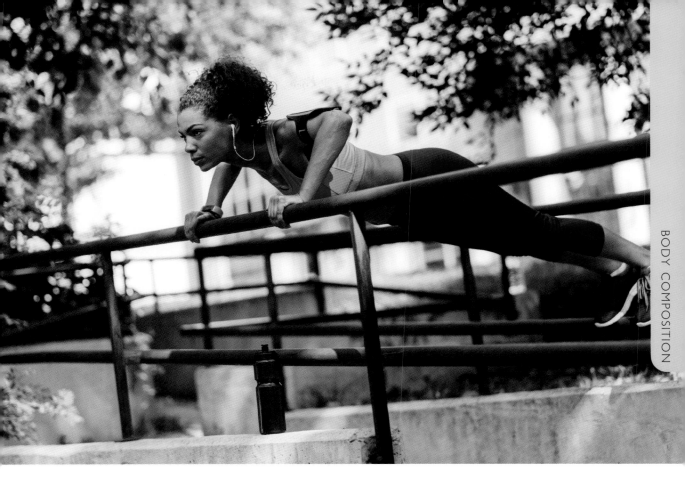

uses air displacement within an enclosed chamber (BOD POD) rather than weight under water. Body volume is indirectly measured by measuring the volume of air displaced in the chamber. Volume and body weight are then used to calculate body density, which allows FFM and FM to be estimated. But, like underwater weighing, it is available only through university exercise science departments and is relatively expensive.

Skinfold measurements

The skinfold measurement method is widely available in gyms, health clubs, clinics and practices. The callipers measure in millimetres the layer of fat just underneath the skin at various places on the body. This is done on three to seven specific places (such as the triceps, biceps, hip bone area, lower back, abdomen, thigh and below the shoulder blade). Using these measurements, scientists have developed mathematical equations that account for age, sex and known body densities to produce a body density value, which another equation then changes into a body fat percentage. Alternatively, skinfold thicknesses themselves can be used as a proxy of body fatness in several regions to look at individual changes over time.

The accuracy of this method depends almost entirely on the skill of the person taking the measurements. Also, it assumes that everyone has a predictable pattern of fat distribution as they age. Therefore, it becomes less accurate with elite athletes, as they tend to have a different pattern of fat distribution compared with sedentary people, and for very lean and obese people. There are different sets of equations to use, which take account of these factors. For the general population (over 15% body fat), the Durnin and Womersley (1974) equations are more suitable. The Jackson–Pollock (1984) equations apply best to lean and athletic people (Pollock and Jackson, 1984)

Kinanthropometry is the term for the recording of skinfold thickness measurements and body girth measurements (e.g. arms, chest, legs etc.) in order to monitor changes in body composition over time. The sites of girth measurements are shown in Figure 9.2.

An alternative is to present the body fat measurement as a 'sum of skinfolds'. This is the sum of the individual skinfold thicknesses from the seven specific sites.

Bioelectrical impedance analysis

Most body fat monitors and scales work using bioelectrical impedance analysis (BIA). These are widely available in gyms, health clubs and clinics, as well as for home use. Here, a mild electrical current is sent through the body between electrodes attached to two specific points of the body (either between the hand and opposite foot, or from one foot to the other). The principle is that lean tissue (such as muscle and blood) contains high levels of water and electrolytes and is therefore a good conductor of electricity, whereas fat creates a resistance. Increasing levels of fat mass result in a higher impedance value and correspond to higher levels of body fat.

The advantages are the machine is portable, simple to operate and testing takes less than 1 minute. The disadvantage is the poor degree of accuracy compared with other methods. For example, changes in body fluid levels and skin temperature will affect the passage of the current and therefore the body fat reading. It tends to overestimate the body fat percentage of lean muscular people by 2–5% and underestimate the body fat percentage of overweight people by the same amount (Sun et al., 2005). It is important that you are well-hydrated when having a BIA measurement; if you are hypohydrated, the current will not be conducted through your lean mass so well, giving you a higher body fat percentage reading.

Dual-energy X-ray absorptiometry

Dual-energy X-ray absorptiometry (DEXA) was originally developed for measuring bone density and diagnosing osteoporosis. However, it can also be used to measure body composition. It produces an accurate body composition map, showing where your fat is distributed around the body (e.g. trunk vs legs and arms). In this method, two types of low-energy X-rays are scanned over the whole body, which are absorbed differently by bone, muscle and fat. The procedure takes about 5–20 minutes, depending on the type of machine.

It is one of the most accurate methods for assessing body fat, although less reliable for lean athletes (Ackland et al., 2012). The disadvantages are the cost and size of the machine, lack of accessibility and exposure to radiation. DEXA machines are found in hospitals and research institutions. It may be possible to request a body fat analysis at your nearest site, but be prepared to pay considerably more than you would for the other methods.

Magnetic resonance imaging (MRI)

An MRI scanner uses magnetic fields and radio waves to produce detailed 3D images of the body. The body is scanned in segments or slices, which are used to predict whole body values. An MRI scan provides the most precise body composition measurement and is regarded as the gold standard method. It can distinguish between visceral and subcutaneous fat. However, MRI scanners are expensive and used mainly for research, so are not a practical method for everyday body composition measurement.

HOW ACCURATE ARE THESE METHODS?

Table 9.2 summarises studies that have assessed the accuracy of the various methods. MRI, DEXA and underwater weighing are regarded as the most accurate methods (Ackland *et al.*, 2012). Skinfold and BIA measurements – provided they are carefully carried out – can estimate body fat percentages with a 3–4% error (Houtkooper, 2000; Lohman, 1992). For example, if the actual body fat percentage is 15% then predicted values could range from 12 to 18% (assuming a 3% error). However, if poor measurement techniques or incorrectly calibrated instruments are used then the margin of error could be greater. Since a relatively high degree of error is associated with these indirect body fat assessment methods, it is not recommended to set a specific body fat goal for athletes. Instead, a range of target body fat values would be more realistic.

WHAT IS THE MINIMUM BODY FAT I NEED?

A fat-free body would not survive. It is important to realise that a certain amount of body fat is

Table 9.2	ACCURACY OF BODY FAT MEASUREMENT METHODS
Method	**Degree of inaccuracy**
DEXA	<2%
Skinfold measurement	3–4%
BOD POD	2–3.5%
Underwater weighing	2–3%
Bioelectrical impedance	3–5%
Near-infrared interactance	5–10%

Source: Ackland et al., 2012.

vital for life. In fact, there are two components of body fat: essential fat and storage fat.

Essential fat includes the fat that forms part of your cell membranes, brain tissue, nerve sheaths, bone marrow and the fat surrounding your organs (e.g. heart, liver, kidneys). Here, it provides insulation, protection and cushioning against physical damage. In a healthy person, this accounts for about 3% of body weight.

Women have an additional essential fat requirement called *sex-specific fat*, which is stored mostly in the breasts and around the hips. This fat accounts for a further 5–9% of a woman's body weight and is involved in oestrogen production as well as the conversion of inactive oestrogen into its active form. So, this fat ensures normal hormonal balance and menstrual function. If stores fall too low, hormonal imbalance and menstrual irregularities result, although these can be reversed once body fat increases (*see* p. 224). There is some recent evidence that a certain amount of body fat in men is necessary for normal hormone production, too. It is commonly suggested that 5% body fat for men and 12% for women is the minimum required for healthy endocrine and immune function (Lohman, 1992).

The second component of body fat, *storage fat*, is an important energy reserve that takes the form of fat (adipose) cells under the skin (subcutaneous fat) and around the organs (intra-abdominal fat). Fat is used virtually all the time during any aerobic activity: while sleeping, sitting, standing and walking, as well as in most types of exercise. It is impossible to spot reduce fat selectively from adipose tissue sites by specific exercises or diets. The body generally uses fat from all sites, although the exact pattern of fat utilisation (and storage) is determined by your genetic make-up and hormonal balance. An average person has

enough fat for 3 days and 3 nights of continuous running – although, in practice, you would experience fatigue long before your fat reserves ran out. So, your fat stores are certainly not a redundant depot of unwanted energy!

WHAT IS A DESIRABLE BODY FAT PERCENTAGE FOR ATHLETES?

There is no 'one size fits all' recommendation. Body fat percentages for athletes vary depending on the particular sport. According to scientists at the University of Arizona, the ideal body fat percentage, in terms of performance, for most male athletes lies between 6 and 15%, and for female athletes, 12 and 18% (Wilmore, 1983). In male athletes, middle- and long-distance runners and bodybuilders have the lowest body fat levels (less than 6%) while cyclists, gymnasts, sprinters, triathletes and basketball players average between

Table 9.3	AVERAGE BODY FAT PERCENTAGES IN VARIOUS SPORTS				
Sport	**Male**	**Female**	**Sport**	**Male**	**Female**
Baseball	12–15%	12–18%	Shot put	16–20%	20–28%
Basketball	6–12%	20–27%	Skiing (X country)	7–12%	16–22%
Bodybuilding	5–8%	10–15%	Sprinting	8–10%	12–20%
Cycling	5–15%	15–20%	Swimming	9–12%	14–24%
Gymnastics	5–12%	10–16%	Tennis	12–16%	16–24%
High/long jumping	7–12%	10–18%	Triathlon	5–12%	10–15%
Ice/field hockey	8–15%	12–18%	Volleyball	11–14%	16–25%
Racquetball	8–13%	15–22%	Weightlifting	9–16%	No data
Rowing	6–14%	12–18%	Wrestling	5–16%	No data

Source: Ackland *et al.*, 2012.

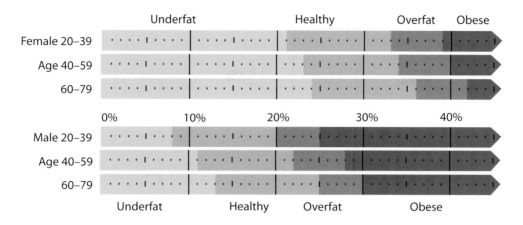

Figure 9.2 Healthy body fat ranges for adults

Source: Gallagher *et al.*, 2000.

6 and 15% body fat (Sinning, 1998). In female athletes, the lowest body fat levels (6–15%) are observed in bodybuilders, cyclists, gymnasts, runners and triathletes (Sinning, 1998).

Physiologists recommend a minimum of 5% fat for men and 12% fat for women to cover the most basic functions associated with good health (Lohman, 1992). However, optimal body fat levels may be much higher than these minimums. The percentage of fat associated with lowest health risk is 13–18% for men and 18–25% for women. Figure 9.2 gives the body fat percentages for standard (non-athletic) adults.

Clearly, there is no ideal body fat percentage for any particular sport. Each individual athlete has an optimal fat range at which their performance improves yet their health does not suffer. For this reason, sports scientists believe that a range of values for body fat percentage should be established, outside of which your performance and/or health is likely to be impaired. Staying below the upper limit should be your target but lower is not necessarily better.

LOWER IS NOT NECESSARILY BETTER

Reducing your body fat may lead to improvements in performance but if the loss is too rapid or too severe then your performance and health may suffer. Women and men who try to attain very low body fat levels, or a level that is unnatural for their genetic make-up, encounter problems. These problems can be serious, particularly for women, who may suffer long-term effects. Collectively known as 'relative energy deficiency in sport (RED-S)', these problems are discussed in greater detail in Chapter 11.

WHAT ARE THE DANGERS FOR WOMEN WITH VERY LOW BODY FAT LEVELS?

One of the biggest problems for women with very low body fat levels is the resulting hormonal imbalance and amenorrhoea (absence of periods).

As explained in more detail in Chapter 11, this tends to be triggered once body fat levels fall below a certain threshold, which varies from one person to another. This fall in body fat, together with other factors such as low energy availability (*see* p. 209), disordered eating behaviour, high-intensity training and volume, and physical and emotional stress is sensed by the hypothalamus of the brain, which then decreases its production of the hormone (gonadotrophin-releasing hormone) that acts on the pituitary gland. This, in turn, reduces the production of important hormones that act on the ovaries (luteinising hormone and follicle-stimulating hormone), causing them to produce less oestrogen and progesterone. The end result is a deficiency of oestrogen and progesterone and a cessation of menstrual periods (*see* Fig. 9.3).

Amenorrhoea can lead to more serious problems such as bone loss, because low oestrogen

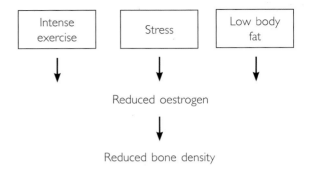

Figure 9.4 Low body fat and bone density

levels result in loss of bone minerals and, therefore, bone density (*see* Fig. 9.4). In younger (premenopausal) women, this is called osteopoenia (i.e. lower bone density than normal for age), which is similar to the osteoporosis that affects postmenopausal women, where bones become thinner, lighter and more fragile. Amenorrhoeic athletes, therefore, run a greater risk of stress fractures. The British Olympic Medical Centre has reported cases of athletes in their 20s and 30s with osteoporotic-type fractures.

Low body fat levels also upset the metabolism of the sex hormones, reducing their potency and thus fertility. Therefore, a very low body fat level drastically reduces a woman's fertility. However, the good news is that once your body fat level increases over your threshold and your training volume is reduced, your hormonal balance, periods and fertility generally return to normal.

WHAT ARE THE DANGERS FOR MEN WITH VERY LOW BODY FAT LEVELS?

Body fat and testosterone are interlinked. Studies on competitive male wrestlers 'making weight' for contests found that once body fat levels fell below 5%, testosterone levels decreased, causing

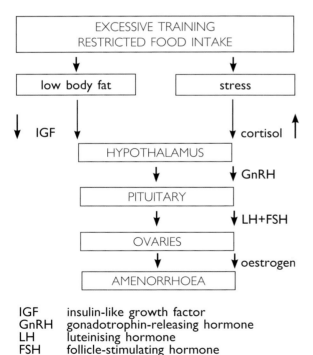

IGF	insulin-like growth factor
GnRH	gonadotrophin-releasing hormone
LH	luteinising hormone
FSH	follicle-stimulating hormone

Figure 9.3 The development of amenorrhoea

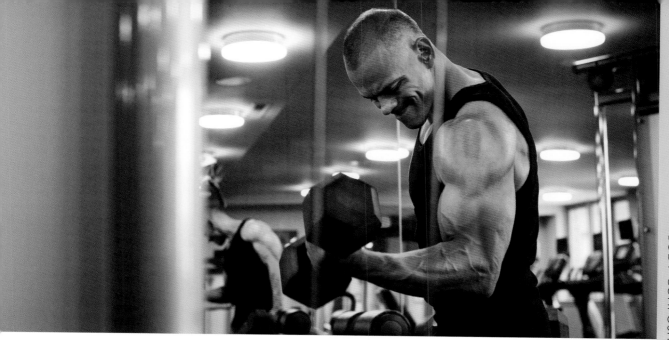

a drastic fall in sperm count and libido (Strauss *et al.*, 1985). Similar correlations were reported in a study that tracked a natural bodybuilder for 6 months as he prepared for a competition (Rossow *et al.*, 2013). His body fat reduced from 14.8% to 4.5%, but he also experienced an 80% drop in testosterone levels and an increase in 'mood disturbances'. A study of male road cyclists measured higher levels of fatigue, illness, injury (including fractures), a drop in cycling performance and a less successful race season in those who intentionally restricted their dietary intake (Keay *et al.*, 2019). Low testosterone levels can cause a decrease in libido, bone loss, muscle loss, fatigue, sleep disruption, mood changes and infertility. However, testosterone levels and libido return to normal once body fat increases.

Thyroid hormone, growth hormone, IGF-1, metabolic rate and the immune system are all severely reduced when body fat levels drop too low. Cortisol levels rise drastically, especially during periods of intense training.

Summary of key points

- Excess body fat is a disadvantage in almost all sports and fitness programmes, reducing power, speed and performance.
- Very low body fat does not guarantee improved performance either. There appears to be an optimal fat range for each individual, which cannot be predicted by a standard linear relationship.
- There are three main components of body fat: 1) essential fat (for tissue structure); 2) sex-specific fat (for hormonal function); and 3) storage fat (for energy).
- The minimum percentage of fat recommended for men is 5% and for women, 10%. However, for normal health, the recommended ranges are 13–18% and 18–25% respectively. In practice, many athletes fall below these recommended ranges.
- Very low body fat levels are associated with hormonal imbalance in both sexes, and amenorrhoea, infertility, reduced bone density and increased risk of osteoporosis in women.

Weight //Management

10

Many athletes and active individuals wish to lose weight, either to improve health and performance, make a competitive weight category or for aesthetic reasons. However, inappropriate weight loss methods and rapid weight loss can have serious health and performance consequences, leading to a drop in performance, low energy availability and disordered eating. A knowledge of safe weight loss methods is, therefore, essential. Since 95% of dieters fail to maintain their weight loss within a 5-year period, lifestyle management is the key to long-term weight management.

This chapter examines the effects of weight loss on performance and health, and highlights the health risks of rapid weight loss methods. Research on appetite control and metabolism is presented, along with guidance for losing fat and retaining muscle mass. It considers the evidence behind different dietary approaches, from low carbohydrate to low fat, and gives an evidence-based, step-by-step strategy for successful fat loss.

On the other hand, many athletes want to gain weight. This is usually a desire to increase muscle mass in order to improve strength and sports performance, although muscle and strength are also associated with good health and longevity.

This chapter explains the science of muscle growth and gives an evidence-based diet and exercise strategy to achieve weight gain.

WILL DIETING AFFECT MY HEALTH OR PERFORMANCE?

Reducing body fat levels can be advantageous to performance in many sports (*see* p. 168 'Does body fat affect performance?'). However, it is important to achieve this through scientifically proven methods. Unfortunately, rapid weight loss can have serious health consequences, and lead to a marked reduction in performance.

To make weight for a competition (e.g. boxing, bodybuilding, judo), athletes may resort to rapid weight loss methods, such as fasting, hypohydration, exercising in sweatsuits, saunas, diet pills, laxatives, diuretics or self-induced vomiting. Weight losses of 4.5 kg in 3 days are not uncommon. In a study of 180 female athletes, 32% admitted they used more than one of these methods (Rosen *et al.*, 1986). In another, 15% of young female swimmers said they had tried one of these methods (Drummer *et al.*, 1987). Clearly, an athlete may achieve a desirable weight category or appearance, but to the detriment of his or her performance.

Hypohydration results in a reduced cardiac output and stroke volume, reduced plasma volume, slower nutrient exchange and slower waste removal, all of which have an impact on health and performance (Fogelholm, 1994; Fleck and Reimers, 1994). In moderate-intensity exercise lasting more than 30 seconds, even hypohydration of less than 5% body weight will diminish strength or performance, although it does not appear to affect exercise lasting less than 30 seconds. So, for athletes relying on pure strength (e.g. weightlifting), rapid weight loss may not be as detrimental.

Rapid weight loss results in a diminished aerobic capacity (Fogelholm, 1994). A drop of up to 5% has been measured in athletes who had lost just 2–3% of body weight through hypohydration. A loss of 10% can occur in those who lose weight through strict dieting. Anaerobic performance, strength and muscular endurance are also decreased, although researchers have found that strength (expressed against body weight) can actually improve after gradual weight loss (Tipton, 1987).

Prolonged dieting can also have serious health consequences. In female athletes, low body weight and body fat have been linked with menstrual irregularities, amenorrhoea and stress fractures (see pp. 177–8); in male athletes, with reduced testosterone production (see pp. 178–9). It has also been suggested that the combination of intense training, food restriction and the psychological pressure for extreme leanness may precipitate disordered eating and clinical eating disorders in some susceptible athletes (Sundgot-Borgen 1994 (a) and (b)).

There is a fine line between dieting and obsessive eating behaviour, and many female athletes, in particular, are under pressure to be thin and improve their performance. The warning signs and health consequences of eating disorders are discussed in Chapter 11.

IS REPEATED WEIGHT LOSS HARMFUL?
Repeated weight loss, weight cycling or yo-yo dieting has been linked with an increased risk of heart disease, secondary diabetes, gall bladder disease and premature death. However, studies are divided as to whether it makes you more likely to regain weight and develop obesity. One review of 31 studies concluded that there is little detrimental effect of weight cycling on current and future obesity and metabolic risk (Mackie et al., 2017). Contrary to popular belief, there is no evidence that weight cycling permanently slows your metabolism (it returns to its original levels once normal eating is resumed) (Muls et al., 1995). But yo-yo dieting can be harmful for your psychological health. Each time you regain weight, you experience a sense of failure, which can lower your confidence and self-esteem.

WHAT MAKES YOUR RESTING METABOLIC RATE HIGH OR LOW?
Resting metabolic rate (RMR) is the energy burned at rest and makes up the largest component of your total daily energy expenditure (TDEE), on average between 60 and 75% (see p. 17). The most important factor that determines your RMR is your body weight. The more you weigh, the higher your RMR, because the larger your body, the more calories it needs for basic maintenance. The amount of fat-free mass you have (muscle, bone and vital organs) also affects RMR. This is calorie-burning tissue, so the more fat-free mass you have, the higher your RMR will be.

High-intensity exercise (greater than 60% VO_2max) that's sustained for at least 30 minutes temporarily raises your RMR as your body pays off the oxygen debt, replenishes its energy reserves (PC and ATP) and repairs muscle tissue. This post-exercise increase in RMR is called the excess post-exercise oxygen consumption (EPOC) and comes chiefly from the body's fat stores. The longer and more intense the workout, the greater the EPOC. However, the increase in RMR is usually temporary and relatively small, returning to baseline within a few hours.

It is a myth that overweight people have a lower RMR than lean people (except in clinical conditions such as hypothyroidism or Cushing's syndrome). Numerous studies have shown a linear relationship between total body weight and metabolic rate, i.e. the RMR increases proportionally with increasing body weight. Genetics undoubtedly play a role – some people have genes that can increase appetite and reduce metabolism, which can predispose them to gain excess weight. However, this does not mean that obesity is inevitable; it can be prevented by effective nutrition, physical activity and behavioural strategies.

CAN DIETING SLOW MY RMR?

When you restrict your calories, this has a knock-on effect on energy expenditure. Feedback regulation occurs resulting in a compensatory increase in appetite and drop in RMR, non-exercise activity thermogeneisis (NEAT) and exercise activity thermogenesis (EAT) (see p. 17) as the body tries to resist weight loss and preserve its energy stores (Polidori et al., 2016). This explains why most people find it difficult to adhere to weight loss diets for long periods and regain weight after dieting.

Definition of terms

Metabolism is the term given to all processes by which your body converts food into energy. The *metabolic rate* is the rate at which your body burns calories. Your *basal metabolic rate (BMR)* is the rate at which you burn calories on essential body functions, such as breathing and blood circulation during sleep, and measured in a fasted state. In practice, the *resting metabolic rate (RMR)* is more frequently used, as it can be measured while you are awake and in a non-fasting state. It accounts for 60–75% of the calories you burn daily.

This slowdown of RMR is called 'adaptive thermogenesis' (Rosenbaum and Leibel, 2010; Dulloo and Jacquet, 1998). The more severe the fat loss, the greater the decrease in your RMR. Generally, the RMR decrease is between 10 and 30%. Essentially, it's your body's way of conserving energy and maintaining normal body weight when energy is in short supply (Tremblay et al., 2013). One study found that when people were put on a restricted calorie diet, they had a lower RMR than could be explained by their weight loss (Heilbronn et al., 2006). Adaptive thermogenesis can be triggered within 3 days of dieting but RMR is thought to be restored once people become weight stable (Ostendorf et al., 2018).

Also, when you create a large calorie deficit, protein oxidation increases and this can lead to loss of lean muscle tissue. Muscle burns around 15–25 calories per kilogram each day, so when you lose muscle through dieting your RMR will further slow down. This means you will need fewer calories than you did previously.

When you lose body fat, fat cells shrink and produce less leptin, signalling to your brain a reduction in the body's energy stores. Leptin normally inhibits appetite and increases RMR, but when leptin levels fall, RMR slows and hunger increases in an attempt to preserve the body's fuel stores.

HOW CAN I LOSE BODY FAT WITHOUT LOSING MUSCLE?

The key to losing body fat while retaining muscle is to reduce your usual calorie intake by a relatively modest amount of 15% (or 10–20%). This will minimise the metabolic slowdown that is associated with more severe calorie reductions. If you cut calories more severely, it will not make you lose fat faster. Instead, it will cause your body to lower its metabolic rate in an attempt to conserve energy stores. Research has shown that a relatively modest rate of weight (around 0.7% loss of BW/week) in combination with resistance training preserves muscle mass while improving strength gains (Garthe *et al.*, 2011).

In theory, 0.45 kg (1 lb) of fat can be shed when a deficit of 3500 kcal/week is created. However, in practice, it may not work exactly like this because it depends on your initial calorie intake. For example, athlete A normally eats 3000 kcal/day and athlete B normally eats 2000 kcal/day. If both athletes reduced their calorie intake by 3500 kcal/week (or 500 kcal/day), athlete A now eats 2500 kcal/day and athlete B now eats 1500 kcal/day. The two athletes will, in practice, get very differ-

WEIGHT MANAGEMENT

Are all calories equal?

Thermodynamics dictate that a calorie is a calorie regardless of the macronutrient composition of the diet. However, when food is consumed, there is a difference in the amount of energy from protein, carbohydrate and fat that can be utilised by the body for fuel. Some of the energy consumed will be used up digesting and absorbing the food and converting it into available fuel. This is called the thermic effect of food (TEF). TEF represents approximately 10% of total daily energy expenditure, although the TEF for each macronutrient is different. Protein has a higher TEF than the other macronutrients, equating to 25–30% of total calories (Jéquier, 2002). In other words, for every 100 calories of protein consumed, 25–30 of these calories will be used up digesting, absorbing and metabolising it, leaving only about 70–75 available to the body. In contrast, the TEF of carbohydrate is 6–8% and the TEF of fat is 2–3%. This means that protein is the least efficient source of energy, while fat is the most efficient fuel source. Additionally, protein has a higher satiating effect than carbohydrate or fat, so it can help you achieve a negative energy balance. This also explains why high-protein low-carbohydrate diets may produce greater weight loss (at least in the short term) compared with other diets: protein makes you feel less hungry so you spontaneously eat less. However, in studies where calories are rigorously controlled, there is no significant difference in weight loss between high- and low-carbohydrate diets.

ent results in terms of their body composition. Athlete A will likely lose around 0.45 kg fat/week because they have created a modest 15% reduction. Athlete B may lose 0.45 kg fat/week initially, but they will also lose significant amounts of muscle tissue. That's because they cut their calories by 25%, which is too severe. In general, calorie reductions of greater than 15% will lead to a metabolic slowdown and muscle loss, making fat loss slower. Furthermore, neither athlete will continue losing 0.45 kg fat/week indefinitely; the rate of loss will slow down or plateau as body weight drops and fewer calories are needed for weight maintenance. To continue losing body fat, progressively greater reductions in calorie intake or greater increases in calorie expenditure are required.

Reducing calorie intake by approximately 15% will lead to fat loss without appreciably slowing the metabolism. Chapter 18, shows you how to calculate your calorie, carbohydrate, protein and fat requirements to lose body fat at an effective rate.

WILL I STILL BE ABLE TO TRAIN HARD WHILE LOSING WEIGHT?

The problem with most weight loss diets is they do not provide enough calories or carbohydrate

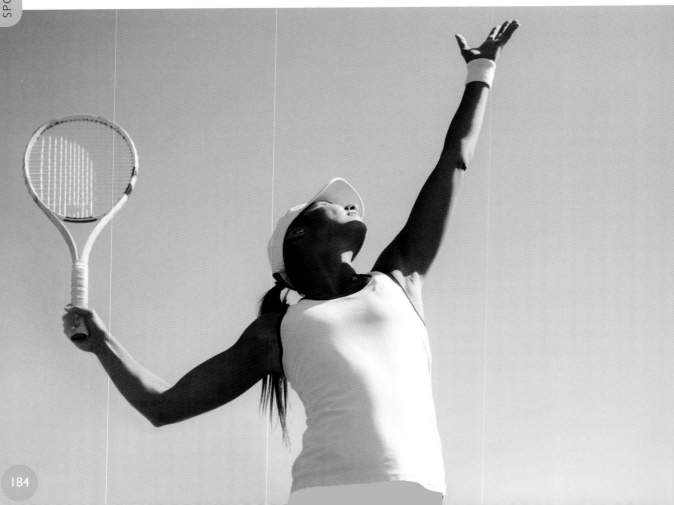

to support intense training. When energy intake is too low or energy expended through exercise is too high, this can lead to low energy availability (LEA) (*see* p. 209), leaving you with depleted muscle glycogen stores, persistent fatigue, poor performance, loss of lean body mass and insufficient energy to support essential functions such as metabolic and immune function, bone health and the menstrual cycle in female athletes. LEA is a major cause of relative energy deficiency in sport (RED-S), which can have detrimental effects on health and performance (*see* pp. 213–17).

It is possible to continue training hard while losing weight provided you reduce your calorie intake by no more than 15% on some training days, not all of them. Any more than this risks LEA. Additionally, increasing protein intake to 1.8–2.0 g/kg/day is recommended in order to prevent lean mass losses during periods of energy restriction (Phillips and Van Loon, 2011).

One consistent finding from studies is that an adequate carbohydrate intake (>3 g/kg BW/day) is critical for preserving muscular strength, endurance, and both aerobic and anaerobic capacity. A lower intake can result in glycogen depletion and increased protein oxidation (muscle loss). Retaining lean mass is also vital for losing fat. The less muscle you have, the lower your resting metabolic rate and the harder it is to lose fat.

If you compete in weight-category or weight-sensitive sports (*see* p. 211), you should aim to lose any excess weight during the base phase of training rather than during the build or competition phase, when training intensity is higher.

WEIGHT LOSS DIETS

Most diets work in the short term, but not all are healthy and most are not sustainable in the long term. The more extreme the diet, the lower the chance of adhering to it.

Low-carbohydrate diets

There is no universal definition of a low-carbohydrate diet (LCD) but the consensus is that it involves a carbohydrate intake <130 g/day (Feinman *et al.*, 2015). Very low-carbohydrate diets (VLCDs), or ketogenic diets, are defined by their ability to raise ketone levels in the bloodstream – a state called ketosis – which is attained by restricting carbohydrate to a maximum of 50 g/day (Westman *et al.*, 2007). The idea behind ketogenic diets is that they force the body to burn fat preferentially instead of carbohydrate. When you severely restrict carbohydrate, fats are broken down in a different way – a process called ketogenesis – into ketones (D-β-hydroxybutyrate, acetone and acetoacetate), which can then be converted into energy.

Proponents of low-carbohydrate diets claim that people lose weight more effectively when insulin levels are kept as low as possible. According to the 'insulin theory', carbohydrate causes a rise in blood insulin levels, which in turn, encourages the body to store fat. Over time, body cells become unresponsive to the actions of insulin ('insulin resistance') and, as a result, the pancreas produces more of it, further pushing the body into fat-storage mode. The solution, according to low-carbohydrate proponents, is to cut carbohydrate intake dramatically and force the body to go into ketosis. The resulting low insulin levels inhibit fat storage and promote fat oxidation.

However, LCDs have been criticised by eminent researchers who state that it is not the insulin that makes people put on weight; the opposite is more likely to be true. In most cases, it's having high levels of body fat that makes people insulin resistant. When people lose weight, insulin control usually returns to normal.

LCDs may result in short-term weight loss, partly due to depletion of glycogen stores (and the accompanying water), and partly because they create a calorie deficit. If you cut carbohydrate, you automatically restrict the foods you can eat. It's difficult to overeat high-protein foods such as meat and eggs and with fewer choices most people end up consuming fewer calories. Also, the high protein and fat content of LCDs and VLCDs (rather than the low carbohydrate content) makes them more satiating so you feel less hungry and spontaneously eat less (Soenen *et al.*, 2012). It's a simple negative energy balance equation.

In randomised controlled trials, LCDs and low-fat diets both produce similar (modest) long-term weight loss results. Most meta-analyses show that weight loss differences between the two diets are minimal at 12 months, although LCDs usually produce slightly greater weight loss at 6 months (Johnston *et al.*, 2014). The US National Lipid Association Nutrition and Lifestyle Task Force concluded that LCD and ketogenic diets are not superior to other dietary approaches for weight loss and, while they may have advantages related to appetite control, are difficult to maintain in the long term (Kirkpatrick *et al.*, 2019). In one of the largest studies to date, the Diet Intervention Examining The Factors Interacting with Treatment Success (DIETFITS), researchers found no significant difference in weight loss between a low-fat vs a low-carbohydrate diet after 12 months (Gardner *et al.*, 2018). A systematic review of randomised control trials showed no difference in weight loss between LCDs and low-fat diets (Churuangsuk *et al.*, 2018).

A meta-analysis of 32 controlled feeding studies (where all food was provided to the subjects as opposed to self-selected intake) with isocaloric (having similar caloric value) substitution of carbohydrate for fat found that both energy expenditure and fat loss were greater with lower-fat diets (Hall and Guo, 2017). In other words, LCDs do not have any thermic or fat loss advantage, as is often claimed by LCD proponents. In fact, the opposite may hold, according to a rigorous study at the National Institutes of Health, US (Hall *et al.*, 2015). In the study, 19 obese adults were confined to a metabolic ward for two 2-week periods and given diets that cut their calorie intake by a third, by reducing either carbohydrates or fat. Researchers analysed the amount of oxygen and carbon dioxide breathed out to calculate precisely the chemical processes taking place inside the body. After 6 days on each diet, those on the low-fat diet lost 80% more body fat than those on the LCD.

These conclusions apply equally to athletes and the general population. A review of studies conducted between 1921 and 2021 concluded that ketogenic diets do not have any benefits over other diets in terms of weight or body fat loss for athletes (Ashtary-Larky *et al.*, 2021). What's more, ketogenic diets can cause a loss of lean mass in resistance-trained individuals.

If there is any advantage of LCDs over other diets for weight loss, it is potentially their ability to reduce hunger and increase satiety. However, this is likely due to their high protein or fat content rather than restriction of carbohydrate. The potential benefits and disadvantages of LCDs for endurance performance are covered in Chapter 3 (*see* pp. 55–63).

Low-fat diets

Low-fat diets can be defined as providing 20–35% energy from fat (Aragon *et al.*, 2017). This is consistent with the dietary recommendations by Public Health England for the general population (Public Health England, 2011) as well as those by major health organisations.

A review of 32 randomised control trials showed an association between the proportion of energy from fat in the diet and body weight in the general population (Hooper *et al.*, 2015(a)). Researchers found that cutting down on the proportion of fat consumed (compared to usual intake) led to a decrease in body weight, BMI, body fat and waist circumference. Low-fat diets are likely to cause weight loss by creating a calorie deficit. Since fat is the most energy dense nutrient, cutting fat is likely to cause a significant reduction in calorie intake, thereby reducing body fat over time. Experiments that have covertly manipulated the fat content of the diet so that it looks and tastes the same show that low-fat diets result in greater weight loss and vice versa (Lissner *et al.*, 1987).

It is recommended that athletes should consume a minimum of 20% energy from fat (Thomas *et al.*, 2016). Very low-fat diets (VLFDs) providing less than 20% energy from fat can leave you deficient in a variety of nutrients and increase the risk of health problems. You will certainly be missing out on the essential fatty acids (linoleic acid and linolenic acid) found in vegetable oils, seeds, nuts and oily fish (*see* pp. 87–90).

VLFDs are likely to be low in fat-soluble vitamins A, D and E. More importantly, fat is needed to enable your body to absorb and transport them, and to convert beta-carotene into vitamin A in the body. Although you can get vitamin D from UV light and vitamin A from beta-carotene in brightly coloured fruit and vegetables, getting enough vitamin E can be much more of a problem. It is found in significant quantities only in vegetable oils, seeds, nuts and egg yolk.

Chronically very low-fat diets often result in a low calorie and low nutrient intake overall. Low-calorie diets may result in depleted glycogen stores, resulting in poor energy levels, reduced capacity for high-intensity exercise, fatigue, poor recovery between workouts and low energy availability (*see* p. 209). They can also increase protein breakdown – causing loss of muscle mass and strength or a lack of muscle growth.

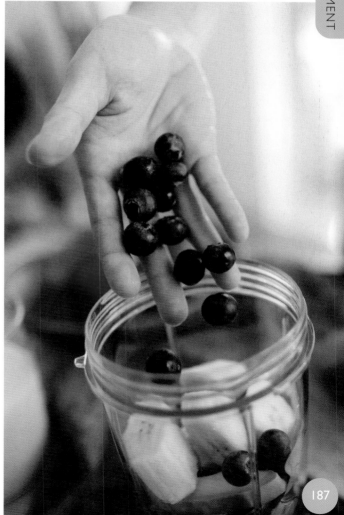

Time-restricted eating

Time-restricted eating (TRE) is a form of intermittent fasting that involves a fasting period of 12–16 hours and an eating period of 8–12 hours each day. The idea is that aligning your eating to your circadian rhythm (internal body clock) will help your body work more efficiently, resulting in improved health and weight loss. Studies show that circadian rhythm disruption has a negative impact on hormones that control appetite, energy expenditure and blood glucose (Ruddick-Collins et al., 2020).

Most of the studies to date have been done with fruit flies and mice (Hatori et al., 2012; Chaix et al., 2014). The evidence for TRE with humans is limited and, to date, only a small number of studies have shown positive results for weight loss. One US study found that people who reduced their eating window from 14 hours to 10–11 hours lost an average 3 kg over 16 weeks (Gill and Panda, 2015). Another showed similar results but no further weight loss benefits when people cut down to an 8-hour eating window (Gabel et al., 2018). A UK study found that people who ate breakfast 90 minutes later than usual and dinner 90 minutes earlier than usual consumed fewer calories and lost more body fat than those who maintained their usual eating habits (Antoni et al., 2018). However, TRE does not necessarily result in greater weight loss than other diets. A review of 11 studies comparing TRE with traditional calorie-restricted diets showed no differences in weight or body fat loss between groups (Rynders et al., 2019).

It's not known at the moment whether there is an optimum window or how critical timing is. One study suggests that an early eating window (8 a.m. to 2 p.m.) may be advantageous as it reduces appetite and subsequent food intake (Ravussin et al., 2019). This echoes the findings from a US study, which found that eating within a 6-hour window before 3 p.m. decreased hunger and lowered type 2 diabetes risk factors in men with pre-diabetes (Sutton et al., 2018).

The weight loss benefits of TRE may be explained by the fact that when people have less time to eat, they tend to consume fewer calories. TRE may also reinforce the body's circadian rhythm by preventing late-night eating. However, it is not appropriate for athletes with high energy demands or those who train twice a day as it would not allow time to refuel and recover properly. Competitive swimmers, for example, often train early in the morning and again late in the evening. Eating within a narrow window isn't realistic for them.

Summary: which diet is best for weight loss?

On balance, provided you eat fewer calories, all diets produce similar weight loss results in the long run. It is unimportant whether the calorie deficit comes from carbohydrate or fat. In other words, the most effective diet is one people can stick to and sustain. The key to losing weight and keeping it off is to eat more healthily, increase your activity and make sustainable changes to your lifestyle that you are comfortable with and will be able to adopt long term. Failing to keep to a diet can not only affect your health and metabolism but can also cause psychological problems. A 2-year study at the University of California found that overweight women who did not follow a set diet, but who simply ate more healthily and listened to hunger and satiety cues, improved their health (e.g. blood pressure and choles-

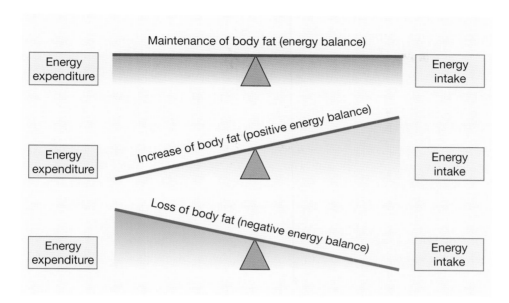

Figure 10.1 The role of energy balance

terol levels) and had higher self-esteem (Bacon *et al.*, 2005). In contrast, those who dieted for 6 months regained their weight and reported significant drops in confidence and self-esteem.

WEIGHT LOSS STRATEGY

Your balance of energy intake versus expenditure determines your weight. To lose body fat, you have to expend more energy than you consume over time. In other words, you have to achieve a negative energy balance, or energy deficit (*see* Fig. 10.1). However, energy balance is a dynamic state; if you change one side of the equation, for example reduce your energy intake, this influences the other side of the equation and causes a compensatory drop in energy expenditure (RMR, NEAT and EAT) as the body tries to resist weight loss and preserve its energy stores.

Research has shown that a combination of diet and activity is more likely to result in long-term success than diet or exercise alone. Unfortunately, there are no miracle solutions or short cuts. The objectives of an effective weight loss strategy are to:

- achieve a modest negative energy (calorie) balance
- maintain lean tissue
- gradually reduce body fat percentage
- avoid a significant reduction in your resting metabolic rate
- achieve an adequate intake of nutrients.

Step 1: Set realistic goals

Before embarking on a weight loss plan, write down your goals. Research has proven that by writing down your intentions, you are far more likely to turn them into actions.

These goals should be specific, positive and realistic ('I will lose 5 kg of body fat') rather than hopeful ('I would like to lose some weight'). Try to allow a suitable time frame to lose 15 kg one month before a summer holiday is, obviously, unrealistic! Tracking your progress, for example by using an app that logs your food and exercise, may help to maintain your motivation and increase the chances of success.

Step 2: Monitor your progress

You can track your progress by measuring your waist circumference and weight once a week. Avoid too frequent weighing because this can lead to an obsession with weight. Bear in mind that weight loss in the first week may be as much

as 2 kg, especially if your carbohydrate intake drops drastically, but this is mostly glycogen and its accompanying fluid (glycogen is stored with up to three times its weight of water). Afterwards, aim to lose no more than 0.5 kg fat/week. Faster weight loss usually suggests a loss of lean tissue.

The best way to ensure you are losing fat not muscle is to measure your body composition regularly. The simplest method is to use a combination of girth or circumference measurements (e.g. chest, waist, hips, arms, legs), as shown in Figure 10.2, and skinfold thickness measurements, obtained by callipers (*see* pp. 173–4). Exercise physiologists recommend keeping a record of the skinfold thickness measurements rather than converting them into body fat percentages. This is because the conversion charts are based on equations for the average, sedentary person and may not be appropriate for sportspeople or very lean or fat individuals. Monitoring changes in measurements at specific sites of the body allows you to see how your shape is changing and where most fat is being lost. This is a far better motivator than weighing scales! Alternatively, you can use one of the other methods of body composition measurement described in Chapter 9.

Step 3: Cut your calorie intake by no more than 15%

As explained previously, reducing your calorie intake by approximately 15% (or 10–20%) will allow you to lose body fat without appreciably slowing your metabolic rate. It will also help prevent loss of lean body mass. Although it may be tempting to cut calories further, a more severe calorie deficit reduces the capacity for high-intensity exercise, increases fatigue, and increases the

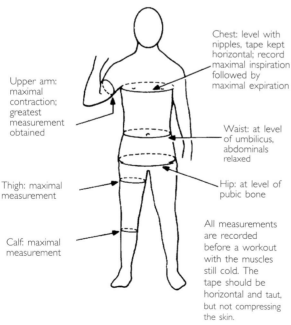

Upper arm: maximal contraction; greatest measurement obtained

Chest: level with nipples, tape kept horizontal; record maximal inspiration followed by maximal expiration

Waist: at level of umbilicus, abdominals relaxed

Thigh: maximal measurement

Hip: at level of pubic bone

Calf: maximal measurement

All measurements are recorded before a workout with the muscles still cold. The tape should be horizontal and taut, but not compressing the skin.

Figure 10.2 Girth measurements

risk of nutritional deficiencies, LEA and disordered eating.

Alternatively, you can estimate your daily calorie target for weight loss by calculating your RMR (from the Mifflin-St Jeor equation, *see* p. 282) and total daily energy expenditure and then reducing this by 15%. A step-by-step guide is given on p. 303. For example, if your total daily energy expenditure is 3000 kcal to maintain your current weight, to achieve a 15% deficit your new daily calorie target would be 2550 kcal. However, as you lose weight, you will need to recalculate your daily calorie target to continue losing fat. The leaner you become, the harder it is to lose fat at the same rate.

Step 4: Keep a food log

Initially, you can log your daily food and drink intake either in a food diary or using one of the many calorie tracking apps available. They can be a good way to evaluate your present eating habits and to find out exactly what, why and when you are eating. A food log will allow you to check whether your diet is well balanced or lacking in any important nutrients, and to take a more careful look at your usual meal patterns and lifestyle. It can also help you to become familiar with the nutritional content of foods. Bear in mind that the calorie content on food labels is an estimation, so you should not place too much importance on calorie tracking. Once you have a good idea of the calorie content of everyday foods, there is no need to continue logging your intake or counting calories as this may lead to an unhealthy obsession. Be aware of calories but focus instead on the nutritional value of foods and opt for fresh whole foods – fruit, vegetables, whole grains, pulses, nuts, seeds, lean meats, fish,

Equations for estimating RMR

Several equations have been developed to estimate RMR from body weight. The classic equations of Harris and Benedict, developed in the early 1900s, have been frequently used, but have been superseded by newer equations, such as the Mifflin-St Jeor equation, which uses an individual's weight, height and age (Mifflin *et al.*, 1990). Studies comparing various predictive equations for RMR have found the Mifflin-St Jeor to be the most accurate (Frankenfield *et al.*, 2005). However, the Mifflin-St Jeor equation does not account for exercise or make any adjustment for body composition, so applies to people with average body composition.

dairy and soya products. These foods are mostly high in fibre, filling and satiate your appetite, so help you naturally eat fewer calories.

Use your food log to evaluate:

- the nutrient-poor foods in your diet, which you need to eliminate – these are likely to be highly processed foods and drinks, high in sugar (e.g. biscuits, cakes, soft drinks, chocolate, crisps and snacks);
- your fibre intake – try to eat more fibre-rich foods such as lentils, oats, whole grains, nuts, seeds, fruit and vegetables in place of highly refined carbohydrates (e.g. white bread, pasta, rice and breakfast cereals);
- the timing of your meals and snacks – eat regularly spaced meals, avoid snacking if not genuinely hungry, and plan your meals around your workout.

The psychology of dieting

Researchers believe that a psychological difference exists between restrained eaters and non-dieters. In restrained eaters, the normal regulation of food intake becomes undermined as normal appetite and hunger cues are ignored. This leads to periods of restraint and semi-starvation, followed by overindulgence and guilt, followed by restraint, and so on.

Psychologists have shown that habitual dieters tend to have a more emotional personality than those who are not preoccupied with weight. They also tend to be more obsessive about food and weight.

At the University of Toronto, dieters and non-dieters were given a high-calorie milkshake, followed by free access to ice cream (Herman and Polivy, 1991). The dieters actually went on to eat more ice cream than the non-dieters. This is due to a phenomenon known as 'counter regulation'; having lost the inbuilt regulation system of non-dieters, they were unable to detect and thus compensate for the calorie pre-load.

Researchers at Penn State University demonstrated that 'weight worriers' appear to lack the internal 'calorie counter' possessed by people who don't worry about their weight (Rolls and Shide, 1992). When given a yoghurt half an hour before lunch, those who worried about their weight ate more for lunch than those who were not weight concerned. It appears that such dieters have poor appetite control and are unable to compensate for previous food intake.

Step 5: Match your carbohydrate intake to your training load

To create a calorie deficit of 15%, you will need to reduce your overall carbohydrate intake. This does not mean embarking on a low-carbohydrate diet; rather reducing carbohydrate to a level that still allows you to train hard but not too low to cause fatigue or a drop in performance. A chronic low-carbohydrate diet combined with high-intensity training can result in LEA, symptoms of overtraining, lowered immunity and reduced performance.

The best way to achieve this is by matching your carbohydrate intake to your training load. So, on days when your carbohydrate needs are higher, for example when performing high-intensity endurance training, aim to consume most of your daily carbohydrate in the 2–4 hour time period before exercise and the 2–4 hour time period after exercise so that your performance won't suffer and you will have enough energy to train hard. Remember, you cannot fuel high-intensity exercise (more than 70% of maximal aerobic capacity) from fat alone (*see* p. 26). Aim for around 50–100 g of carbohydrate pre-exercise, depending on how close your meal is to your workout, and also how long and hard you plan to train. After exercise, consume 1–1.2 g/kg BW, equivalent to 70–84 g for a 70 kg person, but adjust this according to the duration and intensity of your workout. If you have exercised hard for longer than 2 hours you may need more than this, as your glycogen stores will be depleted. If you have exercised for less than an hour, you will need less. Adding 15–25 g protein to your post-exercise recovery drinks and meals will promote optimal muscle recovery after hard training (*see* pp. 71–2).

On days when carbohydrate needs are lower, for example when doing low-intensity sessions (less than 70% of maximal aerobic capacity), training with lower muscle glycogen levels should not adversely affect your performance. Performing low-intensity sessions with low carbohydrate availability not only helps to reduce body fat but also promotes endurance training adaptations, increases rates of fat oxidation and, in some cases, improves exercise capacity (*see* p. 56).

In general, keep free sugars (sugars added to foods during manufacture and processing) and ultra-processed foods to a minimum as they are energy dense, providing lots of calories for relatively few nutrients. The box on p. 194 gives a number of ways to reduce sugar.

Step 6: Don't cut fat too drastically

Reducing the fat content of your diet will help to reduce overall energy density but don't cut it out of your diet completely. You need a certain amount each day to provide essential fatty acids and absorb and transport fat-soluble vitamins. It is also satiating so it gives the body the feeling of being full. Very low-fat diets can lead to deficient intakes of essential fatty acids and fat-soluble vitamins. Aim to consume 20–35% of energy from fat. Unsaturated fatty acids should make up the majority of your fat intake, with saturated fatty acids making up no more than 10% energy and trans fatty acids kept as close to zero as possible (*see* pp. 85–90).

Cut down on highly processed foods that are high in saturated fats, such as sausages, burgers, pastry and pies, cakes, biscuits, puddings and chocolate. Choose leaner meats, poultry and fish instead of fatty meat, and use less oil in cooking.

Step 7: Increase protein to offset muscle loss

A higher protein intake can offset some of the potential loss of muscle when losing weight. Studies suggest that increasing your protein intake to 1.8–2.7 g/kg BW/day (or 2.3–3.1 g/kg fat-free mass) while cutting your daily energy intake by a modest 10–20% can prevent muscle mass loss (Hector and Phillips, 2018; Murphy *et al.*, 2015; Helms *et al.*, 2014(a); Phillips and Van Loon, 2011). This equates to 126–189 g protein/day for an athlete weighing 70 kg. You should distribute your daily protein evenly between meals and snacks, aiming to consume 0.25–0.3 g/kg BW/day or about 20–24 g per meal in order to maximise MPS.

One study found that when athletes ate 1.6 g or 2.4 g protein/kg BW (twice and three times the RDA respectively) they lost more fat and less muscle compared with those who just ate the RDA for protein, 0.8 g/kg body weight (Pasiakos *et al.*, 2013). All three groups lost the same amount of weight but those eating extra protein lost more fat and retained more muscle at the end of the dieting period.

Protein can also help control appetite and reduce hunger. Researchers have shown that it is more effective than carbohydrate and fat for switching off hunger signals and promoting satiety (Westerterp-Plantenga *et al.*, 2012). Protein triggers appetite-regulating hormones in the gut, which tell the appetite control centre in the brain that you are satiated (*see* p. 71). The higher the protein intake, the greater the level of satiety produced (Belza *et al.*, 2013).

A study at the University of Illinois found that women who exercised regularly (5 x 30-minute walking sessions; 2 x 30-minute weight training

How to reduce sugar

Get accustomed to less sweetness – Give your palate time to adjust. Instead of banning sugar, reduce the amount of sugar you add to foods and drinks a little at a time. Over time, you'll get accustomed to the taste of less-sweet foods.

Limit sugary drinks including fruit juice and sports drinks – They are not only a source of empty calories but sugary drinks also show the strongest relationship with tooth decay, obesity and type 2 diabetes. The problem is that it's easier to over-consume calories in liquid form than solid foods. Although fruit juice contains natural sugar, the juicing process means the sugars in the cell wall of the plant are released as 'free sugars', which damage teeth, raise blood sugar levels quickly and provide additional calories. Replace soft drinks, fruit juice and energy drinks with water, low-fat milk or unsweetened tea or coffee.

Minimise ultra-processed foods – Replace ultra-processed sugary foods (e.g. sweets, chocolate, cakes, biscuits and desserts) in your diet with whole-food sources of sugar, such as fruit and vegetables, which have a smaller effect on your blood sugar levels. Ultra-processed foods also stimulate hunger and make it harder to control appetite and body weight.

Don't ban fruit – The sugars that occur naturally in fruit are much less concentrated and they're consumed along with fibre, which helps slow their absorption. Fruit is also a valuable source of vitamins, minerals and phytochemicals.

Read the label – There are many types of sugar so check labels for sucrose, glucose syrup, invert sugar, fructose, dextrose, maltodextrin, fruit syrup, raw sugar, cane sugar and glucose. Even foods disguised as health foods can be loaded with added sugars – agave nectar, honey, organic cane sugar and maple syrup all fall into the same category.

Go for natural sweetness – Opt for fresh fruit instead of sweets, cakes, biscuits and pastries. Add fruit to plain yoghurt or porridge/breakfast cereal instead of sugar. Swap puddings for fresh berries and plain yoghurt or baked bananas. But go easy on dried fruit – it's a concentrated source of sugar and easy to overeat.

Beware of 'low-fat' foods – These often contain more sugar than their 'full-fat' equivalents, since manufacturers replace the fat with other ingredients, including sugar, to improve their taste. These foods may not always satisfy your taste expectations so you may end up eating more of them.

Rethink your breakfast – Many breakfast cereals are loaded with sugar. Opt for porridge, eggs on toast, or plain yoghurt with fresh fruit and nuts – a higher-protein breakfast will keep you feeling fuller for longer.

Adapt recipes – As a rule, you can cut the sugar in most cakes and desserts by one-third without compromising flavour or texture. Try adding sweeter spices such as cinnamon, nutmeg, vanilla, almond extract, ginger or lemon to improve flavour. For cakes, substitute puréed apple or mashed banana for some of the sugar.

sessions per week) while eating a high-protein diet lost more weight compared with those who ate a high-carbohydrate diet containing the same number of calories (Layman *et al.*, 2005). Almost 100% of the weight loss in the high-protein dieters was fat, and much of that was from the abdominal region. In contrast, in the high-carbohydrate group, up to a third of the weight loss was muscle. Researchers suggest that the high-protein diet worked better because it contained a high level of leucine, which works with insulin to stimulate fat-burning while preserving muscle.

Step 8: Blood glucose control

This can be achieved by eating low-GI meals – a balanced combination of carbohydrate, protein and fat, with a focus on high-fibre foods (such as whole grains, fruit and vegetables). This helps improve appetite regulation, increases feelings of fullness and delays hunger between meals. Remember that adding protein, fat or soluble fibre to carbohydrate always reduces the speed of absorption and produces a lower blood sugar rise. In practice, this is easy to achieve if you plan to eat a carbohydrate source (e.g. potatoes) with a high-protein source (e.g. fish) and add vegetables. Better still, include low-GI carbohydrates, such as lentils and beans, in your meals.

Step 9: Eat more fibre

Apart from reducing your risk of certain cancers and heart disease, fibre slows down the emptying of food from your stomach, reduces hunger and helps to keep you feeling full. Fibre also gives food more texture so you need to chew your food more. This slows down your eating speed, reducing the chances of overeating, and increases satiety.

Can I gain muscle while losing fat?

Conventional dogma suggests that you cannot lose fat and gain muscle simultaneously. However, a study at McMaster University found that you can – if you combine a low calorie and high protein intake with a very high-intensity training programme (Longland *et al.*, 2016). The study involved 40 overweight men who performed an intense resistance training programme (6 days a week, including 2 days of circuit resistance training, 2 days of high-intensity intervals on a bike, 1 day of bike time-trial and 1 day of plyometric body weight circuits) for 4 weeks while consuming 40% fewer calories than their calculated requirements. those who consumed a high-protein diet (2.4 g/kg BW/day) lost significantly more body fat (4.8 kg vs. 3.5 kg) and gained significantly more muscle (1.2 kg vs. 0.1 kg) than those who consumed 1.2 g protein/kg BW, which was close to what the volunteers typically consumed (but still higher than the recommended daily intake). However, the exercise regime was exceptionally tough and the weight loss benefits may not be sustainable.

Fibre also slows the digestion and absorption of carbohydrates, resulting in a slow steady energy uptake and stable insulin levels. Non-fluctuating glucose and insulin levels will encourage the use of food for energy rather than for storage as body fat; it also reduces hunger and satisfies the appetite.

Does skipping breakfast increase weight loss?

Studies show that people who skip breakfast are more likely to eat highly palatable high-calorie foods later on (Goldstone et al., 2009) and also eat more at lunchtime (Chowdhury et al., 2015). However, contrary to popular belief, they do not fully compensate for the calories saved at breakfast and generally still go on to consume fewer calories over the course of the day (Betts et al., 2016; Levitsky and Pacanowski, 2013).

A study from the University of Bath, found that people who eat breakfast burn 442 more calories by being active, mainly in the morning after eating, than those who skip breakfast (Betts et al., 2014). It is thought that people who skip breakfast burn fewer calories because they do less spontaneous physical activity.

While occasionally skipping breakfast may help reduce your daily calorie intake (Clayton and James, 2015), it is not a good weight loss strategy if you want to train hard later in the day. Researchers from Loughborough University, found that those who omitted breakfast experienced a 4.5% drop in their performance in a cycling time-trial (after lunch but before dinner) (Clayton et al., 2015).

It is a myth that exercising in a fasted state (e.g. before breakfast) increases fat burning and leads to increased weight loss. For weight loss, the important factor is energy balance (see p. 41) repeated to the point of failure.

The most filling foods are those with a high volume per calorie. Water and fibre add bulk to foods, so load up on foods naturally high in these components. Fruit, vegetables, pulses and wholegrain foods give maximum fill for minimum calories. If you can eat a plate of food that is low in calories relative to its volume, you're likely to feel just as satisfied as eating smaller amounts of high-calorie food.

Step 10: Be flexible

Studies have shown that adopting a flexible approach to dieting and not being too rigid is a more successful strategy for achieving and maintaining weight loss. Not depriving yourself of foods you love and enjoying the occasional indulgence without feeling guilty is important from a psychological standpoint. Many people find that regularly including their favourite foods in small portions satisfies their cravings and keeps them motivated to adhere to their weight loss diet for long periods of time. If you know you can eat a little of your favourite food regularly then you'll stop thinking of it as a forbidden food and won't want to overeat it.

Step 11: Make gradual lifestyle changes that are sustainable

Long-term weight management can only be achieved by making changes to your eating and exercise habits that you are comfortable with and can stick to. If you make too drastic a change, such as cutting out an entire food group or replacing meals with shakes, then it is very unlikely that you will be able to sustain it long term. A weight loss plan should be one that is realistic and sustainable. However, one of the biggest barriers to this is an unwillingness to commit to a few necessary changes in lifestyle. Table 10.1 lists some of the common reasons why many people fail to manage their weight in the long term, together with some suggestions as to how to overcome them.

Step 12: Include regular physical activity

Anyone on a calorie-reduced programme will lose both muscle and fat. On a severe calorie-reduced programme, muscle loss can account for up to 50% of weight loss. However, muscle loss can be minimised by including resistance exercise as well as cardiovascular exercise.

Resistance exercise

The UK government recommends that all adults should undertake activities that increase or maintain muscle strength at least twice a week (Department of Health & Social Care, 2019). The activities chosen should ideally use major muscle groups in both the upper and lower body and be repeated to failure. Examples include body weight exercises, free weights, resistance machines or resistance bands.

Resistance exercise should be included in your fat-loss programme for two reasons. First, your RMR will be elevated for several hours post-exercise, due to the oxidation of body fat (Melby *et al.*, 1993). You won't necessarily burn more calories lifting weights than doing cardiovascular exercise, but the increased muscle mass you develop as a result will increase your resting metabolic rate. One study found that people who did a combination of cardiovascular and resistance exercise lost more body fat than those doing cardiovascular exercise only, but also gained more muscle (Willis *et al.*, 2012).

Second, when resistance exercise is added to a weight loss programme, more muscle is preserved and a greater proportion of weight loss is fat loss.

Table 10.1	LIFESTYLE CHANGES
Lifestyle	**Suggestion**
Not enough time to prepare healthy meals	Plan meals in advance so all ingredients are at hand. Make meals in bulk and refrigerate/freeze portions.
Work shifts	Plan regular meal breaks and take your own healthy food with you.
Work involves lots of travelling	Take portable healthy snacks (e.g. sandwiches, fruit, nuts, protein bars, dried fruit, yoghurt, milk, protein drinks).
Need to cook for rest of family	Adapt favourite family meals (e.g. spaghetti bolognese) to make them healthier. Add extra vegetables and high-fibre ingredients (e.g. beans, wholemeal pasta).
Overeat when stressed	Use stress management and relaxation techniques.
Eat out frequently	Choose healthier options in restaurants (e.g. salads, fish, vegetable-based dishes).

Resistance training acts as a stimulus for muscle retention and growth.

Cardiovascular (CV) exercise

For health, the UK government guidelines recommend a minimum of 150 minutes of moderate-intensity activity (such as brisk walking or cycling) or 75 minutes of vigorous activity (such as running) per week (Department of Health & Social Care, 2019). This is in line with the Physical Activity Guidelines for Americans (U.S. Department of Health and Human Services, 2018) and the American College of Sports Medicine (Donnelly *et al.*, 2009). These 150 minutes can be accumulated in bouts of any length. For weight loss and weight maintenance, though, the UK government and ACSM both recommend more than 150 minutes per week together with dietary restriction.

Cardiovascular activity not only increases total energy expenditure but may also help offset some of the muscle loss that occurs in a calorie deficit. However, you should not rely on CV exercise exclusively. Without resistance training, you could still lose substantial amounts of muscle tissue – some studies have estimated as much as 40% (Aceto, 1997). This is because CV exercise does not act as sufficient stimulus to ensure muscle retention while you are in calorie deficit. Muscle loss will subsequently result in a lowering of your metabolic rate.

Despite what many people believe, low-intensity, long-duration aerobic exercise is not the most effective method for reducing body fat. Research indicates that not only does high-intensity aerobic exercise burn fat more effectively but it also increases EPOC. What matters most is the number of calories expended per unit of time. The more calories you expend, the more fat you break down. For example, walking (i.e. low-intensity aerobic exercise) for 60 minutes burns 270 kcal, of which 160 kcal (60% calories) comes from fat. Running (i.e. high-intensity aerobic exercise) for the same amount of time burns 680 kcal, of which 270 kcal (40% calories) comes from fat. Therefore, high-intensity aerobic exercise results in greater fat loss over the same time period. This principle applies to everyone, no matter what your level

The science of muscle growth

To build muscle you need to combine a resistance training programme with an adequate intake of energy and nutrients. The idea is to train or load the muscles just hard enough during your workout to break down muscle proteins. This mechanical loading of the muscle triggers muscle protein synthesis (MPS), or muscle growth (Wackerhage *et al.*, 2019; Rennie and Tipton, 2000). After your workout, the muscle releases cytokines (hormone-like molecules) that signal muscle repair for up to 48 hours. These activate various pathways such as the mammalian target of rapamycin complex 1 (mTORC1), a molecular switch that turns on the machinery that manufactures muscle proteins (Bodine *et al.*, 2001). These pathways enable amino acids to pass from the bloodstream into the muscle cell, and then to be transported within the cell to areas where they will be assembled into new muscle proteins. These new proteins are then added to the muscle fibres, making the muscle stronger and denser.

Training for muscle gain

Certain compound exercises, such as dead lifts, clean and jerks, snatches and squats, not only stimulate the 'prime mover' muscles, but also have a powerful anabolic ('systemic') effect on the whole body and the central nervous system. These are the classic mass builders and should be included once a week in any serious muscle/strength training programme.

To stimulate the maximal number of muscle fibres in a muscle group, select one to three basic exercises and aim to do 4–12 total sets for that muscle group. Latest research suggests that doing fewer sets (4–8) but using heavier weights (80–90% of your 1-rep maximum – i.e. the maximum weight that can be lifted through 1 complete repetition) results in faster size and strength gains. If you exercise that muscle group to exhaustion, you will need to allow up to 7 days for recuperation before repeating the same workout. So, aim to train each muscle group once a week (on average). In practice, divide your body parts (e.g. chest, legs, shoulders, back, arms) into three or four, and train one part per workout.

Always use strict training form and, ideally, have a partner to 'spot' for you so that you can use near-maximal weights safely. Always remember to warm up each muscle group beforehand with light aerobic training (e.g. exercise bike) and some relevant stretches. Ensure you also stretch the muscles after (and, ideally, in between each part of) the workout to help relieve soreness.

of fitness – exercise intensity is always relative to the individual. Walking at 6 km/h may represent high-intensity exercise for an unconditioned individual; running at 10 km/h may represent low-intensity exercise for a well-conditioned athlete.

High-intensity interval training (HIIT)
High-intensity interval training (HIIT) has been shown to be more effective than steady-state training for promoting fat loss as well as for improving cardiovascular fitness, blood glucose control, insulin sensitivity and blood vessel function. The basic concept of HIIT is to train at different speeds for a number of intervals. Researchers at Laval University in Quebec, Canada, found that nine times more fat was lost in the group that used HIIT, compared to the group that used traditional steady-state CV exercise (Tremblay *et al.*, 1994). It also increases your metabolic rate for longer. In other words, your body's fat-burning process remains elevated for a few hours after your workout, even when you are at rest.

HIIT can be performed with a variety of activities– running, swimming, cycling, elliptical training or skipping ropes. Ensure you warm up properly to prevent injury. Be aware of your own limits, and work out accordingly. A 2:1 work/rest ratio, composed of 20 seconds of work and 10 seconds of recovery (a type of workout sometimes called Tabata), is thought to be the most efficient ratio to improve the cardiovascular system. However, including a variety of work-recovery cycles is best.

How can I gain weight?

Muscle weight gain can be achieved by combining a consistent well-planned resistance training programme with a balanced diet. Resistance training provides the stimulus for muscle growth while your diet provides the right amount of energy (calories) and nutrients to enable your muscles to grow at the optimal rate. One without the other would result in only minimal lean weight gain.

WHAT TYPE OF TRAINING IS BEST FOR GAINING MUSCLE?

Resistance training (weight training) is the best way to stimulate muscle growth (hypertrophy) and strength. The current recommendation is to train with 40–80% of your 1 repetition maximum (1RM, i.e. the maximum weight that can be lifted once) for hypertrophy, or with at least 60% of your 1 RM for strength (Schoenfeld *et al.*, 2017(a)). Additionally, you should perform multiple sets and rest for at least 2 minutes in-between sets (Morton *et al.*, 2018). However, studies have shown that resistance training with lighter weights (<60% 1RM) to failure can also result in a similar degree of muscle hypertrophy as higher weights (>60%1RM) (Schoenfeld *et al.*, 2017(a)).

Concentrate on the 'compound' exercises, such as bench press, squat, shoulder press and lat pull-down, as these work the largest muscle groups of the body together with neighbouring muscles that act as assistors or synergists. These types of exercises stimulate the largest number of muscle fibres in one movement and are therefore the most effective and efficient way to gain muscle mass. Keep the smaller isolation exercises, such as biceps concentration curls or tricep kickbacks, to a minimum; these produce slower mass gains and should be added to your workout only occasionally for variety.

HOW MUCH WEIGHT CAN I EXPECT TO GAIN?

The amount of muscle weight you can expect to gain depends on several genetic factors, including your body type, muscle fibre mix, the arrangement of your motor units and your hormonal balance, as well as your training programme and diet.

Your genetic make-up determines the proportion of different types of fibres in your muscles. The fast-twitch (type II) fibres generate power and increase in size more readily than the slow-twitch (type I or endurance) fibres. So, if you naturally have plenty of fast-twitch fibres in your muscles, you will probably respond faster to a strength training programme than someone who has a higher proportion of slow-twitch fibres. Unfortunately, you cannot convert slow-twitch into fast-twitch fibres – hence two people can follow exactly the same training programme, yet the one with lots of fast-twitch muscle fibres will naturally gain muscle faster than the other.

Your natural body type also affects how fast you gain muscle mass. An ectomorph (naturally slim build with long lean limbs, narrow shoulders and hips) will find it harder to gain weight than a mesomorph (muscular, athletic build with wide shoulders and narrow hips) who tends to gain muscle readily. An endomorph (stocky, rounded build with wide shoulders and hips and an even distribution of fat) gains both fat and muscle readily.

People with a higher natural level of the male (anabolic) sex hormones, such as testosterone, will also gain muscle faster. That is why women cannot achieve the muscle mass or size of men unless they take anabolic steroids.

However, no matter what your genetics, natural build and hormonal balance, everyone can gain muscle with resistance training.

HOW FAST CAN I EXPECT TO GAIN WEIGHT?

Mass gains of 20% of starting body weight are common after the first year of training. However, the rate of weight gain will gradually drop off over the years as your muscle adapts to increasingly larger workloads and you approach your genetic potential. In one study, experienced male and female lifters gained an average 0.99–1.06 kg muscle mass over 8 weeks (Thomas and Burns, 2016). Male beginners may expect to gain 1–1.5% total body weight per month and experienced athletes 0.25–0.5% BW/month. Women usually experience about 50% of the gains of men – i.e. 0.25–0.75% BW/month for beginners, and 0.125–0.25% BW/month for experienced

Tips for increasing energy intake

Make eating and drinking a priority – This may mean rescheduling other activities. Plan your meal and snack times in advance and never skip or rush them, no matter how busy you are.

Increase your meal frequency – Eat at least three meals with three or four nutrient-dense snacks in between. It can sometimes be easier for those with a poor appetite to graze on smaller portions instead of consuming a big meal.

Eat larger portions at mealtimes – Adding an extra portion of toast at breakfast, an extra slice of cheese to your sandwich, and an extra spoonful of pasta or an extra potato at dinner is an easy way to increase overall intake.

Plan ahead – Schedule your meals and snacks around your training, work and social commitments so you always have access to suitable foods and drinks.

Eat consistently – Never skip meals and avoid long intervals between meals.

Include nutrient-dense snacks – These include yoghurt, nuts, dried fruit, granola or fruit and nut bars, protein bars, cheese and crackers, hummus and breadsticks, and avocado on toast. Consume these between meals.

Add energy-dense, nutritious foods – Try adding cheese, nuts, seeds, nut butter, avocado, dried fruit and olive oil to meals. Scatter grated cheese on vegetables, soups, potatoes, pasta dishes and hotpots. Mix nuts, seeds and dried fruit into porridge and yoghurt. Spread bread, toast or crackers with peanut butter or hummus. Drizzle olive oil, dressing or mayonnaise over veggies and salad.

Include liquid nutrition – Drink milk, milk-based drinks, meal replacement or protein supplements or smoothies once or twice a day. Using whole milk in drinks and plain Greek yoghurt in smoothies is an easy way to increase calorie intake.

Incorporate healthy fats and oils into your diet – These include olive (or rapeseed) oil, oily fish (such as salmon, sardines and mackerel), olives, avocado, nuts, seeds and nut butters.

athletes – partly due to their smaller initial body weight and smaller muscle mass, and partly due to lower levels of anabolic hormones. Monitor your body composition rather than simply your weight. If you are gaining more than 1 kg per month on an established programme then you are likely to be gaining fat!

HOW MUCH SHOULD I EAT?

To gain lean weight and muscle strength at the optimal rate, you need to be in positive energy balance, i.e. consuming more calories than you need for maintenance on a daily basis. This cannot be stressed too much. These additional calories should come from nutrient-dense foods and drinks rather than sugar- or saturated fat-laden foods. This will improve overall health and well-being.

1. Calories

Consuming 20% more calories per day than your body requires should lead to a steady gain of muscle mass. Estimate your maintenance calorie intake using the formulae in Steps 1–4, Chapter 18. Next, multiply your maintenance calories by 1.2 (120%).

Example:

If your maintenance calorie requirement is 2700 kcal, you will need to eat 2700 x 1.2 = 3240 kcal.

In practice, most athletes will need to add roughly an extra 500 kcal to their daily diet. Not all of these extra calories are converted into muscle – some will be used for digestion and absorption, given off as heat or used for physical activity. Increase your calorie intake gradually, say 200 a day for a while, then after a week or two,

increase it by a further 200 kcal. Slow gainers may need to increase their calorie intake by as much as 1000 kcal a day.

2. Carbohydrate

In order to gain muscle, you need to train very hard, and that requires a lot of fuel. The key fuel for this type of exercise is, of course, muscle glycogen. Therefore, you must consume enough carbohydrate to achieve high muscle glycogen levels. If you train with low levels of muscle glycogen, you risk excessive protein (muscle) breakdown, which is just the opposite of what you are aiming for.

In a 24-hour period during low- or moderate-intensity training days, you should consume 5–7 g/kg of body weight.. As your calorie needs increase by 20%, so should your usual carbohydrate intake. In practice, aim to eat an extra 50–100 g carbohydrate/day.

3. Protein

As explained in Chapter 4, dietary protein provides an enhanced stimulus for muscle growth and strength (Phillips *et al.*, 2011; Phillips, 2012). To build muscle, you must be in 'positive nitrogen balance', which means your body retains more dietary protein than is excreted or used as fuel. A suboptimal intake of protein will result in slower gains in strength, size and mass, or even muscle loss, despite hard training.

For building or maintaining muscle mass, the IAAF recommend 1.3–1.7 g/kg BW/day (Witard *et al.*, 2019). For example, if you weigh 70 kg then you will need 91–119 g protein a day. A review of 49 studies shows that increasing your intake above this level produces no further gains in muscle mass (Morton *et al.*, 2018).

4. Fat

Fat should comprise between 20 and 35% of total calories, or the balance of calories once you have met your needs for carbohydrate and protein. Most of your fat should come from unsaturated sources, such as olive oil and other vegetable oils, avocado, oily fish, nuts and seeds.

Example:
If you consume 3000 kcal a day, your fat intake should be:

- (3000 x 20%) ÷ 9 = 66 g
- (3000 x 35%) ÷ 9 = 117 g

i.e. between 66 and 117 g fat per day.

NUTRIENT TIMING

The timing of your food intake around exercise is important. You can optimise glycogen recovery after training by consuming 1–1.2 g carbohydrate/kg BW during the 2-hour post-exercise period (Burke *et al.*, 2011). So, for example, if you weigh 70 kg you need to consume 70–84 g carbohydrate within 2 hours after exercise. This is particularly important if you have less than 8 hours between workouts or competitions.

However, it's not only carbohydrate that aids recovery after training: several studies suggest that taking carbohydrate combined with protein after exercise helps create the ideal hormonal environment for glycogen storage and muscle building (Zawadzki *et al.*, 1992; Bloomer *et al.*, 2000; Gibala, 2000; Kreider *et al.*, 1996). Both trigger the release of insulin and growth hormone in your body. These are powerful anabolic hormones. Insulin transports amino acids into cells, reassembles them into proteins and prevents muscle

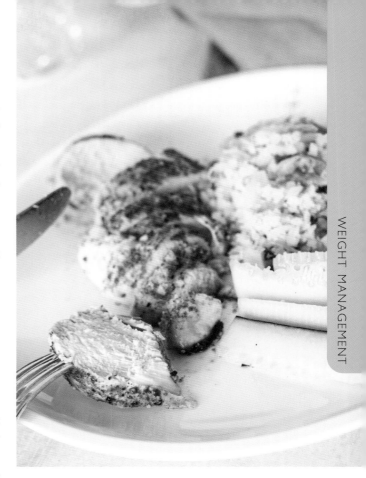

breakdown. It also transports glucose into muscle cells and stimulates glycogen storage. Growth hormone increases protein manufacture and muscle building.

There is evidence that protein consumed early in the post-exercise recovery phase increases the rate of MPS and promotes muscle repair (Van Loon, 2014). The optimal post-exercise protein intake is 0.25–0.4 g/kg BW, equivalent to 17.5–28 g for an athlete weighing 70 kg (Thomas *et al.*, 2016; Phillips and Van Loon, 2011; Moore *et al.*, 2009; IOC, 2011; Rodriguez *et al.*, 2009). When athletes consumed less than this amount of protein they gained less muscle; when they consumed more than this amount they experienced no further muscle gains.

The window for muscle recovery and protein consumption is longer than once thought. It is now known that the anabolic effect of exercise lasts up to 24 hours so the benefits of consuming protein may extend for many hours. In other words, consuming protein immediately after training will increase MPS, but so will protein consumption at any time over the subsequent 24 hours.

For optimal MPS throughout the day, you should also consume 0.25–0.4 g protein/kg body weight at each meal (*see* pp. 71–2). Consuming less than this amount may result in a suboptimal rate of MPS; consuming more will not produce

Post-workout snacks

The following options provide around 20 g high-quality protein:

- **600 ml milk** – Any type of milk will provide the protein needed to maximise muscle adaptation after strength and power training. It also contains the optimal amount of the branched-chain amino acid leucine to promote muscle building after exercise.
- **500 ml recovery milkshake** – Use 500 ml of milk plus yoghurt and fresh fruit (in general, bananas, strawberries, pears, mango and pineapple give the best results) for an excellent mixture of protein, carbohydrate and those all-important antioxidants.
- **450 ml yoghurt** – Choose plain yoghurt after a strength workout, or fruit yoghurt after an endurance session lasting an hour or more. Both contain high-quality proteins that will accelerate muscle repair; fruit yoghurt has added sugar so it has the ideal 3:1 carbohydrate:protein ratio for speedy glycogen refuelling.
- **330–500 ml whey protein shake** – Shakes made up with milk or water are an easy and convenient mini-meal in a glass. Opt for one containing 20 g protein. Powders and ready-to-drink versions generally contain a balanced mixture of carbohydrate (usually as maltodextrin and sugar), protein (usually whey), vitamins and minerals.
- **50 g almonds or cashews plus 250 ml yoghurt** – Nuts provide not only 10 g of protein but also B vitamins, vitamin E, iron, zinc, phytonutrients and fibre. Yoghurt supplies another 10 g of protein. The fat in the nuts may reduce insulin a little, but will not affect muscle building.
- **250 ml strained plain Greek yoghurt** – This is also perfect after a strength workout, because strained Greek yoghurt is more concentrated, containing about twice the protein of ordinary yoghurt.
- **500 ml ready-to-drink milkshake** – Opt for a shake that contains around 20 g protein for convenient refuelling after exercise. Alternatively, make your own speedy version by mixing 3 tsp milkshake powder with 500 ml milk.
- **A 'protein' bar** – Bars containing a mixture of carbohydrate and whey protein are a convenient option after workouts. Opt for one containing around 20 g protein.

greater strength or mass gains. Excess protein will be oxidised and used as a fuel source. It is better to evenly distribute your protein throughout the day, consuming similar amounts at breakfast, lunch and dinner, rather than eating most of your protein at dinner (Mamerow *et al.*, 2014; Areta *et al.*, 2013).

Consuming some of your protein before sleep may also increase MPS and muscle mass gains. A study at Maastricht University found that athletes who consumed a pre-bed protein drink containing 28 g protein had greater increases in strength and muscle mass after 12 weeks compared with those who did not (Snijders *et al.*, 2015).

WHICH TYPE OF PROTEIN IS BEST FOR MUSCLE GAIN?

Milk, whey, casein, egg, meat, fish, and soya provide all the essential amino acids at levels that closely match the body's needs. Studies have shown that these types of protein stimulate muscle growth more than other types of protein (*see* pp. 72–3).

These foods are also rich in the amino acid leucine, which has been shown to be a critical element in regulating protein manufacture in the body as well as playing a key role in muscle recovery after exercise (*see* p. 74). In combination with the other essential amino acids (EAAs), it triggers protein manufacture, which in turn leads to increased muscle size and strength.

However, plant protein sources, such as beans, lentils, nuts, soya and (to a smaller degree) grains, also contribute amino acids to your diet and will count towards your total daily protein intake.

Liquid forms of protein (such as milk and whey protein drinks) are particularly beneficial for MPS immediately after exercise as they are digested and

How does creatine cause weight gain?

Weight gain is due partly to water retention in the muscle cells and partly to increased muscle growth. Researchers have found that urine volume is reduced markedly during the initial days of supplementation with creatine, which indicates the body is retaining extra water (Hultman *et al.*, 1996).

Creatine draws water into the muscle cells, thus increasing cell volume. In one study with cross-trained athletes, thigh muscle volume increased 6.6% and intracellular volume increased 2–3% after a creatine-loading dose (Ziegenfuss *et al.*, 1997). It is thought that the greater cell volume caused by creatine supplementation acts as an anabolic signal for protein synthesis and therefore muscle growth (Haussinger *et al.*, 1996). It also reduces protein breakdown during intense exercise.

The fact that studies show a substantially greater muscle mass even after long-term creatine supplementation indicates that creatine must have a direct effect on muscle growth. In studies at the University of Memphis, athletes taking creatine gained more body mass than those taking the placebo, yet both groups ended up with the same body water content (Kreider *et al.*, 1996). If creatine allows you to train more intensely, it follows that you will gain more muscle mass. For more details on creatine supplement doses, see pp. 126–9.

absorbed more rapidly than solid foods (Burke *et al.*, 2012). Milk consumed immediately after resistance exercise has been shown to increase muscle growth and repair, reduce post-exercise muscle soreness, improve body composition and rehydrate the body better than commercial sports drinks (Elliot *et al.*, 2006; Hartman *et al.*, 2007; Wilkinson *et al.*, 2007; Karp *et al.*, 2006).

Milk and whey protein are particularly rich sources of leucine, so both represent ideal post-workout foods for promoting muscle growth. You can get 20 g protein from 500–600 ml of cow's or soya milk. This volume of milk also provides 30 g of carbohydrate, which will help replenish muscle glycogen stores and build muscle. The type of milk (skimmed or whole milk) is unimportant as far as MPS is concerned. A milkshake, hot chocolate, coffee latte and other drinks made with milk are also suitable recovery options.

WILL WEIGHT GAIN SUPPLEMENTS HELP?

There are literally dozens of supplements on the market that claim to enhance muscle mass, although many of the claims are not supported by scientific research, lack safety data, and some have even been found to contain illegal substances! For more information on supplements, *see* Chapter 7. However, some supplements may be worth considering for weight gain:

- **Creatine** – This may help increase performance, strength and muscle mass. Dozens of studies since the mid-1990s show significant increases in lean mass and total mass, typically 1–3% lean body weight (approx. 0.8–3 kg) after a 5-day loading dose, compared with controls. *See also* pp. 126–9.
- **All-in-one supplements** – Ones containing protein, maltodextrin, vitamins and minerals provide a convenient alternative to solid food. They will not necessarily improve your performance but can be a helpful and convenient addition (rather than replacement) to your diet if you struggle to eat enough whole food, you need to eat on the move or you need the extra nutrients they provide.
- **Protein supplements** – These may benefit you if you have particularly high protein requirements or cannot consume enough protein from food alone (e.g. you follow a vegetarian or vegan diet) (*see* pp. 140–3).

> ## High-calorie, nutrient-dense foods
>
> - Nuts – peanuts, almonds, cashews, brazils, pistachios
> - Dried fruit – raisins, sultanas, apricots, dates
> - Wholegrain sandwiches and wraps with cheese, chicken, tuna, falafel, avocado or egg
> - Yoghurt, cheese and eggs
> - Milk, milkshakes and flavoured milk
> - Porridge, granola, muesli or wholegrain cereal with milk
> - Healthy oils and dressings – olive oil, rapeseed, mayonnaise
> - Oat-based cereal bars, granola bars, flapjacks, fruit and nut bars
> - Bread or toast with nut butter or cheese
> - Avocado on toast
> - Hummus with breadsticks or crackers

Summary of key points

- In weight-category sports, athletes may resort to rapid weight loss methods to make weight for competition. Rapid weight loss can have an adverse effect on performance and health.
- While repeated weight loss does not slow the RMR, it can be harmful to your psychological health.
- The most important factor that determines your RMR is your body weight.
- RMR decreases in response to weight loss ('adaptive thermogenesis').
- Athletes should not restrict their energy intake too severely to avoid low energy availability and loss of lean tissue.
- A variety of diets can lead to weight loss but what matters most is consistently eating fewer calories. There is no evidence to date that low-carbohydrate diets or time-restricted eating produce greater weight or fat loss in the long term than traditional energy-restricted diets.
- Ultimately, for successful long-term weight loss, a diet plan needs to be sustainable and help you lose fat without compromising your performance.
- To lose body fat, you have to achieve negative energy balance, i.e. expend more energy than you consume.
- Effective fat loss can be achieved by reducing calorie intake by 15% (or 10–20%); this will minimise both lean tissue loss and RMR reduction.
- A higher protein intake of 1.8–2.7 g/kg BW/day (or 2.3–3.1 g/kg fat-free mass) can offset some of the potential loss of muscle when training with a calorie deficit.
- Protein can help control appetite and reduce hunger.

- The main elements of an effective fat-loss strategy include setting realistic goals, monitoring your progress, achieving a calorie reduction of 10–20%, adjusting carbohydrate according to training goals, minimising ultra-processed foods, including healthy fats, eating fibre-rich foods, not banning any food, making gradual lifestyle changes and including both cardiovascular and resistance training.
- To build muscle, a consistent weight training programme must be combined with a balanced intake of calories, carbohydrate, protein and fat.
- The amount of lean weight you gain depends on your genetic make-up, body type and hormonal balance.
- To gain lean weight, you need to achieve positive energy balance. Increase both your maintenance calorie and carbohydrate intake by approximately 20%.
- A protein intake of 1.6 g/kg body weight is recommended for muscle hypertrophy and strength gains.
- Consume 0.25–0.4 g protein/kg BW immediately after training and include 0.25–0.4 g/kg BW in each meal throughout the day.
- Proteins containing all eight essential amino acids and high levels of leucine are particularly beneficial for promoting MPS, e.g. milk and milk-based products.
- To gain weight, put more total eating time into your daily routine, increase meal frequency, eat larger portions and include energy- and nutrient-dense foods e.g. milk, smoothies, yoghurt, nuts, dried fruit, avocado and cheese.
- There are very few supplements that are supported by good evidence; these include protein supplements and creatine.

Relative Energy Deficiency in Sport

11

A lower body weight or lean physique is deemed to be beneficial for performance or aesthetics in many sports. However, the optimal body composition for fitness or sports performance is not necessarily a desirable one from a health point of view. The pursuit of a lower body weight, 'ideal' body composition or body shape to improve performance may result in low energy availability (LEA) and leave an athlete vulnerable to serious health and performance symptoms associated with relative energy deficiency in sport (RED-S).

RED-S more accurately describes the clinical syndrome previously known as the Female Athlete Triad, which was first described during a consensus conference convened by the American College of Sports Medicine in 1992, and documented in a position stand published in 1997 (Otis et al., 1997). In the 2005 IOC Consensus Statement, the Female Athlete Triad was defined as 'the combination of disordered eating (DE) and irregular menstrual cycles eventually leading to a decrease in endogenous oestrogen and other hormones, resulting in low bone mineral density' (BMD) (International Olympic Committee, 2005). In 2007, the American College of Sports Medicine redefined the Triad as a clinical entity that refers to the 'relationship between three interrelated components: energy availability (EA), menstrual function and bone health' (Nattiv et al., 2007).

Since then, researchers have shown that the clinical phenomenon is not a rigid triad of three components, but rather a syndrome underpinned by an energy deficiency relative to the balance between energy intake and energy expenditure required for health and daily living, growth and sporting activities. It is now known that many body systems are affected, and it can occur in males as well as females, Caucasian and non-Caucasian, able-bodied and disabled populations, athletes and non-athletes. In 2014, the IOC published a consensus statement, replacing the term 'Female Athlete Triad' with a broader and more comprehensive term, 'relative energy deficiency in sport' (RED-S) (Mountjoy et al., 2014). An update summarising new research in the field of RED-S was published in 2018 (Mountjoy et al., 2018). The Female Athlete Triad is part of the RED-S continuum. RED-S highlights that there is a broader spectrum of symptoms, affecting multiple systems.

This chapter defines RED-S and describes the underlying causes and prevalence among athletes. Thereafter, risk factors, symptoms and health- and performance-related consequences are presented, followed by a summary of how it can be diagnosed, prevented and treated. It then covers disordered eating, menstrual health and bone health in greater depth, as these are major risk factors for RED-S.

What is RED-S?

Relative energy deficiency in sport (RED-S) refers to the situation in which an athlete or physically active individual has insufficient energy intake relative to energy expenditure, resulting in impaired physiological functioning, including impairments of metabolic rate, menstrual function, endocrine (hormone) function, bone health, immunity, protein synthesis and cardiovascular health. The underlying cause of RED-S is chronic *low energy availability (LEA)* or *energy deficiency*, a state in which the body does not have enough energy left to support all physiological functions needed to maintain optimal health.

WHAT IS 'ENERGY AVAILABILITY'?

The energy required to sustain normal body functions, such as breathing, digestion and brain functioning is equivalent to the resting metabolic rate (*see* pp. 5–6). Exercise requires additional energy. The energy we consume from food is partitioned by the body to cover these two demands. When the energy needed to cover the demands of exercise is subtracted from the energy consumed, the residual energy is called *energy availability (EA)* and is expressed as kcal/kg of fat-free body mass. It is defined as the amount of 'unused' energy remaining to carry out physiological functions after the energy cost of exercise training is subtracted from daily energy intake (Loucks *et al.*, 2011). In research settings, EA is calculated using the following equation:

- (energy intake(kcal) – exercise energy expenditure (kcal)) ÷ kg fat free mass (FFM)

For example, a 60 kg athlete with 15% body fat who consumes 2500 kcal a day and burns 1000 kcal in training has an energy balance of 1500 kcal. If you divide this by the athlete's fat-free mass (55 kg) and you have an EA of 27 kcal/kg FFM/day.

The exact EA value to maintain health varies between individuals, depending on body composition and age. Studies on healthy, sedentary women have defined 45 kcal/kg FFM/day as a threshold at which optimal energy balance and health can be achieved (Loucks and Thuma, 2003). If EA falls below the minimum level required for an individual, the body goes into a state of low energy availability (LEA), essentially energy-saving mode. It has been suggested that 30 kcal/kg FFM/day should be the lower threshold of energy availability in females, below which there will be a disruption of endocrine function (Loucks and Thuma, 2003; Mountjoy *et al.*, 2018). Therefore, LEA is commonly defined as less than 30 kcal/kg FFM/day. For males, a threshold of 25 kcal/kg FFM/day has been suggested (Fagerberg, 2018).

HOW DOES LOW ENERGY AVAILABILITY OCCUR?

LEA may occur when either energy intake is too low or energy expended through exercise is too high, or a combination of both, leaving insufficient energy to support normal physiological functions such as metabolic and immune function, bone health and the menstrual cycle in female athletes.

Fig. 11.1 shows how LEA may arise either *intentionally* or *unintentionally*. The central column shows an athlete who is consuming sufficient energy to cover the energy demands from training, and has sufficient energy available to cover requirements for life processes. The column on the left shows an athlete who has reduced their energy intake but energy demand from training remains the same, resulting in LEA. The column on the right shows that although the athlete has maintained the same energy intake, the training load has increased, resulting in LEA.

Thus intentional LEA can arise when an athlete chooses to make a change to their diet, training load and body composition in order to gain a performance or aesthetic advantage. This stems from a misguided belief that a lower body weight enhances athletic success. Unintentional LEA can arise when an individual is not aware of how much energy is required for the training they are doing,

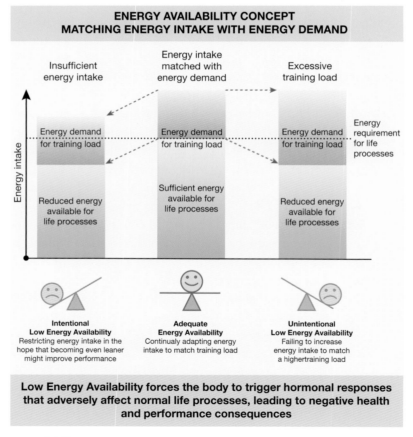

Figure 11.1 Energy availability concept
www.nickykeayfitness.com

or if they increase their training load without adequately increasing energy intake.

WHO IS AT GREATEST RISK OF DEVELOPING RED-S?

Prevalence of RED-S among athletes ranges from 22 to 58% (Logue *et al.*, 2020). However, in one study of 112 female athletes at the Australian Institute of Sport almost all (80%) participants had at least one symptom of RED-S, with 37% having two or three symptoms (Rogers *et al.*, 2021).

Athletes at risk of developing RED-S are those participating in body weight-sensitive (where a high power-to-weight ratio confers a performance advantage), weight-category or aesthetically focused sports. The first category includes distance runners, road cyclists, triathletes, climbers, cross-country skiers and ski jumpers due to the close link between low body weight and performance. Those participating in aesthetic sports such as dance, ice skating, diving, synchronised swimming, bodybuilding and gymnastics are at risk because success depends on body shape as well as physical skill. Athletes competing in weight-category sports such as martial arts, boxing, jockey and lightweight rowing are also more likely to develop eating disorders due to the pressures of meeting the weight criteria.

Although most studies have been done with females, growing evidence suggests body image issues are common in male athletes too (Burke *et al.*, 2018). RED-S is more common in males who compete in sports that place a high emphasis on appearance or leanness or where there is a culture of 'weight cutting' to achieve a competitive edge (Keay *et al.*, 2019; Heikura *et al.*, 2018(a)). However, RED-S is not limited to athletes – it can also affect those who are moderately active but not fuelling sufficiently.

Elite athletes and athletes in a high-performance environment are particularly at risk of RED-S compared to the normal population. Studies suggest that they are more likely to experience body dissatisfaction, a belief that a lower body weight will result in greater performance, or social pressure to look a certain way, which in turn may impact an athlete's eating behaviour and put them at risk for eating disorders and LEA (Wasserfurth *et al.*, 2020; Sundgot-Borgen and Tostveit, 2010). Pressure can also be experienced from the coach, teammates, and through social media platforms. There are particular personality traits that can predispose an athlete to developing RED-S. These include a desire to be the best, obsession, competitiveness, perfectionism, compulsiveness and self-motivation.

HOW CAN RED-S BE IDENTIFIED?

Measuring EA (via energy intake, exercise energy expenditure and FFM) can be time-consuming, inaccurate and impractical outside a research setting. For this reason, it is more commonly identified in the clinical setting using a validated screening tool such as the RED-S clinical assessment tool (RED-S CAT), resting metabolic rate (RMR) assessment, dual-energy X-ray absorptiometry-derived body composition and bone mineral density, venous and capillary blood samples in conjunction with questionnaires, such as the Low Energy Availability in Females Questionnaire (LEAF-Q), Depression, Anxiety and Stress Questionnaire (DASS-21), Generalized Anxiety Disorder (GAD-7), Center for Epidemiological Studies Depression Scale (CES-D) and SCOFF questionnaire for

Table 11.1	THE RISK STRATIFICATION OF RED-S		
	High risk	**Medium risk**	**Low risk**
Energy availability status	Severe low energy availability causing immediate risk to health	Low energy availability insufficient to support health and optimal performance	Adequate energy availability for health and training demands
Symptoms and eating patterns	Eating disorder (disrupted eating patterns with psychological factors)	Disordered eating	Fuelling matched to demand
Body weight	Body weight well below that expected for height	Weight loss, or steady weight below minimal healthy weight for height	Body weight as anticipated for height and minor deviations during season
Growth and development in young athletes	Significant drop from centile on growth charts; arrested puberty	Drop from centile on growth charts; arrested puberty	According to centile charts
Injury/illness	Prolonged and significant injury (especially bone stress fractures) or Illness	Recurrent injury (especially bone stress fractures) or illness	Infrequent injury/illness
Menstrual function	Primary or secondary amenorrhoea	Menstrual disruption	Normal menstrual function
Athletic performance	Impaired athletic performance	Initially maintained athletic performance, then below expectation for training load	Athletic performance as anticipated for training load
Investigations: blood tests	Blood tests support hypothalamic suppression and potentially electrolyte Abnormalities	Endocrine markers show evidence of functional hypothalamic Suppression	No significant abnormalities from investigations
DXA (bone health and body composition)	DXA BMD Z score (age matched) significantly <– I and disrupted body composition	DXA BMD Z score (age matched) <-1 (in particular lumbar spine). Body composition: low body Fat	Body composition and BMD as expected for sport/dance
Management	Address immediate risks to health. No training, no competition	Modification to training	No restrictions on periodised training and competition
	Address nutrition and psychological aspects	Review baseline nutrition, fuelling around exercise and recovery/rest	Fine-tuning of nutrition and training as required
Education, awareness and prevention	Important to raise awareness for all athletes		

Source: www.Health4Performance.co.uk and Mountjoy et al. 2015

disordered eating, which screen for physiological symptoms (Mountjoy *et al.*, 2015). Table 11.1 shows the risk stratification of RED-S.

RED-S is a diagnosis of exclusion. If RED-S is suspected then it is important to contact a medical professional to rule out underlying medical conditions. A sports medicine doctor will then be able to carry out appropriate blood tests to measure hormonal and nutritional markers of LEA.

WHAT ARE THE SYMPTOMS OF RED-S?

Initially, athletes with LEA may not display clinical symptoms or adverse performance effects. Once symptoms do appear, they may be subtle and easy to mistake for other conditions. There are several warning signs to look out for. These include:

Physiological

- Three consecutive missed periods in females (although this can be masked by oral contraception, which produce withdrawal bleeds not periods, or no bleeding at all) or a change to a previously regular cycle
- Low libido in males
- Poor development of muscle mass
- Digestive issues (such as constipation or feeling bloated)

Performance

- Persistent fatigue – beyond that expected for the training load
- A drop in performance or lack of expected improvement in performance
- Poor recovery
- Increased perception of effort during exercise and daily activities
- Recurrent illness and injuries (such as stress fractures)

Psychological and behavioural

- Changes in mood (such as feeling anxious or irritable)
- Reduced social interaction
- Irrational behaviour
- Problematic relationship with food and/or training
- Disrupted sleep patterns

What are the health consequences of RED-S?

RED-S can have detrimental consequences on many aspects of health and sports performance. The body always prioritises movement and so when there is short- or long-term LEA it compensates by going into an energy preservation mode and thus slows down many of the biological processes in the

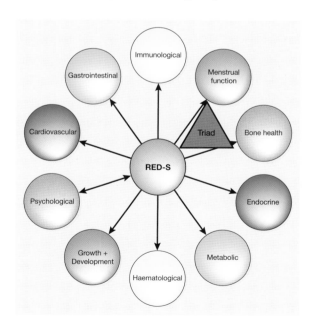

Figure 11.2 Health consequences of relative energy deficiency in sport (RED-S)
Mountjoy *et al*, 2014

body. The body reduces production of hormones in the reproductive system, such as oestrogen and testosterone, which has profound effects on many other systems in the body, including bone health. A study of 1000 female athletes aged 15–30 years showed that those with LEA were more likely to have increased risk of menstrual dysfunction, poor bone health, metabolic issues, haematological detriments, psychological disorders, cardiovascular impairment and gastrointestinal issues than those with adequate EA (Ackerman *et al.*, 2019). Everyone responds differently to LEA – not all athletes with RED-S experience all of these. An individual's experience of RED-S depends on their body composition, age, lifestyle, mentality and LEA severity. The health consequences of RED-S are shown in Figure 11.2, p. 213.

ENDOCRINE

Effects of LEA on the endocrine system in females include disruption of the hypothalamic–pituitary–gonadal axis, alterations in thyroid function, changes in appetite-regulating hormones (e.g. decreased leptin and oxytocin, increased ghrelin, peptide YY and adiponectin), decreases in insulin and insulin-like growth factor 1 (IGF-1), increased growth hormone (GH) resistance and elevations in cortisol (Logue *et al.* 2018, Allaway *et al.*, 2016). Many of these hormonal changes likely occur to conserve energy for more important bodily functions or to use the body's energy reserves for vital processes. In men, reductions in testosterone (Hackney *et al.*, 1988) and other hormone levels (MacConnie *et al.*, 1986) have been measured.

MENSTRUAL FUNCTION

The menstrual cycle is the best indicator of underlying health. If the cycle has become irregu-

lar or even stopped completely, this is a direct reflection of the body's response to nutrition, lifestyle, exercise, hormonal imbalance, or underlying health conditions.

LEA can lead to amenorrhoea, due to disruption of gonadotropin-releasing hormone (GnRH) pulsatility at the hypothalamus, followed by alterations of LH and follicle stimulating hormone release from the pituitary and decreased oestradiol and progesterone levels; this is considered a form of functional hypothalamic amenorrhoea (FHA) (Gordon *et al.*, 2017; Nattiv, *et al.* 2007). However, the duration and severity of LEA needed to create such disturbances is not clear. *See* pp. 224–227 for more information on LEA and menstrual dysfunction.

BONE HEALTH

One of the most severe effects of LEA and amenorrhoea is the reduction in bone mineral density, bone mass and strength and increased risk of early osteoporosis and stress fractures (Papageorgiou *et al.*, 2018). This is partly due to low levels of oestrogen and progesterone, both of which act directly on bone cells to maintain bone turnover (Drinkwater *et al.*, 1984; Misra *et al.*, 2004). LEA induces an increase in bone resorption (the natural breakdown of old bone) and a decrease in bone formation, causing a loss of bone mass and structure.

METABOLIC

As EA declines, physiological adaptations will occur, resulting in a reduction in the resting metabolic rate. One study found that female athletes with a low or reduced EA (<45kcal/kg FFM/day) had a lower resting metabolic rate than those with optimal EA (Melin *et al.*,

2015). A study with female rowers found that a 4-week block of intensified training decreased resting metabolic rate and increased fatigue, likely related to an imbalance between energy intake and output (Woods *et al.*, 2017(b)).

HAEMATOLOGICAL

Iron is essential for making haemoglobin (the oxygen-carrying protein in red blood cells) and myoglobin (the protein that carries and stores oxygen in muscle cells), aerobic energy production (the 'electron transport system' that controls the release of energy from cells) and immune function. Iron deficiency, often seen in female athletes, can contribute directly and indirectly to LEA. This is due to a potential reduction in appetite, decreased metabolic fuel availability and impaired metabolic efficiency, leading to an increase in energy expenditure during exercise and rest. It is also thought that LEA may contribute to iron deficiency (Petkus *et al.*, 2017).

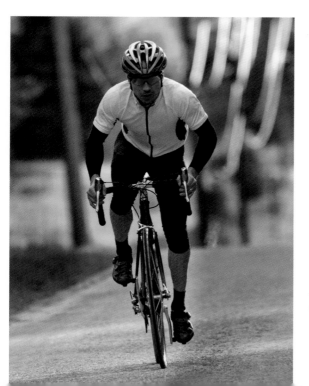

GROWTH AND DEVELOPMENT

LEA can impact growth and development. Studies have shown that adolescents with anorexia nervosa did not achieve their genetic height potential (Lantzouni *et al.*, 2002). This is thought to be related to altered levels of hormones responsible for growth (such as IGF-1 and GH).

CARDIOVASCULAR

Low levels of oestrogen affect the functioning of the cardiovascular system. One study showed that amenorrhea in young endurance athletes is associated with endothelial dysfunction and unfavourable blood lipid levels (Rickenlund *et al.*, 2005).

IMMUNOLOGICAL

The immune system is affected by LEA, which increases susceptibility to illness and infection. During a study of elite Australian athletes preparing for the 2016 Rio Olympic Games, LEA was associated with increased likelihood of illnesses, including those of the upper respiratory tract and gastrointestinal tract, bodily aches and anxiety in the previous month (Drew *et al.*, 2018).

PSYCHOLOGICAL

Psychological problems may be both the cause and consequence of LEA. Traits such as a higher drive for thinness has been linked to altered levels of hormones and disordered eating linked to reduced psychological well-being (De Souza *et al.*, 2007).

GASTROINTESTINAL

In the severe state of LEA of anorexia nervosa, gastrointestinal symptoms such as constipation can develop (Norris *et al.*, 2016).

DISORDERED EATING AND EATING DISORDERS

Disordered eating and eating disorders are more common in athletes with RED-S and these are discussed in more detail on pp. 218–24.

What are the performance consequences of RED-S?

Long-term LEA can impair performance through a variety of mechanisms. These include impaired recovery, glycogen storage and protein synthesis or by preventing consistent high-quality training due to the risk of injury and illness (*see* Fig 11.3). If the body cannot maintain basic health it cannot adapt to and recover from training to perform optimally. Performance variables associated with low EA include decreased training response, impaired judgement, decreased coordination, decreased concentration, irritability, depression and decreased endurance performance (Ackerman *et al.*, 2019).

A study of elite rhythmic gymnasts measured a direct correlation between LEA and sports performance (Silva and Paiva, 2015). Another study found that endurance athletes with functional hypothalamic amenorrhea had lower neuromuscular performance (measured as knee muscular strength and endurance) compared to athletes with normal menstrual cycles. This was linked to lower FFM, oestrogen, thyroid hormones and higher cortisol levels (Tornberg *et al.*, 2017). Although lower body weight and higher power to mass ratio are regarded as beneficial for running performance, this suggests that long-term energy restriction is likely to negatively affect performance and health. In a study of male road cyclists, those who intentionally restricted their dietary intake in an attempt to reduce body weight in the belief that this would improve race results experienced greater fatigue, illness, injury (including fractures), a drop in cycling performance and a less successful race season (Keay *et al.*, 2019). A study of rowers found that 4 weeks of intensified training without a concurrent increase in energy intake resulted in a significant drop in RMR, reduced performance, altered mood and a substantial increase in fatigue (Woods *et al.*, 2017(a)). It was concluded that the rowers developed unintentional LEA, which negatively affected their training and recovery.

However, in many cases, weight loss may mask under-performance in athletes experiencing LEA and may even result in slight performance enhancement. Despite the negative effect of LEA

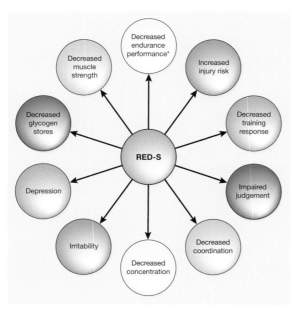

Figure 11.3 Potential performance consequences of relative energy deficiency in sport (RED-S)

Mountjoy *et al.* (2014)

on performance, athletes may appear to perform at the same level if the effects of lower body weight are greater or equal to the negative effect of LEA on performance.

How can RED-S be prevented?

Many athletes don't understand the true negative consequences of RED-S as they may be performing well at the moment, something that prevents many athletes and coaches addressing health issues. However, they aren't reaching optimal training and performance in a state of LEA. It is not possible to maintain performance long term.

Contrary to popular belief, lighter does not always mean faster! The weight at which an individual achieves optimal performance will depend on many factors, including age, gender, genetics and natural build. Instead of trying to attain an unnaturally low body weight or body fat, the aim instead should be attainment of a healthy weight and body composition that allows the individual to perform well without compromising their health.

In certain situations where weight loss or maintenance of a very low body weight is deemed essential for athletic success then the aim should be to preserve lean body mass, as this will help prevent or minimise bone loss (Papageorgiou *et al.*, 2018). This may be achieved by a modest calorie reduction of no more than *approximately 15%* on some training days, but not others. This should produce a relatively modest energy deficit of around 300 calories a day. Any more than this risks LEA. Additionally, increasing protein intake to 1.8–2.0 g/kg/day is recommended in order to prevent lean mass losses during periods of energy restriction (Phillips and Van Loon, 2011).

LEA can begin unintentionally, so if an individual increases their training load, for example undergoing a hard block of training, they should take steps to avoid LEA by being more proactive in planning their food intake. They will need to pay attention to their energy levels, and make a sustained, conscious effort to consume enough energy each day even if they do not always feel hungry. For example, they will need to consume more energy on hard training days, prioritise post-exercise nutrition and avoid going long periods without eating. If this proves difficult then including some lower-fibre (e.g. 'white' instead of wholemeal pasta) options can make this easier. Including plenty of foods rich in healthy fats, such as nuts, seeds, nut butters, avocado and olive and rapeseed oil in meals and snacks will help boost energy intake without adding too much extra volume. If an individual finds it difficult to eat larger portions, they may increase meal frequency and add high-energy snacks, such as nuts, nut butter on toast, and fruit and nut bars between meals.

How can RED-S be treated?

The overall aim of treatment is to restore EA. This may involve *increasing energy intake* and/ or *reducing training load* (e.g. intensity, duration or frequency of training). However, these two things can often be harder than they sound, so consider seeking the help of a professional to get you back on track and support from family and friends. Your GP, sports doctor, sports dietitian or a psychologist will be able to provide assessment and advice.

There are many potential complications, e.g. an individual's desire to stay fit, lean and active may make compliance difficult. It takes time to regain a positive energy balance and, depending the on severity, recovery can take weeks, months or years. An individual's psychological well-being may be dependent on their performance, body image and training, so asking them to stop/reduce training can be difficult.

Once adequate EA has been established, a structured plan for a gradual return to training and nutrition needs to be developed. The initial focus should be on restoring muscle tone, bone health and neuromuscular skills through body weight strength and conditioning. This will help reduce injury risk. A routine of fuelling before, during and after training also needs to be established, with priority given to recovery nutrition within the 2-hour post-exercise window to enable hormonal responses to training.

Once muscle strength has been restored then endurance training may be gradually increased. Energy expenditure will be higher so it is essential that energy intake is increased in line with the energy demands of training. High-intensity and interval training should only be introduced once a good fuelling routine has been established as this places the highest stress on the body and requires the highest energy demand on the individual.

Disordered eating and eating disorders

Many athletes are very careful about what they eat and often experiment with different dietary programmes in order to improve their performance. However, there is a fine line between paying attention to detail and obsessive eating behaviour. The pressure to be lean in order to improve performance or conform to competition regulations that are ill-suited to their physique makes some athletes develop eating habits that not only put their performance at risk but also endanger their health. Furthermore, misconceptions about nutrition, e.g. that carbohydrates make you gain weight, or the avoidance of specific foods are prevalent among athletes and could lead to unhealthy eating behaviours (Martinsen *et al.*, 2010).

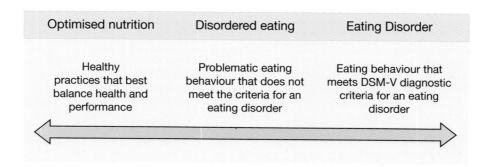

Figure 11.4 The spectrum of eating behaviours, from optimised nutrition to eating disorders.
Wells *et al.*, (2020)

of 'weight cutting' to achieve a competitive edge (e.g. wrestling, boxing and horse racing).

WHO IS AT GREATEST RISK?

There is no single cause of DE but, typically, it stems from a belief that a lower body weight or body fat or high power-to-weight ratio enhances performance. The athlete begins to diet and, for reasons not completely understood, then adopts more restrictive and unhealthy eating behaviour. DE is often a result of an interplay between biological, genetic and environmental factors.

Risk factors include personality traits (such as perfectionism, obsessiveness and strong achievement orientation), early start of sport-specific training, frequent weight cycling, dieting and weight loss at early age, a desire to be lean to increase performance, pressure to lose weight from coaches, overtraining, recurrent injuries and the regulations in some sports (Nattiv *et al.*, 2007). In weight-sensitive sports, comments by coaches on an athlete's body composition are associated with a psychological pressure to diet and there is a common belief that judges are influenced by the body composition of the athlete (Byrne and McLean, 2002). The strongest predictor of DE in athletes seems to be body image dissatisfaction. Athletes who are dissatisfied with their body and athletes who report a desire to be leaner to improve performance are more likely to develop EDs and DE than those who are less dissatisfied.

In addition, pressures on athletes to reduce weight and body fat can create a culture for DE. The result is that in weight-sensitive sports, such as the weight-class, and aesthetically judged sports, there might be an indirectly increased risk for EDs.

It is possible that some people with a predisposition to eating disorders are attracted to certain sports because this environment may normalise what may otherwise be considered disordered. For example, people with DE often exercise to cope with difficult emotions and have very rigid exercise routines, and a sports environment can endorse these behaviours. A study of male and female dancers found the interaction of psychological factors and physical factors put them at risk of LEA and clinical consequences of RED-S (Keay *et al.*, 2020).

WHAT ARE THE WARNING SIGNS AND SYMPTOMS OF DISORDERED EATING?

Athletes with EDs and DE try to keep their disorder a secret. However, there are physical and behavioural signs you can look out for. These are detailed in Table 11.3 on p. 222.

WHAT ARE THE HEALTH AND PERFORMANCE CONSEQUENCES OF DISORDERED EATING?

One of the health risks of DE is the development of RED-S and this can result in impairments of bone health, menstrual function, endocrine, metabolic and haematological status, growth and development, psychological well-being, and cardiovascular, gastrointestinal and immunological systems (Mountjoy *et al.*, 2014; Loucks *et al.*, 2011). The chaotic and restricted eating patterns of disordered eating often result in menstrual and fertility problems. Menstrual dysfunction (*see* pp.224–7) is common among people suffering from anorexia nervosa.

Osteopenia (lower than normal bone density) and osteoporosis and among the most severe

Table 11.3	WARNING SIGNS AND SYMPTOMS OF DISORDERED EATING AND EATING DISORDERS	
Physical/medical	**Psychological/behavioural**	
• Hair loss • Dry skin, brittle hair and nails • Lanugo hair (fine hair on the surface of the skin) • Dorsal hand callus or abrasions • Dental and gum problems • Bradycardia (abnormally low heart rate) • Hypotension (abnormally low blood pressure) • Hypoglycaemia (abnormally low blood sugar levels) • Delayed onset of puberty • Menstrual dysfunction • Reduced bone mass/stress fractures • Swollen parotid (saliva) glands • Constipation, diarrhoea, bloating • Hypohydration (p. 147) • Oedema (swelling) • Electrolyte disturbances • Hypokalemia (low blood potassium levels) • Muscle cramps • Metabolic alkalosis (overly alkaline blood) • Significant weight loss/frequent weight fluctuations • Fatigue • Anaemia • Hypothermia	• Restrictive eating, binging and purging • Avoidance of eating/eating situation • Dissatisfaction with body image (especially in the sport context)/self-critical (especially concerning body, weight and sport performance) • Low self-esteem • Poor coping skills • Mood swings • Extreme performance orientation • Perfectionism • Compulsive and excessive training, even when injured • Restlessness; relaxing is difficult or impossible • Insomnia • Reduced social activities • Poor concentration • Resistance to weight gain or maintenance recommended by sport support staff • Anxiety • Depression	

complications of LEA and EDs (Heikura *et al.*, 2018(b)). The combination of low body fat levels, restricted calorie intake, low calcium intake, intense training and stress can result in stress fractures and other injuries and, ultimately, premature osteoporosis. One study found that DE was associated with low bone mineral density in runners who had regular menstrual cycles (Cobb *et al.*, 2003). Researchers at the University of British Columbia, Vancouver, found that female runners with a recent stress fracture were more likely to have a high degree of dietary restraint compared with runners without a history of stress fractures (Guest and Barr, 2005).

Performance consequences of DE arise from inadequate fuelling and training interruptions due to frequent illness and injury. Endurance is likely to be impaired if glycogen in the liver and muscles become depleted. There can also be reductions in training capacity and maximal oxygen consumption, and inadequate recovery and adaptation.

Without enough protein to maintain and repair muscle, there will be a loss of lean body mass, strength and power. The athlete quickly becomes more susceptible to injury, illness and infection. Deficiencies of vitamins and minerals will eventually develop, and these will affect performance, too, increasing the risk of muscle weakness, injuries and infections.

Athletes who use diuretics or laxatives or self-induce vomiting will become hypohydrated. This quickly results in fatigue and poor performance. It can also have serious effects on health. The reduced blood volume results in decreased blood flow to the skin, which means the body is not able to sweat properly and maintain a normal temperature during exercise. This, in turn, increases core temperature and increases the risk of heat exhaustion and heatstroke.

In summary, athletes with DE and EDs are likely to suffer from nutritional deficiencies, chronic fatigue, hypohydration and a dramatic reduction in performance.

HOW CAN EATING DISORDERS BE IDENTIFIED AND TREATED?

The early identification and appropriate management of DE leads to better outcomes.

Approaching someone you suspect has DE requires great tact and sensitivity. Sufferers are likely to deny that they have a problem; they may feel embarrassed and their self-esteem threatened,

How are athletes with disordered eating able to continue training?

It seems extraordinary that athletes with very low calorie intake continue to exercise and compete, without appearing to be unduly affected by the inadequate nutrition. Undoubtedly, a combination of psychological and physiological factors are involved.

On the psychological side, athletes with EDs are able to motivate and push themselves to exercise, despite feelings of exhaustion. Research shows sufferers are typically strong willed, highly driven and have a strong desire to succeed. Thus, in the short term they are able to continue training and competing, despite their low calorie intake.

On the physiological side, it is likely that the body adapts by becoming more energy efficient, reducing its metabolic rate (10–30% is possible). This would allow the athlete to train and maintain energy balance on fewer calories than would be expected. Some scientists, however, suggest that excessive exercise during dieting may augment the fall in metabolic rate.

To overcome physical and emotional fatigue, many sufferers of anorexia and bulimia use caffeine. However, in the long term, performance ultimately falls.

so it is vital to avoid a direct confrontation about their eating behaviour or physical symptoms. Be tactful, tread very gently – do not suddenly present 'evidence' – and avoid accusations. Talking to them about menstruation, training or injuries can be a less threatening approach than questions regarding body weight, dieting or food.

Various forms of specialist help are available, such as trained counsellors from a self-help organisation or private EDs clinic (*see* p. 406), or treatment within a core multidisciplinary team of doctors, psychologists and sports dietitians working within sport. The Australian Institute of Sport and National Eating Disorders Collaboration has published practical recommendations on the assessment and clinical management of DE in high-performance sport (Wells *et al.*, 2020).

Menstrual dysfunction

Menstrual dysfunction is defined as irregular, infrequent or absent menstrual cycles. The Royal College of Obstetrics and Gynaecology (RCOG) defines primary amenorrhoea as no menarche (periods) by 16 years of age, secondary amenorrhoea as cessation of periods for longer than six months in a previously regular menstruating woman, and oligomenorrhoea is defined as fewer than nine cycles per calendar year.

This lack of menstrual periods can happen when there is significant weight loss, disordered eating, or intense training or exercise. It's a myth that amenorrhoea is simply a consequence of hard training; it should be regarded as a clinical state of overtraining, because of the adverse effects it has on many systems in the body.

HOW COMMON IS MENSTRUAL DYSFUNCTION IN FEMALE ATHLETES?

A study of adolescent athletes found that 28% suffered menstrual dysfunction (Armento *et al.* 2020). Several studies have found that menstrual dysfunction is more prevalent among female athletes participating in weight-sensitive and aesthetic sports, such as distance running, cross-country, cycling, gymnastics and dancing (Beals and Hill, 2006; Torstveit and Sundgot-Borgen, 2005; Sundgot-Borgen, 1994(a) and (b); Sundgot-Borgen and Larsen, 1993).

In a study at the University of Utah and the University of Indianapolis, significantly more lean-build athletes suffered menstrual irregularities than non lean-build athletes (Beals and Hill, 2006). This may be due to the greater volume of training associated with endurance sports. However, a study at San Diego State University indicates that approximately 20% of female high school athletes, regardless of sport, are at risk of disordered eating or menstrual dysfunction and that the two conditions are often interrelated (Nichols *et al.*, 2007). Nearly 27% of lean-build athletes had menstrual dysfunction, compared with 17% non lean-build athletes.

WHO IS AT GREATEST RISK OF MENSTRUAL DYSFUNCTION?

Studies have shown that female athletes who have consistently LEA are at increased risk of menstrual dysfunction (Loucks, 2003). Contrary to popular belief in the athletic community, menstrual dysfunction is unlikely to develop as a result of exercise alone, nor is there a specific body fat percentage below which regular periods stop. Instead, a combination of factors, including LEA, disordered eating behaviour, intense training before menarche, high-intensity training and volume, low body-fat levels and physical and emotional stress are usually involved. The more of these risk factors that you have, the greater the chance of developing menstrual dysfunction. However, the most important trigger for menstrual dysfunction appears to be LEA.

Girls who begin intense training pre-puberty usually start their periods at a later age than the average. This may be due to a combination of high-volume exercise and low body-fat levels. Some female athletes, particularly runners, may have shorter than average menstrual cycles due to anovulatory cycles, which are cycles during which an egg is not produced. This pattern is linked to low levels of female hormones: oestrogen and progesterone, follicle-stimulating hormone (FSH) and luteinising hormone (LH).

WHY IS MENSTRUAL FUNCTION DISRUPTED IN CERTAIN ATHLETES?

It is thought that menstrual dysfunction is an energy-conserving adaptation by the body to LEA. When energy intake keeps pace with energy expenditure, normal menstrual function is maintained. But when energy intake is insufficient to keep pace with energy expenditure, the body and brain sense a state of net energy deficit, which then results in menstrual dysfunction. From an evolutionary perspective, in this state of energy deficit, energy is conserved for the most vital body functions and the reproductive axis shuts down. In other words, the body tries to save energy by economising on the energy costs of menstruation i.e. shutting down the normal menstrual function.

It is possible that a genetically determined threshold or 'set point' of energy availability (and/or body fat) exists for each individual, below which normal menstrual function ceases.

The body mechanism is as follows: the combination of mental or physiological stress and a chronic LEA increases cortisol production by the adrenals, which disrupts the release of gonadotrophin-releasing hormone (GnRH) from the brain. This, in turn, reduces the production of the gonadotrophin-releasing hormone, luteinising hormone (LH) and follicle-stimulating hormone (FSH), oestrogen and progesterone (Loucks et al., 1989; Edwards et al., 1993). Leptin – a hormone produced by fat cells in adipose tissue – also plays a key role in the regulation of GnRH. When levels fall (due to low body fat levels), this signals to the hypothalamus to reduce release of GnRH, thus downregulating the reproductive system.

WHAT ARE THE HEALTH CONSEQUENCES OF MENSTRUAL DYSFUNCTION?

One of the most severe effects is the reduction in bone density, and increased risk of early osteoporosis and stress and non-stress fractures. This is partly due to low levels of oestrogen and progesterone, both of which act directly on bone cells to maintain bone turnover (Drinkwater et al., 1984). When hormone levels drop, the natural breakdown of old bone exceeds the speed of formation of new bone. The result is loss of bone minerals and a loss of bone density. Training, then, no longer has a positive effect on bone density: it cannot compensate for the negative effects of low oestrogen and progesterone. Athletes with menstrual dysfunction are more prone to musculoskeletal injuries in general, and stress fractures in particular.

In addition, high levels of cortisol, ghrelin (the 'hunger hormone') and low levels of leptin and IGF-1 – both linked to menstrual dysfunction – are also thought to contribute to bone loss and low bone density (Carbon, 2002). Canadian researchers have found that disordered eating is correlated with menstrual irregularities and increased cortisol levels, all of which are risk factors for stress fractures (Guest and Barr, 2005).

Studies have found that the bone mineral density in the lumbar spine can be as much as 20–30% lower in amenorrhoeic distance runners compared with normally menstruating runners (Cann et al., 1984; Nelson et al., 1986). A study of elite distance runners found that those with amenorrhoea or low testosterone were four-and-a-half times more likely to suffer a bone injury than eumenorrhoeic runners (Heikura et al., 2018(b)).

Amenorrhoeic dancers have been shown to have significantly lower bone mineral density at the lumber spine compared with eumenorrhoeic dancers, putting them at greater risk of osteoporosis (Keay et al., 1997).

Whether bone mineral density 'catches up' once menstruation resumes is not known for certain. One long-term study found that bone mass increased initially, but in the long term, it remained lower compared to active and inactive women (Drinkwater, 1986).

WHAT ARE THE PERFORMANCE CONSEQUENCES OF MENSTRUAL DYSFUNCTION?

Menstrual dysfunction results in many performance-hindering effects, all of which are linked to very low oestrogen levels. These include an increased risk of soft tissue injuries, stress fractures, prolonged healing of injuries and reduced ability to recover from hard training sessions (Lloyd et al., 1986). For example, low oestrogen levels result in a loss of suppleness in the ligaments, which then become more susceptible to injury. Low oestrogen levels slow down bone adaptation to exercise and micro-fractures occur more readily and heal more slowly.

A study of female runners found that those with amenorrhoea spent significantly more days injured and ran less over the course of a year than the athletes who had a regular menstrual cycle (Ihalainen et al., 2021). The researchers found that increased annual running volume was associated with improved athletic performance, and only the athletes who were having a regular period saw an improvement in performance over the course of a year.

The good news is that performance will most likely improve once menstruation resumes. Studies show that when amenorrhoeic athletes improve their diet and restructure their training programme to improve energy balance, normal menstruation resumes within about 3 months and performance improves consistently (Dueck et al., 1996). This is perhaps the most persuasive reason to seek treatment if you have amenorrhoea.

HOW CAN MENSTRUAL DYSFUNCTION BE TREATED?

It is important to seek medical advice if an athlete has suffered amenorrhoea for longer than 6 months. An initial consultation with a GP will rule out medical causes of amenorrhoea. They should then get a referral to a specialist, such as a gynaecologist, sports physician, endocrinologist or bone specialist. As part of their treatment they should consider advice from a sports nutritionist, exercise physiologist or sports psychologist. Treatment will centre on increasing EA by increasing energy intake and/or reducing training load. For example, they may have to reduce their training frequency, volume and intensity or change their current programme to include more cross-training. They may need to increase food intake in order to bring their body weight and body fat within the normal range. If they have some degree of disordered eating, they will need help in overcoming this problem (*see* pp. 223–4).

If amenorrhoea persists after this type of treatment, hormone therapy may be prescribed to prevent further loss of bone mineral density. Doses of oestrogen and progesterone, similar to those used for treating postmenopausal women, are usually used. Supplements containing calcium, vitamin D, magnesium and other key minerals may be advised simultaneously.

Summary of key points

- Relative energy deficiency in sport (RED-S) refers to the impaired physiological function including metabolic rate, menstrual function, bone health, immunity, protein synthesis and cardiovascular health caused by relative energy deficiency or low EA in male and female athletes.
- RED-S is underpinned by low energy availability (LEA), a mismatch between an athlete's energy intake and the energy expended in exercise, leaving insufficient energy to support all physiological functions needed to maintain optimal health and performance.
- Athletes at risk of developing RED-S are those involved with weight-sensitive sports, which can be divided into three categories: 1) gravitational sports, 2) weight-class sports and 3) aesthetically judged sports. Dancers and recreational exercisers are also potentially at risk.

- The optimal EA for healthy physiological function in females is **45 kcal/kg FFM/day**; LEA is commonly defined as **<30 kcal/kg FFM/day**, below which health impairment may occur.
- Health consequences of RED-S include impaired menstrual function/libido, metabolic rate, bone health, immunity, protein synthesis and cardiovascular health, all of which can contribute to impaired sports performance.
- Symptoms of RED-S include weight loss/low body weight, amenorrhoea or menstrual dysfunction, reduced libido, persistent fatigue, recurrent illness and injuries, poor recovery, reduced performance and mood changes.
- Eating disorders (EDs) include anorexia nervosa and bulimia nervosa and are defined by the American Psychiatric Association's Diagnostic & Statistical Manual of Mental Disorders (DSM-V). Disordered eating (DE) is defined as any eating behaviour that is not optimised.
- EDs and DE are more common in athletes in weight-sensitive sports
- Menstrual dysfunction is defined as irregular, infrequent or absent menstrual cycles.
- Menstrual dysfunction develops due to a combination of factors, such as LEA, disordered eating, the commencement of intense training before menarche, high training intensity and volume, low body fat levels and physical and emotional stress.
- Menstrual dysfunction has an adverse effect on many systems in the body, including a reduction in bone density, putting you at risk of early osteoporosis and stress fractures; soft tissue injuries; prolonged healing of injuries and reduced ability to recover from hard training sessions.

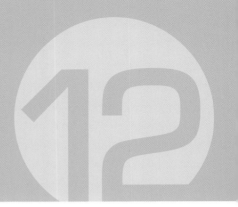

//Gut Health

Your gut health has a huge impact on many aspects of your health and there is a growing body of research that suggests it may also affect your sports performance and recovery. It is now known that elite athletes have a unique make-up of gut microorganisms that reflect their fitness and may be partly responsible for their performance. At the same time, regular exercise affects the composition of the gut microorganisms, increasing microbial diversity and improving health.

This first part of this chapter looks at the effect of exercise on the gut microbiota (the community of trillions of microorganisms in our gut) and the effect of the gut microbiota on performance and recovery. It also considers whether changing your microbiota through diet may help to improve performance.

The second part of this chapter looks at the potential causes of gut problems experienced by many athletes during high-intensity endurance exercise and explores practical nutritional strategies that may alleviate them.

What is the gut microbiota?

Your gut is home to trillions of microorganisms – bacteria, yeasts, fungi and viruses – collectively known as the gut microbiota, estimated to weigh around 200 g in a 70 kg individual (Sender *et al.*, 2016). They affect your gut's health as well as your health and performance. The vast majority live in the colon, with comparatively few living in the small intestine and stomach. It has been estimated that there are more microorganisms in the gut than there are cells in the human body. This gut microbiota contains 150–200 times more genes then the human genome. These genes are referred to as the gut microbiome.

Everyone has a unique microbiota, with the diversity and abundance of microorganisms within this influencing our health. A healthy microbiota is linked to better immunity, cardiovascular health and mental health, a lower risk of chronic diseases, and is thought to help combat gut symptoms associated with high-intensity endurance exercise. Many factors, such as age, genetics, stress and diet affect the gut microbiota and there's a growing body of research suggesting that regular exercise and diet also have a major effect. In addition, our gut microorganisms are thought to affect exercise performance and thus by changing the diversity and composition of our gut microbiota it may be possible to enhance several aspects of your performance.

HOW DOES THE GUT MICROBIOTA AFFECT HEALTH?

The microorganisms in the colon play a crucial role in digestion, vitamin synthesis, energy metabolism and immunity. A high population of health-promoting gut microorganisms will ensure that most of the attachment sites on the surface of the cells lining the gut will be filled with these beneficial bacteria and prevent pathogenic bacteria from gaining a foothold.

Our gut microbiota can also help us break down dietary components – namely fibre and resistant starch – that are otherwise indigestible by human enzymes. In doing so, they produce beneficial substances, including vitamins (folate, riboflavin and vitamin K) and short chain fatty acids (SCFAs), such as acetate, propionate and butyrate. These SCFAs provide fuel for your intestinal, liver and muscle cells, and promote a healthy gut barrier. SCFAs also play an important role in various signalling pathways involved with appetite control, inflammation, gut motility and energy expenditure. Butyrate also has anti-cancer and anti-inflammatory effects and may help protect against oxidative stress.

In contrast, imbalances in our gut microorganisms are associated with the development of chronic diseases, including obesity and type 2 diabetes; bowel diseases such as irritable bowel syndrome and inflammatory bowel disease; allergies, asthma, eczema, depression, anxiety and autism. They can even have an impact on our mental health. These imbalances in gut microorganisms can happen if you have a poor diet or when you take antibiotics, which can kill the healthy bacteria in your gut.

There is no scientific consensus as to what constitutes a 'healthy' gut microbiota, but one consistent observation is that there is increased species diversity among healthy individuals. It is thought that maintaining the balance and diversity of your gut microorganisms is vital for physical and mental well-being.

ARE THERE DIFFERENCES IN GUT MICROBIOTA COMPOSITION BETWEEN ATHLETES AND SEDENTARY PEOPLE?

There's evidence that the gut microbiota of athletes feature more health-promoting bacteria (such as *Akkermansia* and *Prevotella*) and increased diversity compared to sedentary people. For example, a study of 33 professional and amateur competitive cyclists found that 30 had *Akkermansia* present (Peterson *et al.*, 2017). This genus is associated with positive metabolic function and may reflect better fitness. Additionally, the longer the amount of time spent exercising each week, the greater the abundance of the genus *Prevotella*, which correlated with increased branch chain amino acid (BCAA) metabolism, which forms part of muscle protein synthesis and facilitates recovery.

A study led by researchers at the University College Cork in Ireland that compared 40 professional rugby players with sedentary people found that the rugby players had a much greater diversity of gut microorganims and higher than average numbers of the health-promoting strains (Clarke *et al.*, 2014). This microbial diversity is linked to better immunity, higher resistance to upper respiratory tract illness and lower rates of obesity. Additionally, those with a low Body Mass Index (BMI) had a higher amount of *Akkermansia* than those with a high BMI.

These findings were confirmed in a more recent study, which measured higher levels of microbial-produced SCFAs in professional rugby players compared with sedentary people (Barton *et al.*, 2018). SCFAs are associated with enhanced fitness and overall health.

In a study of 37 international-level athletes, researchers were able to identify distinctive differences in the gut microbiota between different types of sport (2020).

Body composition also seems to play a part in determining the ratio of beneficial vs pathogenic microorganisms in the gut. It has been found that lean and obese people have very distinct bacterial population profiles (Valdes *et al.*, 2018).

How does exercise affect the gut?

A review published in the *Journal of the International Society of Sports Nutrition* concluded that regular exercise increases microbial diversity and stimulates the proliferation of microorganisms that increase performance and health (Mohr *et al.*, 2020). Adaptations to exercise may create an environment in the GI tract that allows for more diversity of gut bacteria and greater metabolic function in turn, such as increased production of SCFAs (Mitchell *et al.*, 2019). One study showed a positive correlation between cardiovascular fitness (as measured by VO_2 peak) and greater microbial diversity and metabolic function and having more of the SCFA butyrate (Estaki *et al.*, 2016). This seems to suggest that cardiovascular fitness is a good predictor of gut microbial diversity, which in turn seems to be associated with better health. Scientists at the University of Illinois at Urbana-Champaign found that 6 weeks of endurance exercise improved the diversity of volunteers' gut microbes (Allen *et al.*, 2018). When they stopped exercising, their microbiomes reverted to what they had been at the start of the study. These studies provide compelling evidence that exercise can induce changes in the gut microbiota independent of diet.

Prolonged intense exercise also stimulates positive changes in gut microbial diversity. A study with ultra-endurance rowers before, during and after a 33-day trans-oceanic rowing event saw an increased abundance of SCFA-producing species and species associated with improved metabolic health, which persisted 3 months after the event (Keohane *et al.*, 2019). It is thought that these adaptations might help to compensate for the physiological damage associated with prolonged exercise.

However, single bouts of prolonged endurance exercise have been shown to increase intestinal permeability (also known as 'leaky gut', *see* p. 236). This has a negative effect on gut health through the release of endotoxins into the bloodstream, which stimulates an inflammatory response. Having high levels of the SCFA butyrate may help to prevent such damage, therefore undertaking regular exercise that stimulates the growth of SCFA-producing gut bacteria, supported by a diet that also encourages the abundance of these bacterial species, is likely to be important for good gut health.

How does the gut affect performance?

A review of studies published in 2020 suggests that the gut microbiota may influence performance and having a more diverse microbiota may be beneficial (Hughes, 2019). The exact mechanisms are not fully understood but it is likely that there are several indirect effects that boost performance. These include increased immunity, less oxidative stress – all key factors necessary for performance and muscle recovery after exercise (Trapp *et al.*, 2010; Mach and Fuster-Botella, 2017).

A review of 33 studies with athletes concluded that the gut microbiota plays a key role in controlling oxidative stress and inflammatory responses as well as improving metabolism and energy expenditure during endurance exercise (Mach and Fuster-Botella, 2017). With better immunity, you're less likely to suffer illnesses and gut problems that can hamper your training. And with less oxidative stress and lower inflammation, you will have less muscle damage and faster recovery. Additionally, the short chain fatty acids produced by gut microorganisms help regulate energy metabolism, appetite hormones and body composition. In other words, a healthy gut microbiota is critical for optimal performance and recovery as well as health.

How does diet affect the gut microbiome?

It is well established that diet affects the composition of the gut microbiota. A US study showed that you can achieve significant alterations in your gut microbiota within as little as 24 hours of a dietary change (David *et al.*, 2014).

A diet rich in plant-based foods is linked with the presence and abundance of health-promoting gut microorganisms that are associated with a lower risk of developing conditions such as obesity, Type 2 diabetes and cardiovascular disease, according to results from PREDICT 1,

What is oxidative stress?

Oxidative stress occurs during intense exercise when the number of free radicals (reactive oxygen species, ROS) produced exceeds the ability of your body's antioxidant defence system to neutralise them. This is not a problem at low levels and can even be beneficial for promoting muscle adaptations but, if sustained, it can damage cell membranes and DNA, impair muscle function and hasten fatigue. By consuming a diet rich in antioxidant nutrients, you will strengthen your body's antioxidant defences and help reduce the damage associated with oxidative stress.

What is inflammation?

Inflammation is the body's natural response to protect itself against harm. There are two types: acute and chronic. Acute inflammation occurs in response to an injury or illness; your immune system sends out white blood cells to surround and protect the area, creating visible redness and swelling. In these situations, inflammation is essential and beneficial. Chronic inflammation, on the other hand, is not beneficial. It is a longer-lasting immune response that persists over months or years, and not only puts you at greater risk of chronic diseases such as heart disease, stroke and type 2 diabetes but can also increase fatigue during endurance exercise and hamper your recovery afterwards.

a large-scale international study (Asnicar *et al.*, 2021). The researchers found that people who ate a diet rich in plant-based foods were more likely to have high levels of specific gut micro-organims. For example, having a microbiota rich in *Prevotella copri* and *Blastocystis* species was associated with maintaining a favourable blood sugar level after a meal.

A meta-analysis of studies found that people who consumed a vegetarian or vegan diet for at least 2 years had lower levels of inflammation (as measured by lower blood levels of C-reactive protein) than those who ate meat, suggesting that such diets have an anti-inflammatory effect on the body (Haghighatdoost *et al.*, 2017). A 2019 review of studies points to the potential benefits of foods rich in anthocyanins (a subclass of polyphenols found in fruit and vegetables) for increasing the population of beneficial gut organisms, while at the same time inhibiting the harmful species (Igwe *et al.*, 2019).

Carbohydrates and dietary fibre are the main nutrients that provide carbon and energy to the intestinal microorganisms. In particular, adequate intake of dietary fibre increases the diversity of gut microbiota. In a study of 33 cyclists, higher intakes of carbohydrates and dietary fibre were associated with increased abundance of the health-promoting species *Prevotella* (Peterson *et al.*, 2017). This is likely to be beneficial for athletes since increased production of SCFAs could improve muscle insulin sensitivity, reduce inflammation and improve satiety.

A study with distance runners found that those with low fibre and high protein intakes had reduced microbial diversity and a decrease in SCFA-producing microorganisms (Jang *et al.*, 2019). In other words, a low fibre intake or high protein intake – such as that associated with keto and low carbohydrate diets – may counteract the benefits of exercise that would otherwise increase gut microbial diversity.

Animal and plant proteins have different effects on the gut microbiota. The presence of *Bacteroides* species are highly associated with animal proteins, whereas *Prevotella* species are associated with plant-based diets (Wu et al., 2011). Plant proteins are incompletely digested in the small intestine, with a larger proportion passing to the colon where they are metabolised by the microbiota.

How can you improve your gut health?

Increasing the diversity of your gut microbiota through diet and exercise may improve your over-all health, sports performance and post-exercise recovery. The most effective way to increase the diversity of your gut microbiota – and potentially gain a performance advantage – is by consuming a wide range of foods rich in fibre, polyphenols, probiotics (*see* pp. 139–40) and prebiotics (*see* p. 223). These components are fermented by the health-promoting gut microorganisms to produce SCFAs, enabling them to grow and multiply. Therefore, a high intake of plant foods tends to increase health-promoting species of bacteria and decrease disease-promoting species.

- **Eat a wide range of plant foods** – Try to get as many different kinds of fruit, vegetables, whole grains, beans, lentils, nuts and seeds in your diet as possible. Variety is key because each contains different nutrients that the gut microorganims thrive on. The American

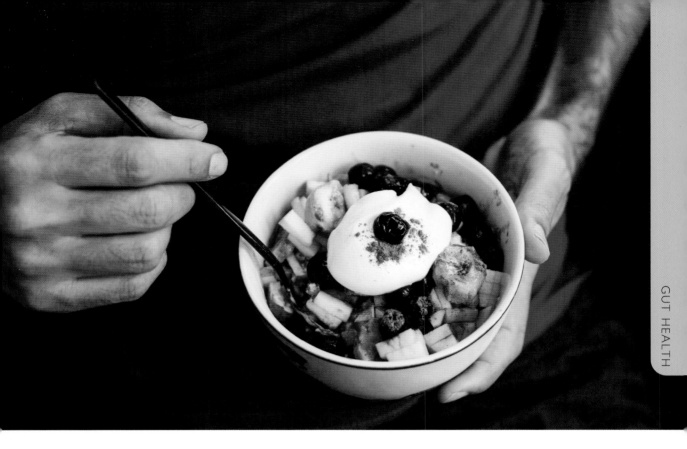

Gut Project, a large-scale study that analysed microbiome samples from more than 10,000 people, showed that people who eat around 30 different plants each week have much greater microbial diversity than those who eat just 10 (McDonald *et al.*, 2018).

- **Eat plenty of fibre** – There are many types of fibre and the more types you eat the greater the benefit. Aim for a minimum of 30 g fibre a day (SACN, 2015). Fibre encourages the growth of health-promoting gut micororganisms.

- **Include polyphenol-rich foods** – Colourful fruit and vegetables, especially berries, as well as nuts, red wine and dark chocolate are rich in polyphenols that encourage the growth of health-promoting microorganisms.

- **Include fermented foods containing probiotics** – these are the live bacteria found in non-dairy yoghurt, sauerkraut (fermented cabbage), miso (fermented soya bean paste), tempeh (fermented soya beans), kombucha (fermented tea) and kimchi (fermented Chinese cabbage), and will have a short-term beneficial effect on your gut microbiota (it lasts only as long as you are eating these foods regularly).

- **Avoid heavily processed foods** – these contain ingredients, such as emulsifiers, that either suppress health-promoting microorganisms or increase 'unhealthy' species.

- **Focus on prebiotics** – these are a type of dietary fibre that feed the 'good' microorganims in your gut. Consuming more of them will increase the proportion of 'good' microorganims. Foods rich in prebiotics include beans, lentils, chickpeas, Jerusalem artichokes, onions, garlic, asparagus and leeks.

How common are gut problems in athletes?

Gut, or gastrointestinal (GI), problems, are relatively common among athletes participating in endurance events such as cycling, triathlon and distance running. It is estimated that 30–50% of endurance athletes experience symptoms such as diarrhoea, an overwhelming need to evacuate the bowels, abdominal pain and cramping, belching, bloating, nausea, heartburn, flatulence and vomiting (de Oliveira *et al.*, 2014). In a study of recreational runners, 43% reported symptoms in the 7 days prior to a marathon and 27% during the race (Pugh *et al.*, 2018). A study of 145 runners found that males and females experienced moderate to severe GI symptoms on 14% and 22% of their runs respectively over a 30-day period (Wilson, 2017).

Gut problems can be debilitating and often impair performance or subsequent recovery. Research shows that the longer the duration of exercise, the greater the incidence of gut symptoms (Pillay *et al.*, 2021); exercising for 2 hours or longer at 60% VO_2max appears to increase the

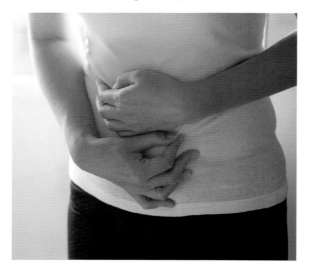

likelihood of developing symptoms, irrespective of fitness status (Costa *et al.*, 2017(a)). Exercising in the heat exacerbates symptoms as blood is redirected to the skin to cool you down.

What causes gut problems?

We don't know for certain why gut problems occur but they are likely to have physiological, mechanical, psychological and nutritional causes.

Physiological: Reduced blood flow to the digestive organs, known as gastrointestinal ischemia, is the most common explanation for gut symptoms (Otte *et al.*, 2001). During prolonged, high-intensity exercise blood is diverted away from digestive organs to the muscles in order to provide the increased oxygen and nutrient requirements. Less blood flow and less oxygen delivery result in the gut slowing down, reducing the gut's ability to digest food and absorb nutrients. It also increases the permeability of the gut wall ('leaky gut'), allowing toxins to pass into the bloodstream and causing symptoms such as cramping.

Psychological: Many athletes experience anxiety and stress before a competition. This triggers the body's 'fight or flight' response, in turn diverting the body's functions and energy to facing the perceived stressor. Consequently, stress hormones (cortisol, adrenaline and noradrenaline) are released, heart rate and blood pressure increase, and blood is diverted away from the gut to the muscles. Digestion slows or even stops altogether, which can result in abdominal discomfort, cramping or diarrhoea. What's more, exercise itself can exacerbate the stress response – the longer and harder you are exercising, the greater the rise in stress hormones. Additionally, some people simply have a more sensitive gut (visceral hypersensitivity) than others, and are therefore more susceptible to gut symptoms.

Mechanical: The repetitive 'jostling' of the intestines during running may lead to gut symptoms such as diarrhoea, urgency to defecate and blood in stools. Being in the 'aero' position during cycling may cause pressure on the abdomen and trigger GI symptoms.

Nutritional: Certain foods and drinks may irritate the gut, for example consuming a drink that is too concentrated in carbohydrate during endurance exercise (de Oliveira and Burini, 2014). Undigested carbohydrate results in bloating, delayed stomach emptying and gas production. High intakes of fibre, fat, protein or fructose may also cause symptoms. Dehydration from heavy sweating reduces blood supply to the gut and can trigger GI symptoms.

Each symptom often has a unique set of causes and therefore different strategies are required to alleviate them.

NAUSEA AND VOMITING

The most common causes include the release of stress hormones that occurs during high-intensity exercise. This can be exacerbated by stress and anxiety before a race, eating too much food before or during exercise (in particular high-fat foods or concentrated drinks), dehydration (which reduces blood flow to the gut), caffeine and hypoglycaemia (low blood glucose). Symptoms may be prevented by reducing exercise intensity (if possible or appropriate), avoiding eating within 30 minutes of exercising (particularly if doing high-intensity exercise), avoiding too many high-fat or high-protein foods before exercise, and avoiding concentrated energy drinks (hypertonic) during exercise. You should also

aim to maintain hydration (or at least minimise dehydration), avoid prolonged periods without eating, and avoid high doses of caffeine if you are sensitive to its side effects.

FULLNESS AND BLOATING

Feeling 'full' is most likely caused by eating too much generally or eating foods high in fat, protein or fibre immediately before or during exercise, or consuming hypertonic drinks, all of which delay stomach emptying. You can avoid symptoms by minimising fat, fibre and protein intake within 1–2 hours of exercise. Bloating is a feeling of distension resulting from the build-up of gas and is often due to consuming excessive fibre and certain carbohydrates, which can be fermented by bacteria in your colon. End products of this fermentation include gases, which can make you feel bloated and uncomfortable. If you are prone to bloating then you may wish to limit your intake of fibre during the day or two before competition. Carbonated drinks may also cause bloating, particularly when consumed with a meal, so you may wish to avoid them. Stress and anxiety are also common causes of gas production and bloating.

STOMACH CRAMP

The most common cause of stomach cramp during exercise is gastrointestinal ischemia (*see* p. 234). This can be exacerbated by high-intensity exercise, stress, anxiety and dehydration. Consuming concentrated sports drinks or over-consuming carbohydrate can also provoke symptoms. When there is a high concentration of carbohydrate in the stomach, water shifts from the bloodstream into the gut to lower the osmolality (number of particles in a given volume of fluid, *see* p. 159).

This can induce a sensation that the brain perceives as cramping, discomfort or pain. Choosing a sports drink with a lower carbohydrate concentration may help prevent stomach cramp. Alternatively, a drink containing multiple carbohydrate sources (e.g. glucose and fructose) may be more appropriate if you plan to consume more than 50 g/hour. For the same reason, care should also be taken not to over-consume carbohydrate from gels, bars and other sports foods during exercise. However, the gut is adaptable and it is possible to train your gut to tolerate carbohydrate consumption during exercise (see p. 237). Nonsteroidal inflammatory drugs (NSAIDS), such as ibuprofen and aspirin, may also cause cramp during exercise as they reduce gut barrier function (and may cause 'leaky gut', see box below).

DIARRHOEA AND DEFECATION

One of the most common causes of mid-race diarrhoea is pre-competition stress and anxiety. Slow deep-breathing techniques, mindfulness and listening to relaxing music before competition help reduce sympathetic nervous system activity and may be beneficial for reducing pre-competition jitters. Consuming concentrated sports drinks or too much carbohydrate can also cause defecation-related symptoms. Unabsorbed carbohydrate entering the colon will draw water from the bloodstream into the gut, leading to diarrhoea. Other potential causes include caffeine, sodium bicarbonate and ketone supplements.

FLATULENCE

Trapped gas and flatulence (expulsion of gas) during exercise can be uncomfortable. It may arise from swallowed air (while eating or drinking), over-consumption of carbohydrate, or the fermentation of foods by gut microorganisms in the colon. When too much carbohydrate is consumed, a small proportion may escape digestion and pass into the colon, where it is fermented by the gut microorganisms residing there. This can result in excessive gas production. If you are regularly troubled by symptoms then reducing your fibre intake and/or limiting your intake of FODMAPS (fermentable oligo-, di- and monosaccharides, and polyols) for 1–2 days before competition can help minimise problems (see pp. 237–8).

What is 'leaky gut'?

Prolonged and high-intensity exercise, especially in the heat, reduces blood flow to the gut and increases permeability, leading to a loss of the tight junctions that normally keep the intestinal cells together (Zuhl et al., 2014). The cells move apart, letting potentially harmful endotoxins produced by gut bacteria enter the bloodstream. This can trigger an inflammatory response (endotoxemia), potentially resulting in GI symptoms such as cramps, nausea and mid-race diarrhoea. Some gut leakiness is inevitable during prolonged exercise but you can minimise the likelihood of endotoxemia by consuming fluid and carbohydrate during exercise. This blunts the passage of large molecules through the gut wall. Increased intestinal permeability may also occur in the non-exercising state and has been linked to irritable bowel syndrome (IBS) as well as various immune-mediated disease states. Athletes with a history of IBS may be more likely to experience GI issues on race day.

How can you prevent or alleviate gut problems?

IDENTIFY YOUR TRIGGERS

Try keeping a food and symptoms diary to help you identify any trigger foods or drinks. Common culprits include foods that are high in fibre, fat or protein; spicy foods, concentrated sports drinks, caffeine and ketone supplements, so you may want to avoid them before and during an important event. It typically takes 1–2 days for fibre to pass through the gut, so start cutting down on fibre and switching to white versions of bread, rice and pasta, about 2 days beforehand.

TRAIN YOUR GUT

The gut is a very adaptable. This means that it can respond to nutritional training during exercise. In other words, you can train your gut – much like any other muscle in your body – to tolerate and absorb more carbohydrate and fluid while exercising.

What's required is a structured and consistent approach to fuelling and drinking on the move. A study with 25 endurance runners showed that 2 weeks of gut training not only improved runners' gut symptoms but also improved their running performance (Costa *et al.*, 2017(b)). The idea is to start with small quantities and increase slowly over time. With practice, the stomach will learn to accommodate a greater volume of fluid and food and empty faster, so you start to feel less full and experience fewer GI symptoms while exercising. Consuming increasingly greater quantities of carbohydrate during exercise will increase the number and activity of glucose transporters in the gut (e.g. SGLT1), allowing greater carbohydrate absorption and utilisation during exercise (Jeukendrup, 2017; Cox *et al.*, 2010).

It is possible to train the gut to absorb up to 90 g carbohydrate/hour by consuming a mixture of glucose (or maltodextrin) and fructose (Jeukendrup, 2014). This may be in the form of sports nutrition products (e.g. energy drink or gels) or whole foods (e.g. bananas or fruit purées). The length of time it takes to train the gut is very individual. One study showed benefits after 28 days (Cox *et al.*, 2010), so it is likely that most people will experience an improvement after a few weeks.

A number of gut-training strategies have been proposed (Jeukendrup, 2017):

1. Drinking regularly during training to 'train the stomach' and encourage faster stomach emptying.
2. Training immediately after a meal to get used to exercising with food in the stomach.
3. Training with a relatively high carbohydrate intake.
4. Simulate the race with a race nutrition plan. Practise consuming the same foods and drinks that you plan to use in the race.
5. Increase the overall carbohydrate content of your diet.

TRY A LOW-FODMAP DIET BEFORE COMPETITION

FODMAPs are short chain carbohydrates found in a wide range of foods, including fruit, vegetables, grains, legumes, dairy and confectionery. They are poorly absorbed and increase the osmotic load in the small intestine. This means that water will be drawn into the intestine and, in sensitive individuals, this can cause diarrhoea. Undigested carbohydrates pass into the colon, where they are fermented by bacteria that reside there, creating gas. Symptoms include bloating, flatulence, cramping and watery, loose stools, and are similar to those experienced by irritable bowel syndrome (IBS) sufferers.

If you don't suffer from IBS but experience GI symptoms only during exercise, you may gain relief by following a low-FODMAP diet just before a competition. This has been shown to significantly reduce daily GI issues in runners with exercise-associated GI symptoms (Lis *et al.*, 2018; Lis *et al.*, 2016). Examples of high-FODMAP foods commonly consumed by athletes include milk, yoghurt, apples, cherries, dates, watermelon, honey, dried apricots, grains, beans, lentils, sports drinks and gels containing fructose. Avoiding these foods or simply cutting fructose and lactose for just 24–72 hours before competition may be enough to avoid GI problems during the event. A study with endurance runners showed that following a low-FODMAP diet for 24 hours reduced the severity of GI symptoms during 2 hours of moderate-intensity running in the heat (Gaskell *et al.*, 2020).

However, following a low-FODMAP diet on a long-term basis could result in low intakes of fibre and important nutrients, which may adversely affect your gut microbiota. If you are considering a low-FODMAP diet it is advisable to seek guidance from a FODMAP-specialised practitioner.

TRY PROBIOTIC SUPPLEMENTS

There is some evidence that probiotic supplementation prior to competition may reduce gut symptoms (*see* pp. 139–40 for more details on probiotics). Recreational triathletes who took probiotic supplements for 12 weeks prior to a long-distance triathlon race experienced fewer GI symptoms (Roberts *et al.*, 2016). Researchers at Liverpool John Moores University, showed that runners who took probiotic supplements for 28 days before a marathon experienced fewer and less severe gut symptoms in the latter stages of racing compared with those who did not take supplements (Pugh *et al.*, 2019).

Summary of key points

- The gut microbiome plays an important role in health and sports performance.
- A diverse gut microbiota benefits performance and recovery.
- Gut microorganisms produce substances, including vitamins and short chain fatty acids (SCFAs), that are beneficial to health, performance and recovery.
- The gut microbiota of athletes feature more health-promoting species of microorganisms and increased diversity compared to those of sedentary people.
- Exercise appears to increase the abundance and diversity of health-promoting species of gut bacteria.
- A diet rich in plant foods, fibre, polyphenols, probiotics and prebiotics increases the diversity of the gut microbiota, which in turn may improve performance and recovery.
- The consumption of animal and plant-derived proteins appears to have different effects on the composition of the gut microbiota.
- Gut problems are common among endurance athletes and are likely to have wide-ranging physiological, mechanical and nutritional causes.
- Some gut problems may be alleviated by avoiding trigger foods or supplements, managing stress and anxiety, gut training or following a low-FODMAP diet prior to competition.

Immune Health and Recovery from Injury

Illness and injury are an inevitable part of sport. Both can result in missed training sessions and competition. Whatever level of sport or activity you do, no one likes to take time off from training for longer than is necessary. So, when illness or injury strike, good nutrition becomes more critical than ever. It can support and speed up recovery and return to play. On the other hand, poor nutrition can set back recovery and lengthen the time out of competition.

A survey of British Olympic athletes found that 35% of athletes get at least one illness per season, with each illness resulting in 7 days of training lost (Palmer-Green *et al.*, 2013). Respiratory illness is the most common, with upper respiratory infection (URI), such as the common cold, accounting for 44% of all illnesses. Additionally, 43% of athletes will get at least one injury per season, some suffering multiple injuries, with each injury causing on average 17 days lost to training and one competition to be missed. The most common injuries are tendon and muscle tears, ligament injuries, concussion, bone fractures and dislocation. Most will result in reduced physical activity although more serious injuries will necessitate immobilisation of a limb. This, in turn, can result in a substantial increase in body fat and a significant loss of muscle mass – representing a significant training setback.

This chapter comprises two parts: 1) Immune health and 2) recovery from injury. Part 1 explains the key role of nutrition in supporting immunity and preventing illness and provides practical strategies to reduce infection risk. Part 2 provides practical advice on how to avoid weight loss or gain during recovery from injury, minimise muscle loss and promote faster healing. Although there is little direct research on nutrition for the prevention and treatment of injuries, it is possible to make recommendations from studies using indirect models, such as limb immobilisation or bed rest with healthy non-injured volunteers.

Immune health

The immune system is a network of connected cells that protect the body from potentially harmful microorganisms. It broadly comprises three main lines of defence. The first line of defence consists of physical and chemical barriers (e.g. the skin), which stop bacteria and viruses entering the body. The second line of defence is comprised of *innate immunity*, which is made up of phagocytes (e.g. neutrophils and natural killer cells), which ingest and kill pathogens and damaged cells. The third line of defence is *adaptive immunity*, which is learned over time, and comprises T and B lymphocytes. These cells work together to combat infection, but they have quite different functions that enable them to deal with a huge variety of threats. B cells make antibodies that neutralise infections. T cells are broadly divided into two types: 1) T helper cells and 2) cytotoxic T cells. T helper cells support the functioning of B cells and cytotoxic T cells; cytotoxic T cells kill viruses and cells that viruses have infected. Once the adaptive immune system has defeated the invader, a pool of long-lived memory T and B cells is made. These memory lymphocytes remain dormant until the next time they encounter the same pathogen, when they produce a much faster and stronger immune response. Regular exercise is thought to strengthen the adaptive immune system, reduce immunosenescence – the immune system deterioration associated with ageing – and augment the immune system response to vaccines.

Risk factors for infection

- Autumn and winter (common cold and flu season).
- Poor hygiene and exposure to sick people.
- Long-haul air travel across multiple time zones.
- Low energy availability.
- High levels of stress.
- Poor sleep (quantity or quality).
- Increases in training load, e.g. training camp.

Source: Walsh, 2019

What are the risk factors for infection?

There are two main factors that affect your risk of infection: 1) your degree of exposure to pathogens and 2) the health of your immune system. Recent studies suggest that the main risk factors that increase infection risk in athletes include: winter time (common cold and flu season), poor hygiene and exposure to sick people; long-haul travel; low energy availability; high levels of stress (causing depression and anxiety); poor sleep quantity or quality; and increases in training load (Walsh, 2018; Gleeson, 2016). The health of your immune system is also affected by age and genetics.

Does strenuous exercise suppress the immune system?

For many years it was thought that prolonged, strenuous exercise, such as marathon running, temporarily suppressed the immune system, leading to an 'open window' that left athletes more susceptible to infection. This stemmed from studies in the 1980s and 1990s where athletes reported an increase in URI symptoms in the days and weeks after an event. Scientists attributed this increased risk of infection to a suppressed immune system. More recently, this theory has been thrown into question. First, most symptoms reported after marathons are not true infections and may be due to other factors, such as allergies (Spence *et al.*, 2007). Second, the original data was collected at mass participation events (e.g. marathons) where post-race infection risk was high. In particular, close proximity to other people at mass sporting events or while travelling on public transport increases infection risk. Additionally, long-haul airline travel or pre-event anxiety may lead to sleep disruption, which is another risk factor for infection.

Another reason why scientists thought that immunity was suppressed after strenuous exercise was because some studies reported a drop in immune cell numbers in the bloodstream after exercise. However, researchers now believe that immune cells are not lost or destroyed, rather they are redistributed in the body to areas that are likely to become infected, such as the lungs (Simpson *et al.*, 2020). This is called immune surveillance, and exercise can make it happen more efficiently.

In summary, strenuous exercise does suppress the immune system, albeit for a few hours, but it is not clear whether this increases susceptibility to infection.

How can I reduce the risk of infection?

While there are certain factors (such as age and genetics) that are beyond your control, there is still plenty you can do to reduce your susceptibility to infection. These can broadly be divided into two strategies: 1) reducing your exposure to pathogens and 2) maintaining healthy immune function. The former strategy can be achieved by avoiding contact with ill people, avoiding crowded places, washing your hands regularly with soap and water, using an antimicrobial hand gel or foam, avoiding touching your eyes, nose and mouth with your hands, wearing a face covering, disposing of tissues after blowing your nose, avoiding sharing personal items and practising good food hygiene. The second strategy can be achieved by ensuring a healthy diet, taking

regular physical activity, getting enough sleep, not smoking and managing stress.

Practical nutrition advice to support your immune health

CONSUME A BALANCED DIET

A varied diet with appropriate amounts of energy, protein, vitamins and minerals is essential to maintain an effective immune system (Maggini *et al.*, 2018). Protein is needed for making immunoglobulins, cytokines and antibodies. Deficiencies of protein, energy and certain micronutrients (including iron, zinc, magnesium, manganese, vitamins A, C, D, E, B6, B$_{12}$ and folic acid) must be avoided as these will weaken your immune system and make you more susceptible to infection. Each of these micronutrients has been shown to play multiple roles in supporting immune function and reducing the risk of infection. Research has found a link between having an impaired immune system and having low amounts of many vitamins and minerals (Calder, 2020; Gombart *et al.*, 2020). Focus on fresh fruit, vegetables, whole grains, lean proteins, beans, lentils, nuts and seeds, while limiting highly processed foods.

CONSIDER VITAMIN D SUPPLEMENTATION

Vitamin D is important not only for bone health but we now know that it also involved in many aspects of health, including maintaining the immune system (*see* pp. 96–8). Vitamin D receptors are present in cells of the immune system. Studies have associated vitamin D deficiency with increased incidence of URI and a consequent decrease in performance – even when factoring in variables such as age, sex and body mass (Halliday et al., 2011; He et al., 2013). However, the optimal level of vitamin D for immune function is not known.

Several studies suggest that vitamin D deficiency is widespread among athletes, particularly those in northern latitudes who train mainly indoors or get little sun exposure, or who do not consume vitamin D-rich foods (Owens et al., 2015; He et al., 2013) (see pp. 96–8). Meeting vitamin D requirements is not hard to accomplish in the summertime by safely being exposed to sunlight; however, daily supplementation with 25 mcg (1,000 IU)/day vitamin D is recommended in the winter months to maintain adequate vitamin D status (Harrison et al., 2021; Carswell et al., 2018; Gleeson, 2016). However, there is insufficient evidence that vitamin D supplemen-

tation can prevent or treat COVID-19 symptoms (Stroehlein at al., 2021). Vitamin D is also contained in oily fish (such as salmon, sardines and mackerel), liver and egg yolks, and fortified foods such as spreads and non-dairy milks.

MATCH ENERGY INTAKE TO ENERGY EXPENDITURE

To maintain immune health, you should aim to match your energy intake and expenditure, avoid crash dieting and avoid short- and long-term energy deficits. Restricting your calorie intake during periods of hard training can result in low energy availability (LEA), which increases cortisol levels and lowers immune function, making you more prone to infections. A study of Olympic athletes in the lead-up to the 2016 Olympic

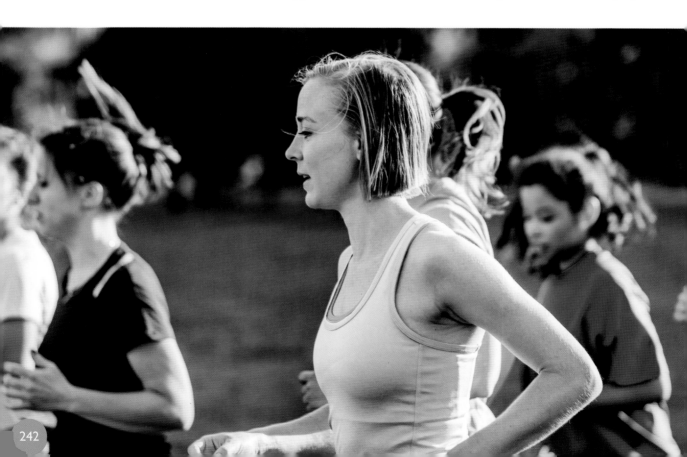

Games found that females with LEA were more likely to have URI than those without LEA (Drew *et al.*, 2018; Drew *et al.*, 2017). Even short-term dieting that results in a loss of a few kilograms over the course of a few weeks can impair immune function and make you more susceptible to URI (Bermon *et al.*, 2017; Shimizu *et al.*, 2011). Paradoxically, carbohydrate periodisation, such as 'train high, sleep low' (*see* p. 61) may benefit training adaptations but it may also result in lowered immunity and increased infection risk (Walsh, 2018).

CONSUME CARBOHYDRATE DURING INTENSE TRAINING

Carbohydrate is a fuel for immune cells. During prolonged and intense endurance exercise, glycogen stores become depleted and levels of stress hormones (adrenaline, noradrenaline and cortisol) rise, resulting in suppression of your immune cells. Studies have also shown that consuming a low-carbohydrate diet (typically less than 10% of energy from carbohydrate) results in a greater stress hormone response and lowered immunity, while a high-carbohydrate diet (typically more than 70% of energy from carbohydrate) produces a lower stress hormone response (Bishop *et al.*, 2001).

However, carbohydrate intake during exercise is thought to be the most effective strategy for preventing immune impairment (Bermon *et al.*, 2017). It has been shown to reduce the rise in stress hormone levels and the associated drop in immunity following exercise (Bishop *et al.*, 2002). The ideal intake during intense exercise lasting longer than 1 hour is 30–60 g carbohydrate/hour (Gleeson *et al.*, 2004). This may be in the form of sports drinks, whole foods such as bananas or sports supplements.

CONSIDER VITAMIN C SUPPLEMENTATION DURING PERIODS OF HEAVY TRAINING

Vitamin C is a powerful antioxidant that quenches reactive oxygen species (*see* pp. 104–5). It also enhances immune cell function in the process of microbial killing, and augments proliferation and differentiation of T cells and B cells that are responsible for making antibodies. A Cochrane review of 29 studies found that, while vitamin C supplementation does not reduce the chance of getting a cold in the general population, it might alleviate the symptoms and duration of a cold (Hermila and Chalker, 2013). Moderate doses of vitamin C supplements (250–1000 mg/day) have been shown to reduce the incidence of URI by 52% in athletes during periods of severe physical stress, such as during heavy training blocks or before and after competition. In one study of ultra-marathon runners, those who took daily vitamin C supplements (1500 mg) 7 days prior to a race had lower levels of stress hormones following the race, which suggests greater protection against infection (Peters *et al.*, 2001).

However, there is no benefit in taking megadoses of vitamin C supplements. It is a water-soluble vitamin, which means that any excess will be excreted through the urine and therefore wasted. In very high amounts, there may be side effects such as diarrhoea, abdominal cramps and kidney stones.

CONSIDER PROBIOTICS DURING PERIODS OF INCREASED INFECTION RISK

Probiotics may be useful during periods of increased infection risk, such as in the weeks before and during international travel and major competition. Probiotics are live microorganisms that can increase the number of beneficial bacteria in the gut, potentially improve immune function and reduce the risk of URI and gastrointestinal illness (*see* pp. 139–40). Some common symptoms associated with gastrointestinal illness include abdominal cramps, acid reflux, nausea, vomiting, diarrhoea and URI. Probiotics are thought to increase immunity by inhibiting the growth of harmful bacteria in the gut and reducing their potentially harmful effects, reinforcing the gut barrier, and by enhancing both innate and acquired immune function.

Probiotics are found in fermented foods such as yoghurt, cheese, sauerkraut, kefir, tempeh, kombucha and sourdough bread, although concentrations are relatively low. The most common types of probiotics include lactic acid bacteria and bifidobacteria. There is evidence that probiotic supplements at daily doses of 10^{10} live bacteria may help protect against and reduce symptoms of URIs (King *et al.*, 2014; Hao *et al.*, 2015; Gleeson, 2008). A Cochrane review of 12 studies found that probiotics reduce the incidence of URIs by 47% and the duration of illness by nearly 2 days (Hao *et al.*, 2015).

Another way to increase the beneficial bacteria in your gut is to eat a varied diet rich in fibre, aiming for around 20–30 different fruit, vegetables, whole grains and pulses a week. Including fermented foods containing probiotics will also help. Eating prebiotic foods (e.g. onions, garlic, lentils, beans, asparagus and leeks) will help promote 'good' gut microorganisms.

TAKE ZINC LOZENGES AT THE ONSET OF A COLD

Zinc lozenges (equivalent to a daily dose of at least 75 mg elemental zinc) have been shown to reduce the duration of the common cold by 44%, or about 3 days when taken within 24 hours after the onset of symptoms, and for the duration of illness (Hermila, 2017; Hermila, 2011). Both zinc acetate and zinc gluconate are effective but it's important you take zinc in lozenge form (not swallowed as tablets) as it needs to dissolve in the mouth and act directly on the cells lining the pharynx. However, the optimal dose is not yet established by studies. Zinc is thought to act as an antiviral agent by increasing interferon gamma (a molecule that helps the body fight viral infections) and reducing the ability of cold viruses to bind with cells. Side effects of zinc lozenges include an unpleasant taste in the mouth and nausea.

CONSUME PLENTY OF POLYPHENOLS

Polyphenols, the natural chemical compounds that give fruits and vegetables their bright colours, have potent anti-inflammatory and antioxidant properties. High intakes are associated with a longer life span, and a reduced risk of cardiovascular disease, type 2 diabetes and hypertension. Polyphenols bind receptors on immune cells and help regulate your immune response. They also act as prebiotics, meaning they increase the growth of health-promoting bacteria in the gut. These bacteria produce compounds that help maintain the mucosal layer that protects the intestinal lining.

Although further research is required, there is some evidence for the positive role played by flavonoids, which make up about 50% of the polyphenol family, on immunomodulatory components of the immune system such as natural killer cells, T cells and macrophages (Bermon *et al.*, 2017). Blue, purple, red and orange fruit and colourful vegetables are rich in flavonoids, as are nuts, herbs, tea, dark chocolate and red wine. A meta-analysis showed that flavonoids play an essential role in the respiratory tract's immune defence system (Somerville *et al.*, 2016). Supplements containing 0.2–1.2 g/day decreased URI incidence by 33% and reduced the duration of illness by 40%. However, the optimal dose is not yet known.

OTHER SUPPLEMENTS

There is some evidence that glutamine supplements, colostrum, beta-glucans, echinacea and quercetin may reduce the risk of infections but more evidence is needed before clear recommendations can be made.

Glutamine levels can fall by up to 20% following intense exercise, putting the immune system under greater strain (Antonio and Street, 1999). In one study, athletes who took glutamine supplements immediately and 2 hours after intense exercise had a lower risk of URI in the 7 days following (Castell *et al.*, 1996).

Echinacea taken for up to 4 weeks during a period of hard training may reduce the risk of URI by stimulating the body's own production of immune cells (Karsch-Völk *et al.*, 2014).

Quercetin supplements (1000 mg/day) taken during periods of intense training may reduce the risk of upper respiratory illness (Nieman *et al.*, 2007).

How does nutrition influence immunity?

Our understanding of how nutrition influences the immune system has changed in recent years. It was once thought that nutrients and supplements work by strengthening immunity

Recommendations to avoid infection and maintain immune health in athletes

1. Try to avoid contact with sick people, particularly in the autumn and winter.
2. Ensure good hand hygiene and appropriate vaccination.
3. Avoid self-infection by touching the eyes, nose and mouth.
4. Do not train or compete if you suffer from 'below-the-neck' symptoms.
5. Monitor and manage all forms of stress, including physical and psychosocial.
6. Carefully manage increments in training stress.
7. Replace overly long training sessions with more frequent spike sessions.
8. Plan recovery or an adaptation week every second or third week.
9. Aim for at least 7 hours of sleep each night.
10. Eat a well-balanced diet and avoid chronic low energy availability.

Source: Walsh, 2018

and increasing the body's *resistance* to infection (i.e. making it better able to destroy microbes). However, it is now known that not all nutrients and supplements work this way. Some exert their effects by dampening immune responsiveness (i.e. preventing an overly exuberant immune response to infection) and making the body more *tolerant* to microorganisms (Walsh, 2019). This results in less severe or shorter periods of infection and explains why your body can tolerate the microorganisms in your gut (gut microbiota) rather than mounting an attack against them. In other words, it is now thought that the body maintains a delicate balance of resistance and tolerance, which allows it to fight infection while maintaining a healthy relationship with the gut microbiota. Examples of these two mechanisms are shown in Table 13.1. The box on p. 245 gives 10 practical recommendations to avoid infection and maintain immune health.

Recovery from injury

Recovery from injury can be divided into three main stages:

1. **Inflammation** – Following any injury, blood flow and oxygen become disrupted, which results in cell damage. In an attempt to remove the damaged cells and start rebuilding new cells, the body initiates an inflammatory response, which typically lasts from a few hours to several days. Inflammation is characterised by pain, swelling, redness and heat.
2. **Proliferation** – After damaged cells have been removed and inflammation subsides, new blood vessels are formed and the body is able to start building temporary tissue (scar tissue).
3. **Remodelling** – Scar tissue is replaced with collagen, which is a stronger, permanent tissue that will restore the injury site to its original strength.

HOW CAN I AVOID GAINING OR LOSING WEIGHT WHILE INJURED?

Injury recovery usually means time off from training or reduced physical activity, which results in decreased energy expenditure and energy

Table 13.1	NUTRITIONAL SUPPLEMENTS FOR IMPROVING IMMUNE RESISTANCE AND TOLERANCE IN ATHLETES		
Supplements that may improve resistance		**Supplements that may improve tolerance**	
Supplement	**How it works**	**Supplement**	**How it works**
Carbohydrate drinks and gels during exercise	Inhibit cortisol rise during exercise	Probiotics	Increase beneficial gut bacteria
Glutamine	Counters post-exercise drop in glutamine	Vitamin C	Antioxidant: quenches ROS
Zinc lozenges	Prevents viral adherence	Vitamin D	Anti-inflammatory: increases antimicrobial protein production
Echinacea	Stimulates macrophages	Polyphenols	Anti-inflammatory antioxidant and anti-pathogenic effects

Source: Walsh, 2019

requirement. However, during the initial recovery phase, resting metabolic rate increases by 15–50%, depending on the type and severity of injury, and effectively counteracts some of the drop in energy output from physical activity (Tipton, 2015). Nevertheless, many athletes are keen to avoid unwanted weight gain when they are not exercising and will often compensate for their reduced energy expenditure by eating less. While it is important to match energy intake and expenditure, care should be taken not to over-restrict food intake when injured as the body needs adequate nutrition to heal an injury. Being in energy deficit, or under-eating, hinders the process, delays healing and reduces muscle protein synthesis (MPS) (Pasiakos *et al.*, 2010). Similarly, a large energy surplus can also delay recovery (Biolo *et al.*, 2008).

In practice, most athletes will probably need to consume less than when in training but more than their sedentary baseline intake. Of course, this is easier said than done as it may take a while for your appetite to readjust if you are used to consuming, say, 3000 or 4000 calories. Replacing processed snacks such as cakes, biscuits and crisps with fruit, vegetables and nuts, which are more nutritious and are naturally more filling, is a good place to start.

HOW CAN I MINIMISE MUSCLE LOSS?

Loss of muscle mass (atrophy) is perhaps the biggest problem during recovery from injury, especially those that require immobilisation of a limb or result in a severe reduction in mobility. Even short periods (1–2 weeks) of muscle disuse can cause substantial loss of muscle mass and strength (Wall *et al.*, 2014). Most of this is due to a decline in muscle protein synthesis (MPS) as the muscles become more resistant to the anabolic effects of dietary protein and take up amino acids from the bloodstream less readily (Wall *et al.*, 2013 (a)).

To minimise muscle loss, it is crucial to consume sufficient protein while injured. Although you're not exercising as much, your body needs additional protein for healing. It provides amino acids, which are required for the formation and repair of body tissues. A suboptimal intake of protein or a drastic reduction from pre-injury levels will impair healing and provoke muscle loss.

There are no official protein recommendations for recovery but higher intakes (2–2.5 g/kg BW/day) may be appropriate (Tipton, 2015). It would also be wise to include a minimum of 20–25 g at every meal and to include protein in snacks (*see* pp. 71–2). Distributing your protein evenly across your meals can promote muscle protein synthesis or mitigate anabolic resistance. High-quality proteins that are naturally high in leucine can help increase protein manufacture, particularly during periods of inactivity when the muscles are less sensitive to muscle-building stimuli. These include whey protein supplements, dairy products, eggs, meat and fish. Leucine supplementation may help counter or ameliorate anabolic resistance and loss of muscle mass but the most important strategy is getting enough protein (English *et al.*, 2016; Wall *et al.*, 2013(b)).

WHICH SUPPLEMENTS MAY PROMOTE RECOVERY FROM INJURY?

Some evidence suggests *creatine* supplementation may help you regain muscle faster during recovery following immobilisation (*see* pp. 126–9). One study found that volunteers who took creatine supplements during a 10-week resistance training rehabilitation programme regained significantly more muscle mass and strength than those taking a placebo (Hespel *et al.*, 2001). However, it is unclear whether taking a creatine supplement is of benefit during shorter periods of rehabilitation or for all types of workouts.

There is growing evidence that taking *omega-3 supplements* (*see* pp. 137–8) during recovery from injury may help to reduce inflammation and promote wound healing (Calder *et al.*, 2013). The optimal dose is not known but including omega-3-rich foods such as oily fish, walnuts, rapeseed oil, chia seeds and ground flaxseed is also likely to help the healing proces.

While deficiencies of micronutrients such as *vitamin C* and *zinc* are likely to impede healing, there is no evidence currently that supplementation speeds up the process.

Collagen (*see* pp. 124–5) is the main protein in tendons, bones, ligaments and cartilage and scientists are currently investigating whether collagen supplementation can prevent or treat musculoskeletal injuries. A joint US-Australian study showed that taking 15 g of vitamin C-enriched gelatine (a food form of collagen) 1 hour before high-intensity exercise (skipping) increased collagen manufacture (Shaw *et al.*, 2017). But it is early stage research and the functional benefits and the effects on injury recovery in elite athletes are not currently known.

Summary of key points

- You can reduce the risk of infection by reducing your exposure to pathogens and maintaining healthy immune function.
- Key strategies to maintain healthy immunity include consuming a healthy diet (containing sufficient energy, protein, vitamins and minerals), regular physical activity, getting enough sleep, not smoking and managing stress.
- Vitamin D supplementation of 25 mcg (1,000 IU/day) is recommended in the winter months to maintain adequate vitamin D status and immune function.
- Aim to match energy intake and expenditure, avoid crash dieting and avoid short- and long-term energy deficits.
- Certain supplements improve immunity either by increasing the body's *resistance* to infection or increasing the body's *tolerance* to microorganisms.
- Supplements that may improve immune resistance include energy drinks and gels during exercise, glutamine, zinc lozenges and echinacea.
- Supplements that may improve tolerance to microorganisms include probiotics, vitamin C, vitamin D and polyphenols.
- During recovery from injury, weight gain or loss can be avoided by adjusting energy intake to expenditure.
- Loss of muscle mass while injured may be minimised by increasing protein intake (2–2.5 g/kg BW/day), including 20–25 g per meal, and including foods with a high leucine content.
- Supplements that may promote faster recovery from injury include creatine and omega-3 supplements. The benefits of collagen are not currently known.

The Young //Athlete

Like adults, young athletes need to eat a balanced diet to maintain good health and achieve peak performance. While there has been relatively limited research performed with adolescent athletes, it is possible to adapt nutritional guidelines for the non-athletic population to the specific demands of exercise and sport as well a tos extrapolate some of the research on adult athletes. This chapter covers the energy, protein and fluid needs for young athletes as well as meal timing, travelling and competing. Weight is also an important issue for some young athletes. Being overweight not only affects their health but also reduces their athletic performance and their self-esteem. Similarly, some young athletes struggle to keep up their weight or put on weight because of the high energy demands of their sport. This chapter details some key strategies to help parents and coaches manage these issues.

HOW MUCH ENERGY DO YOUNG ATHLETES REQUIRE?

The energy intake of young athletes should be sufficient to cover both their requirements for growth and development and the energy demands of their training and daily physical activity. There is no specific data on energy requirements for young athletes since individual requirements vary considerably. You can get a rough estimate using the values in Tables 14.1 and 14.2 on the following pages. These show the estimated average requirements for children for standard ages published by the Department of Health. However, these figures do not take account of regular exercise or sport, so you will need to make an allowance for this.

More relevant to young athletes are the figures shown in Table 14.3 on p.252, which shows energy requirements according to body weight and physical activity level (PAL). PAL is the ratio of overall daily energy expenditure to BMR based on the intensity and time spent being active. PAL estimates are given on p. 306. Sedentary children generally have a PAL of 1.4, while active children are likely to have a PAL between 1.6 and 2.0.

Young athletes should be encouraged to adapt their energy intake to meet the different fuel demands of their training on different days. For example, on days when their training load is higher, their fuel needs will be higher and so they will need to consume more energy in the hours before and after training, for example consuming larger portions and including additional healthy snacks to meet the energy demands of their specific training sessions.

Table 14.1	DIETARY REFERENCE VALUES FOR BOYS 4–18 YEARS				
	Dietary Reference Value (DRV)	**4–6**	**7–10**	**11–14**	**15–18**
Energy	EAR	1715 kcal	1979 kcal	2220 kcal	2755 kcal
Fat	Max 35% energy	67 g	77 g	86 g	107 g
Saturated fat	Max 11% energy	21 g	24 g	27 g	34 g
Carbohydrate	Min 50% energy	229 g	263 g	296 g	367 g
Added sugars*	Max 11% energy	50 g	58 g	65 g	81 g
Fibre **	8 g per 1000 kcal	14 g	16 g	18 g	22 g
Protein		19.7 g	28 g	42 g	55 g
Iron		6.1 mg	8.7 mg	11.3 mg	11.3 mg
Zinc		6.5 mg	7.0 mg	9.0 mg	9.5 mg
Calcium		450 mg	550 mg	1000 mg	1000 mg
Vitamin A		500 ug	500 ug	600 ug	700 ug
Vitamin C		30 mg	30 mg	35 mg	40 mg
Folate		100 ug	150 ug	200 ug	200 ug
Salt***		3 g	5 g	6 g	6 g

Source: Department of Health Dietary reference values for food energy and nutrients for the United Kingdom (1991). London: HMSO.

EAR = Estimated Average Requirement

* Non-milk extrinsic sugars

** Proportion of adult DRV (18 g) i.e. 8 g/1000 kcal

*** Scientific Advisory Committee on Nutrition (2003): Salt and Health. London: HMSO.

Table 14.2	DIETARY REFERENCE VALUES FOR GIRLS 4–18 YEARS				
	Dietary Reference Value (DRV)	4–6	7–10	11–14	15–18
Energy	EAR	1545 kcal	1740 kcal	1845 kcal	2110 kcal
Fat	Max 35% energy	60 g	68 g	72 g	82 g
Saturated fat	Max 11% energy	19 g	21 g	23 g	26 g
Carbohydrate	Min 50% energy	206 g	232 g	246 g	281 g
Added sugars*	Max 11% energy	45 g	51 g	54 g	62 g
Fibre **	8 g per 1000 kcal	12 g	14 g	15 g	17 g
Protein		19.7 g	28 g	41 g	45 g
Iron		6.1 mg	8.7 mg	14.8 mg	14.8 mg
Zinc		6.5 mg	7.0 mg	9.0 mg	7.0 mg
Calcium		450 mg	550 mg	800 mg	800 mg
Vitamin A		500 ug	500 ug	600 ug	600 ug
Vitamin C		30 mg	30 mg	35 mg	40 mg
Folate		100 ug	150 ug	200 ug	200 ug
Salt***		3 g	5 g	6 g	6 g

Source: Department of Health Dietary reference values for food energy and nutrients for the United Kingdom (1991). London: HMSO.

EAR = Estimated Average Requirement

* Non-milk extrinsic sugars

** Proportion of adult DRV (18 g) i.e. 8 g/ 1000 kcal

*** Scientific Advisory Committee on Nutrition (2003) Salt and Health. London: HMSO.

Table 14.3	ESTIMATED AVERAGE ENERGY REQUIREMENTS OF CHILDREN AND ADOLESCENTS ACCORDING TO BODY WEIGHT AND PHYSICAL ACTIVITY LEVEL					
	Weight (kg)	BMR kcal/d	PAL				
			1.4	1.5	1.6	1.8	2.0
Boys	30	1189	1675	1794	1914	2153	2368
	35	1278	1794	1914	2057	2297	2559
	40	1366	1914	2057	2177	2464	2727
	45	1455	2033	2177	2320	2632	2919
	50	1543	2153	2321	2464	2775	3086
	55	1632	2297	2440	2608	2943	3253
	60	1720	2416	2584	2751	3086	3445
Girls	30	1095	1531	1651	1746	1962	2201
	35	1163	1627	1715	1866	2081	2321
	40	1229	1722	1842	1962	2201	2464
	45	1297	1818	1938	2081	2344	2584
	50	1364	1913	2033	2177	2464	2727
	55	1430	2009	2153	2297	2584	2871
	60	1498	2105	2249	2392	2703	2990

Source: Department of Health Dietary reference values for food energy and nutrients for the United Kingdom (1991). London: HMSO.

SHOULD YOUNG ATHLETES LOSE WEIGHT FOR THEIR SPORT?

Some young athletes may feel pressurised to lose weight to improve their performance or appearance. Additionally, they are often influenced to lose weight by the successes of thinner teammates or by the remarks of a well-meaning coach. As a result, young athletes may engage in inappropriate dieting and exercise strategies in the belief these will help them lose weight and give them a competitive advantage. Unfortunately, adolescents are particularly susceptible to weight loss and restrictive practices that may result in low energy availability (*see* p. 209).

Prolonged periods of LEA in young athletes may have a number of health consequences including delayed puberty, menstrual irregularities, poor bone health, risk of development of eating disorders and increased risk of injury (Nattiv *et al.*, 2007). Be vigilant for early warning signs of LEA, such as poor recovery, underperformance, recurrent illness and injuries, and changes in mood. The development of LEA puts them at risk of developing Relative Energy Deficiency in Sport (*see* pp. 209–18).

There is an increased prevalence of disordered eating and RED-S in body weight-sensitive sports (e.g. distance running and road cycling), weight-category sports (e.g. martial arts and lightweight rowing) and aesthetically focused sports (e.g. gymnastics). Early warning signs for RED-S include overtraining even when unwell, lack of recreational activities outside sport, low self-esteem, perfectionism, dieting behaviours and misconceptions about nutrition. Chapter 11 provides more details on the prevalence, causes, symptoms and management of RED-S.

Dos and don'ts for encouraging healthy eating in young athletes

- Do build young athletes' self-esteem.
- Don't restrict a young athlete's calorie intake.
- Don't tell a young athlete that they are 'greedy' or 'lazy'.
- Do tell them that you recognise how hard it is to make healthy choices at times.
- Don't make a young athlete feel guilty about their eating habits.
- Do praise them when you see them eating healthily.
- Do set a good example.
- Don't use food as a reward.
- Don't ban any foods.

Therefore, young athletes should not be encouraged to lose weight for performance. If they are unhappy about their weight, the problem may be one of poor self-esteem or being ill-matched to their sport. The position statement of Sports Dietitians Australia advises against weight loss for young athletes (Desbrow *et al.*, 2014b).

The best thing you can do is to encourage a balanced diet. Talk to young athletes about healthy eating and exercise, teach by example and let them make their own decisions about food.

DO YOUNG ATHLETES BURN FUEL DIFFERENTLY FROM ADULTS?

Studies suggest that during exercise children use relatively more fat and less carbohydrate than do adolescents or adults (Martinez and Haymes, 1992; Berg and Keul, 1988). This applies to

Table 14.4	DAILY PROTEIN REQUIREMENTS OF CHILDREN	
Age	Boys	Girls
4–6 years	19.7 g	19.7 g
7–10 years	28.3 g	28.3 g
11–14 years	42.1 g	41.2 g
15–18 years	55.2 g	45.0 g

Source: Department of Health Dietary reference values for food energy and nutrients for the United Kingdom (1991). London: HMSO.

both endurance and short, higher-intensity activities, where they tend to rely more on aerobic metabolism (in which fat is a major fuel). The nutritional implications are not clear, but there is no reason to recommend they should consume more than the recommended maximum for fat for the general population (35% of energy).

HOW MUCH PROTEIN SHOULD YOUNG ATHLETES CONSUME?

Because young athletes are growing and developing, they need more protein relative to their weight than adults. The Reference Nutrient Intakes for protein published by the Department of Health give a general guideline for boys and girls of different ages. These are given in Table 14.4. However, the published values do not take account of exercise, so are not appropriate for young athletes who will almost certainly need more protein than the general population.

Adolescent athletes are likely to have similar protein requirements to those set for adult athletes (between 1.2 and 2.0 g/kg BW/day), depending on the specific goals of the training programme (Desbrow et al., 2014b). Additionally, consuming 0.25–0.4 g protein/kg BW, or approximately 20 g protein early in the post-exercise recovery phase will promote muscle recovery (see pp. 71–2). Since recovery extends at least 24 hours after exercise, there are further benefits to be gained by distributing protein evenly between meals throughout the day, not only in the post-workout meal. In practice, this means including protein-rich foods such as milk, eggs, meat, fish, poultry, tofu, beans and lentils at every meal, including breakfast. Suitable high-protein snack options include yoghurt, nuts and nut butter.

SHOULD YOUNG ATHLETES USE PROTEIN SUPPLEMENTS?

Protein supplements, such as protein shakes and bars, may offer convenience but are unnecessary for young athletes. Even the very active should be able to get enough protein from a well-planned diet. Whole foods are generally a better option than supplements. Not only do they supply protein, but they also supply other nutrients that are important for growth, development and muscle recovery. The International Association of Athletic Federations recommends whole-food sources of protein rather than supplements (Burke et al., 2019). It is important that young athletes learn how to plan a balanced diet incorporating whole foods.

HOW MUCH CARBOHYDRATE SHOULD YOUNG ATHLETES CONSUME?

There are no specific recommendations for young athletes. However, those previously detailed for adults would be appropriate for this age group

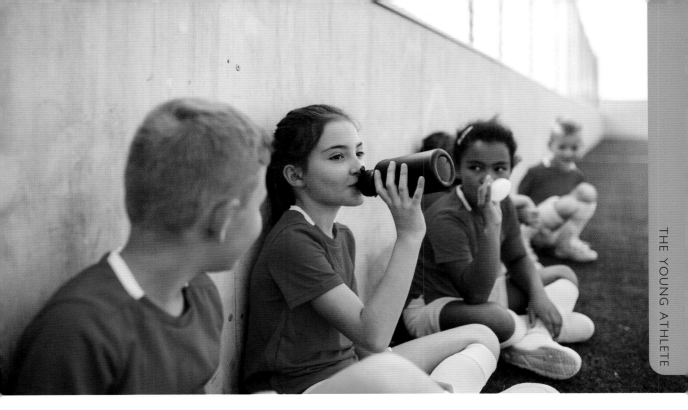

downside, sports drinks are relatively expensive. It's cheaper to make your own version by diluting fruit juice (one part juice to one or two parts water) or squash (diluted one part squash to six parts water). The important thing is that young athletes drink enough fluid. Therefore, the taste is important. If they don't like it, they won't drink it! So, experiment with different flavours until you find the ones they like. A little trial and error may be needed to find the best strength drink, too. If it's too concentrated, it will sit in their stomachs and make them feel uncomfortable.

SHOULD YOUNG ATHLETES TAKE SUPPLEMENTS?

Young athletes should not need vitamin supplements if they are eating a well-balanced diet and a wide variety of foods. The exception is vitamin D, which is difficult to obtain in sufficient amounts from dietary sources. Public Health England recommends everyone over the age of one take a 10 mcg (400 IU) supplement from October to April (*see* p. 97). Vegetarians and vegans may need to consider supplementation with omega-3s and vitamin B_{12} (*see* pp. 273–4).

Many sports organisations believe that it is inappropriate for young athletes to take supplements for performance enhancement. This is partly because supplement use over-emphasises the ability of supplements to improve performance; young athletes stand to benefit more from maturation and experience in sport as well as adherence to consistent training practices and consuming a balanced diet. Importantly, there is a lack of research to support the use of ergogenic sports supplements in young athletes; the side effects and long-term risks are therefore unknown (Unnithan *et al.*, 2001). As dietary supplements are not regulated, there is no guarantee of their safety or efficacy, and a possibility that they may contain impurities that would cause a positive drug test (*see* pp. 108–10).

IS STRENGTH TRAINING APPROPRIATE FOR YOUNG ATHLETES?

A well-designed strength training or weight training programme will improve a young athlete's strength, reduce their risk of sports injuries and improve their sports performance. Contrary to the belief that strength training can damage the growth cartilage or stunt their growth, recent studies suggest that it can actually make bones stronger. In fact, there are no reported cases of bone damage in relation to strength training. Young athletes who strength train tend to feel better about themselves as they get stronger, and have higher self-esteem. But strength training is not the same as power lifting, weightlifting or bodybuilding, none of which is recommended for children under 18 years old.

Bulking up should not be the goal of a strength training programme. Children and teenagers should tone their muscles using a light weight (or body weight) and a high number of repetitions, rather than lifting heavy weights. Only after they have passed puberty should children consider adding muscle bulk. Younger children should begin with body weight exercises such as push-ups and sit-ups. More experienced trainees may use free weights and machines.

Sports scientists say that a well-designed strength training programme can bring many fitness benefits for children and can complement

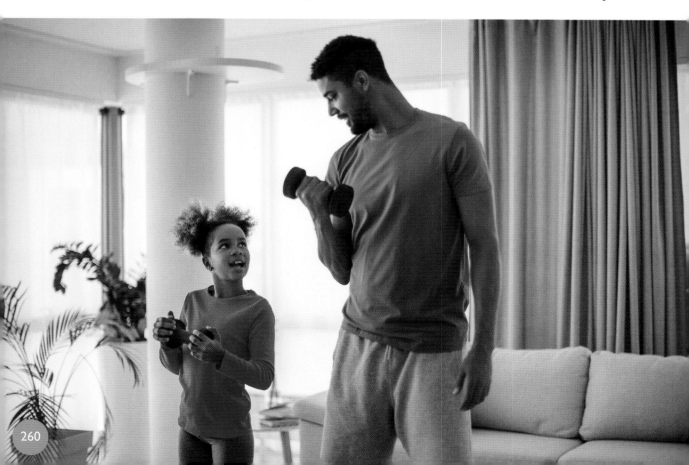

an existing training programme. Indeed, the American Academy of Paediatrics Committee on Sports Medicine endorses it. Here are some guidelines:

- Children should be properly supervised during training sessions.
- They should use an age-appropriate routine (adult routines are not suitable) – typically 30-second intervals with breaks in between, with a thorough warm-up and cool-down period.
- Ensure the exercises are performed using proper form and technique.
- Children should start with a relatively light weight and a high number of repetitions.
- No heavy lifts should be included.
- The programme should form part of a total fitness programme.
- The sessions should be varied and fun.

Summary of key points

- Young athletes expend approximately 25% more calories for any given activity compared with adults.
- Young athletes need more protein relative to their weight than adults – about 1 g/kg BW (adults need 0.75 g/kg BW). Protein supplements are not necessary.
- If young athletes will be exercising continually for less than 90 minutes, they won't need to eat anything during exercise but should be encouraged to take regular drink breaks, ideally every 15–20 minutes.
- After exercise, give young athletes a drink straight away – water or diluted fruit juice are the best drinks – followed by a high-carbohydrate,

high-GI snack to stave off hunger and promote recovery.
- Young athletes are more susceptible to hypo-hydration and overheating than adults.
- Encourage them to drink six to eight cups (1–1.5 litres) of fluid during the day, then top up with 150–200 ml (a large glass) of water 45 minutes before exercise.
- During exercise, they should aim to drink 75–100 ml every 15–20 minutes.
- After exercise, they should drink freely until no longer thirsty, plus an extra glass, or drink 300 ml for every 0.2 kg weight loss.
- As with adults, plain water is best for most activities lasting less than 90 minutes, other-wise a flavoured drink will encourage them to drink enough fluid (*see* p. 258).
- Young athletes should not need supplements if they are eating a well-balanced diet and a wide variety of foods, but a children's multi-vitamin and mineral supplement may provide assurance.
- There is no research to support the use of sports supplements in young athletes and the long-term risks are unknown. The ACSM specifically warn against the use of creatine in athletes under 18.
- If an athlete has a genuine weight problem, seek professional advice. Talk to young athletes about healthy eating and exercise, teach by example and let them make their own deci-sions about food.
- Young athletes who struggle to keep up their weight or put on any weight should be encour-aged to eat more frequent meals and snacks and focus on energy and nutrient-rich foods (*see* pp. 255–6).

The Plant-based Athlete

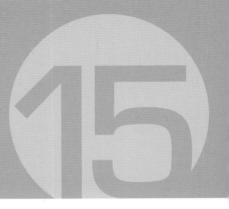

Many athletes choose to follow a vegetarian or vegan diet or avoid red meat for ethical, health or environmental reasons or, increasingly, in the belief that such a diet will improve performance. It is estimated that 13% of people in the UK are vegetarian, with a further 21% identifying as 'flexitarian' or semi-vegetarian (Waitrose, 2018–2019). Large-scale prospective dietary surveys have found that vegetarians and vegans have higher intakes of fruit and vegetables, fibre, antioxidant nutrients and phytonutrients, and lower intakes of saturated fat than do omnivores, as well as a lower risk of death from heart disease and lower rates of certain cancers and type 2 diabetes (Kim *et al.*, 2018; Davey *et al.*, 2003; Key *et al.*, 1996). The question is whether the benefits of a plant-based diet extend to enhanced physical fitness and performance. This chapter considers the research in this area and covers the key nutritional considerations for plant-based athletes. It also provides practical advice to help plant-based athletes meet their requirements.

WHAT ARE THE HEALTH BENEFITS OF A PLANT-BASED DIET?

The British Dietetic Association states that 'Well-planned plant-based diets can support healthy living at every age and life-stage' (BDA, 2021). Large-scale studies have shown that vegetarians and vegans are less likely to suffer from chronic diseases such as heart disease, certain cancers, type 2 diabetes, obesity and high blood pressure than omnivores (Kim *et al.*, 2018; Lassale *et al.*, 2015; Singh *et al.*, 2003; Appleby *et al.*, 1999). For example, researchers at Loma Linda University, found that people following a vegetarian diet had a 12% lower risk of death from any cause in a 6-year follow-up, compared with non-vegetarians (Orlich *et al.*, 2013).

An analysis of three prospective studies of Seventh Day Adventists in North America found that both vegetarians and vegans lived longer and had lower risks for heart disease, stroke and certain cancers than people who ate meat (Le and Sabaté, 2014).

A review of studies published in in 2019 concluded that vegan and vegetarian diets can help protect against chronic metabolic diseases and certain cancers with links found between plant protein intake and healthier markers of heart health, management of type 2 diabetes and improved weight management (Ahnen *et al.*, 2019).

The EPIC-Oxford study of 45,000 people found that vegetarians were 32% less likely to develop heart disease compared with omnivores (Crowe *et al.,* 2013). They were also significantly less likely to be overweight or have type 2 diabetes, and had lower blood pressure and LDL-cholesterol levels.

Bowel cancer is less common among vegetarians. A report by the World Cancer Research Fund (WCRF) found that eating red meat and processed meats increases the risk of bowel cancer (WCRF, 2018). The World Health Organization's International Agency for Research on Cancer (WHO/AIRC) states that processed meat 'definitely' causes cancer and that red meat 'probably' causes cancer (Bouvard *et al.,* 2015). A review of large-scale prospective studies concluded that eating red and processed meat increases colorectal cancer by 20–30% (Aykan *et al.,* 2015). The WCRF recommends eating no more than 350–500 g of red meat a week, and cutting processed meat altogether.

Generally, vegetarians have a lower Body Mass Index (BMI) than meat-eaters (Spencer *et al.,* 2003). This is partly due to healthier lifestyles but also due to the fact that plant-based diets typically have a lower energy density than omnivorous diets.

The health benefits of plant-based diets may be partly due to the absence of meat and partly to the higher consumption of plant foods, such as fruit and vegetables, whole grains, beans, lentils, chickpeas, nuts and seeds. A diet rich in plant foods is typically higher in fibre, unsaturated fats, polyphenols and phytochemicals, all of which are linked to improved gut health, better immunity and lower risk of chronic disease. Fibre and polyphenols feed your 'good' gut microorganisms, helping them grow and multiply (*see* pp. 232–3).

Plant-based diets also tend to be lower in saturated fat, added sugar and ultra-processed foods.

Definitions of plant-based diets

Plant-based diets encompass a number of different patterns of eating, including:

- **Lacto-ovo vegetarian** – eat dairy and eggs but not meat or fish
- **Lacto vegetarian** – eat dairy but not eggs, meat or fish
- **Vegan** – don't eat any foods of animal origin at all, including honey
- **Flexitarian** – eat meat and fish occasionally
- **Pescatarian** – eat fish

It is possible that other lifestyle factors may also play a role – vegetarians and vegans typically exercise more, and are less likely to smoke and drink excessive alcohol, all of which may account for some of the reduction in disease risk.

CAN A PLANT-BASED DIET SUPPORT ATHLETIC PERFORMANCE?

Many people imagine that a plant-based diet cannot fulfil an athlete's nutritional requirements, that meat is necessary for building strength and endurance, and that vegetarian athletes are smaller, weaker, less muscular and less powerful than their meat-eating counterparts. There is no evidence to support these misconceptions. On the contrary, the Academy of Nutrition and Dietetics' position paper on vegetarian diets states that well-planned vegan and vegetarian diets are healthy, nutritionally adequate, match dietary guidelines and meet current recommended intakes, provide health benefits for the prevention and treatment of certain diseases, and are appropriate for people of all ages as well as for athletes (Melina *et al.*, 2016). This view is echoed in the American College of Sports Medicine's joint position paper on nutrition and athletic performance, which states 'a vegetarian diet can be nutritionally adequate containing high intakes of fruits, vegetables, whole grains, nuts, soya products, fibre, phytochemicals and antioxidants' (Thomas *et al.*, 2016).

Although relatively few studies have looked directly at the effects of a vegan or vegetarian diet on performance, they all provide compelling evidence that excluding animal products does not put you at a *disadvantage* when it comes to fitness or performance.

Danish researchers tested athletes after they had consumed either a vegetarian or non-vegetarian diet for 6 weeks alternately (Richter *et al.*, 1991). The carbohydrate content of each diet was kept the same (57% energy). Whichever diet they ate, the athletes experienced no change in aerobic capacity, endurance, muscle glycogen concentration or strength.

In a German study, runners completed an endurance event (1000 km in 20 days) after consuming either a vegetarian or non-vegetarian diet containing similar amounts of carbohydrate (60% energy) (Eisinger, 1994). There was no difference in performance between the vegetarians and the non-vegetarians.

In a study by US and Canadian researchers, athletes who followed a vegetarian diet for 12 weeks of resistance training achieved the same strength and muscle size gains as those following a non-vegetarian diet containing exactly the same amount of protein (Haub *et al.*, 2002).

A review of studies by Canadian researchers in 2004 concluded that well-planned vegan and vegetarian diets can support athletic performance (Barr and Rideout, 2004). Provided protein intakes are adequate to meet needs for total nitrogen and the essential amino acids, researchers showed that plant and animal protein sources can provide equivalent support to athletic training and performance.

A more recent analysis by Australian researchers of eight previous studies also concluded that well-planned and varied vegetarian diets neither hinder nor improve athletic performance (Craddock *et al.*, 2016).

A study of endurance athletes at Arizona State University found that vegetarian athletes had similar strength and greater cardiorespiratory fitness than those who ate meat and concluded that a vegetarian diet may even be advantageous for supporting aerobic fitness in athletes (Lynch *et al.*, 2016).

A study of runners following a vegan, vegetarian or meat-based diet found no difference in their maximal power output and exercise capacity (Nebl *et al.*, 2019). They concluded that a vegan diet could support athletic performance in runners.

Together, these studies suggest that a vegetarian or vegan diet, even when followed for several decades, is compatible with successful athletic performance. However, no studies have examined whether a plant-based diet will *improve* athletic performance, so we don't know with certainty the true effects of a plant-based diet on exercise performance.

CAN A PLANT-BASED DIET SUPPORT RECOVERY?

Plant-based athletes tend to have a higher carbohydrate intake than omnivores (Nebl *et al.*, 2019). This would help them meet the recommended

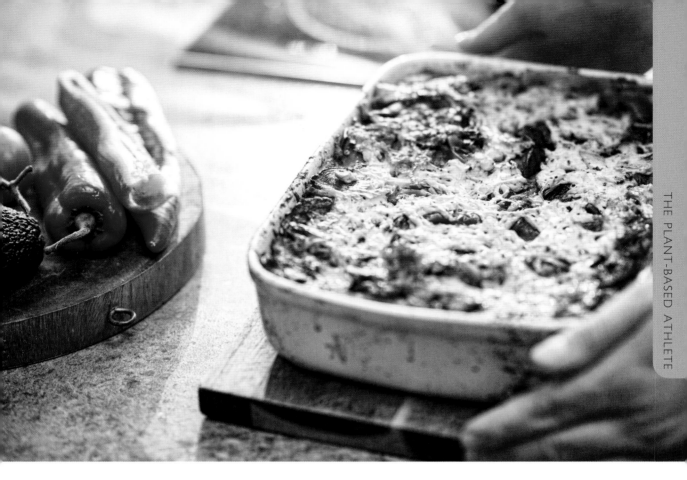

requirement in order to optimise glycogen stores needed for endurance activities.

A typical plant-based diet comprises a wide range of antioxidant-rich foods (e.g. fruit and vegetables), so it is plausible that the consumptions of these foods will result in an enhanced antioxidant system capable to reducing exercise-induced oxidative stress (Trapp *et al.*, 2010).

Plant-based athletes also have higher intakes of fibre and phytochemicals (plant nutrients) that improve gut health. Consuming more fibre – especially a wide variety of different fibre types – and polyphenols means that you're feeding the billions of microorganisms in your gut. This can result in numerous health benefits, including increased immunity, less oxidative stress and lower inflammation – all key factors necessary for optimal performance and recovery (Hughes, 2020).

Studies have found that people who ate a vegetarian diet for at least 2 years had lower levels of inflammation than those who ate an omnivorous diet, suggesting that plant-based diets have an anti-inflammatory effect on the body, which can speed up recovery time (Haghighatdoost *et al.*, 2017).

High intakes of fibre and polyphenols found in plant foods also influence the diversity and balance of gut microorganisms – they encourage healthy gut bacteria to grow and crowd out the unhealthy gut bacteria. Researchers suggest that having a healthy balance of gut bacteria reduces the amount of energy absorbed from food (Spector, 2015).

CAN A PLANT-BASED DIET PROVIDE ENOUGH PROTEIN FOR ATHLETES?

In general, plant-based diets are lower in protein than omnivorous diets but, nevertheless, they tend to meet or exceed the RNI for protein (Sobiecki *et al.*, 2016; Janelle and Barr, 1995). According to the Academy of Nutrition and Dietetics, plant-based diets typically meet or exceed recommended protein intakes when energy needs are also met (Melina *et al.*, 2016). However, since athletes need more protein than the RNI for the general population (1.2–2.0 g vs. 0.75 g/kg BW/day), the question is whether vegetarians can consume enough protein for optimal performance and recovery.

Researchers have concluded that most athletes are able to meet these extra demands from a plant-based diet as long as a variety of protein-rich foods are consumed and energy intakes are adequate (Nieman, 1999; Lemon, 1995; Barr and Rideout, 2004).

Aim for around 20 g per meal, including post-training. Studies by researchers at McMaster University have shown this to be the optimal amount to trigger muscle growth and recovery (*see* pp. 71–2). Good sources of plant proteins include:

- **Legumes** – beans, lentils, peas, chickpeas, peanuts
- **Soya products** – soya milk alternative, soya yoghurt alternative, edamame beans, tofu, tempeh (fermented soya beans), soya mince
- **Grains** – bread, pasta, rice, oats, bulgur (cracked) wheat, teff, freekeh, spelt, seitan (wheat protein)
- **Pseudo-grains** – quinoa, amaranth, buckwheat
- **Mycoprotein** – vegan Quorn
- **Nuts** – walnuts, cashews, almonds, pecans, Brazils, pistachios and nut butters
- **Seeds** – sunflower, sesame, pumpkin, flax, hemp and chia seeds

The protein content of various vegetarian and vegan foods is shown in Table 15.1. Contrary to popular belief, plant proteins do not need to be combined in each meal in order to achieve an adequate intake of amino acids. It is now known that the body has a pool of amino acids, which it draws upon and uses as required. Because of this, you don't have to worry about complementing amino acids at each meal, as long as you consume enough EAAs from a variety of proteins throughout the day. Many foods, including those not considered high in protein, are adding some amino acids to this pool.

ARE PLANT PROTEINS AS GOOD AS ANIMAL PROTEINS FOR BUILDING MUSCLE?

Since the overall protein 'quality' of plant-based diets tends to be lower than animal-based diets, a reflection of a less favourable amino acid profile and have a lower content of leucine and bioavailability (*see* p. 67 for an explanation of protein quality), it is tempting to think that plant proteins are less effective than animal proteins for muscle building. Indeed, studies have suggested that plant proteins produce a smaller MPS response in the 3–5 hour post-exercise period than animal proteins (Wilkinson *et al.*, 2007; Tang *et al.*, 2009; Yang *et al.*, 2012(a)). However, this does not necessarily mean that gains in muscle mass or strength will be less. A meta-analysis of long-term studies (longer than 6 weeks) found that plant proteins are as effective as animal proteins

Table 15.1 THE PROTEIN CONTENT OF VEGETARIAN AND VEGAN FOODS

Food	Portion	Amount of protein (g)*	Food	Portion	Amount of protein (g)*
Protein supplements			**Grains**		
Soya protein isolate powder	1 scoop (25 g)	23	Oats	75 g uncooked	9
Pea protein powder	1 scoop (25 g)	20	Oat milk alternative	1 cup (200 ml)	1
Soya products			Pasta	75 g uncooked (150 g cooked)	9
Soya milk alternative	1 cup (200 ml)	7	Wholewheat noodles	75 g dry uncooked (200 g cooked)	9
Soya yoghurt alternative	1 cup (200 g)	8	Basmati rice	75 g dry uncooked (200 g cooked)	6
Firm tofu	100 g	13			
Tempeh	100 g	21	Wholemeal bread	2 slices (80 g)	8
Soya mince (frozen)	100 g	15	Seitan (wheat protein)	100 g	18
Pulses			**Pseudo grains**		
Red kidney beans (tinned)	125 g drained weight (½ a 400 g can)	9	Quinoa	75 g dry uncooked (200 g cooked)	10
Chickpeas (tinned)	125 g drained weight (½ a 400 g can)	9	Buckwheat	75 g dry uncooked (200 g cooked)	6
Edamame beans (frozen)	125 g	15	**Mycoprotein**		
Green or brown lentils	125 g drained weight (½ a 400 g can)	8	Quorn vegan fillets	1 fillet (63 g)	9
Peas	125 g	7	Quorn vegan pieces	70 g	11
Hummus	2 tbsp (50 g)	3	**Vegetables**		
Falafel	4 falafel (88 g)	8	Potatoes	1 medium (175 g)	3
Nuts			Broccoli	3 florets (80 g)	4
Peanuts	2 tbsp (30 g)	9	**Dairy and Eggs**		
Peanut butter	2 tbsp (30 g)	9	Cheddar cheese	1 slice (25 g)	6
Almonds	2 tbsp (30 g)	6	Eggs	2 eggs	12
Almond milk alternative	1 cup (200 ml)	1	Milk	250 ml	8
Seeds			Plain yoghurt	125 g	6
Sunflower seeds	2 tbsp (30 g)	7	Strained low-fat plain Greek yoghurt	150 g	15
Pumpkin seeds	2 tbsp (30 g)	9			
Chia seeds	2 tbsp (30 g)	6			

* Data from UK *Composition of Foods Integrated Data Set* and UK manufacturers' data

for increasing strength and muscle mass, provided they are consumed in sufficient amounts (Messina *et al.*, 2018). The researchers concluded that soya and whey protein supplements produce similar gains in strength and muscle mass following resistance training. There was no difference in bench press, squat strength or total lean body mass gains between those consuming whey and those consuming soya supplements.

These results support the findings of a previous meta-analysis, which found that provided people consumed sufficient protein, the protein source (soya vs whey) made no difference to their strength and muscle mass gains (Morton *et al.*, 2017). More recently, a study at the University of Sao Paulo and McMaster University compared gains in leg muscle mass and strength between vegans and omnivores consuming 1.6 g protein/day for 12 weeks (Hevia-Larraín *et al.*, 2021). Researchers found no difference in gains between the groups, suggesting that plant proteins are just as effective as animal proteins for building muscle provided they are consumed in sufficient quantity.

Therefore, the lower anabolic potential of plant-based diets can be overcome by:

1. Consuming *larger amounts of protein* – Research suggests that including slightly more protein – an extra 10–22 g daily – will enhance the potential of plant protein to build muscle and strength (Ciuris *et al.*, 2019; Berrazaga *et al.*, 2019; van Vliet *et al.*, 2015). Pulses, tofu, tempeh, grains, nuts and seeds are all good sources.

2. Including *plant foods rich in leucine*, such as tofu, beans, lentils, nuts and seeds. This will increase the overall protein quality of a meal and increase its muscle-building potential. The International Society of Sports Nutrition recommends that acute protein doses should contain between 0.7 and 3 g of leucine (Jäger *et al.*, 2017), equivalent to 49–210 g tofu.

3. Eating a *variety of plant proteins* over the course of a day. This will provide a more balanced amino acid profile and means that the shortfall of EAA in one source will be compensated by higher amounts found in another. Although you do not have to combine proteins in the same meals, many food combinations happen naturally in meals, such as chickpea curry with rice, pasta with lentil ragu, porridge with soya milk alternative, or a falafel wrap.

Vegetarians may benefit more from creatine supplements

Meat is a major source of creatine in the diet – it typically supplies around 1 g per day for non-vegetarians – so vegetarians tend to have lower muscle creatine concentrations than do non-vegetarians (Maughan, 1995). Because initial muscle creatine levels are lower, vegetarians have an increased capacity to load creatine into muscle following supplementation and are likely to gain greater performance benefits in activities that rely on the ATP–PC system (see pp. 22–3), i.e. sports involving repeated bouts of anaerobic activity (Watt *et al.*, 2004).

WHAT ARE THE PITFALLS OF A VEGETARIAN DIET FOR ATHLETES?

As with any dietary change, it is important to plan your diet well and gain as much knowledge about plant-based diets as possible. Some athletes adopt a plant-based diet in order to lose body fat in the belief that such diets are automatically lower in calories. Without proper advice, they may not substitute suitable foods in place of animal products and fail to consume enough protein and other nutrients to support their training. Athletes with disordered eating may omit meat – as well as other food groups – from their diet but disordered eating is certainly not a consequence of plant-based eating!

A very bulky vegan diet that includes lots of high-fibre foods (e.g. vegetables, beans and whole grains) may satiate your appetite before you have consumed sufficient energy to satisfy your body's requirements. If your energy intake does not match the fuel demands of your training load, then, over a period of time you may develop low energy availability (LEA, *see* p. 209). This means you won't have enough energy to support your health and performance, so you may develop serious health problems. To avoid LEA and ensure you eat enough calories, you will need to be more proactive in planning your food and make a conscious effort to consume enough energy, particularly on hard training days. You may need to include lower-fibre sources of carbohydrate (e.g. dried fruit, fruit juice) or include a mixture of both wholegrain and refined grain products (e.g. wholemeal and white bread) in your diet. Include plenty of sources of healthy fats, such as nuts, seeds, nut butters, avocado and olive and rapeseed oil in all your meals and snacks. These foods will help boost your energy intake without adding too much extra volume. Page 206 gives suggestions for high-energy snacks.

The nutrients that are most likely to be lacking in a plant-based diet are protein, iron, omega-3 fatty acids, vitamin B_{12}, calcium, zinc, iodine and vitamin D. Deficiencies of these nutrients will affect

Do plant-based athletes need protein supplements?

Plant-based diets are typically lower in protein than omnivorous diets and can be quite bulky, making it difficult for some athletes to meet their protein requirements from food alone. In these cases, protein supplements can be a convenient option. They may also be useful for athletes training or competing in an environment where their usual foods are not readily available. There is a wide variety of plant protein supplements available, including soya, pea, rice and hemp protein powders. Soya protein is a good option as it contains a balanced amino acid profile and relatively high levels of leucine compared with other plant proteins. Alternatively, opt for blends of plant proteins, such as pea and rice protein, as they contain a more balanced amino acid profile than single plant proteins. Protein powders can be added to shakes, porridge or yoghurt, or used in baking to boost your protein intake.

your performance and health, and increase your risk of illness, fatigue and injury. Knowing how to obtain them from plant-based foods will help you avoid these nutritional pitfalls. How to get enough protein has been covered in the earlier part of this chapter and vitamin D is covered on pp. 96–8.

Iron

Iron is needed for making haemoglobin, the oxygen-carrying protein in red blood cells. Low levels of iron in your diet can result in iron-deficiency anaemia. Early signs include persistent tiredness, pallor, light-headedness and above-normal breathlessness during exercise. According to the Academy of Nutrition and Dietetics, all athletes, whether vegan or not, are at greater risk of developing iron deficiency compared with non-athletes (Melina et al., 2016). That's because aerobic training increases red blood cell manufacture, which in turn increases iron needs (see p. 99). At the same time, iron can be lost from the body via sweat, gastrointestinal bleeding (which sometimes occurs during very strenuous exercise), and foot strike haemolysis (destruction of red blood cells caused by repeated pounding of the feet on hard surfaces). Women in general are more susceptible than men to iron deficiency due to iron losses through menstruation.

Omitting meat may result in lower intakes of iron and, theoretically, an increased risk of iron-deficiency anaemia since iron in plants is less well absorbed than that in meat (1–22% vs.15–35%). The American College of Sports Medicine states that iron deficiency can impair muscle function and limit exercise performance (Thomas et al., 2016). However, there is evidence that the body adapts over time by increasing the percentage of minerals it absorbs from food. Lowered levels of iron in the diet result in increased absorption.

Despite iron from plants being less readily absorbed, research has shown that iron-deficiency anaemia is no more common in vegetarians than in meat-eaters (Alexander et al., 1994; Janelle and Barr, 1995). Even among female endurance athletes, vegetarians are not at greater risk of iron deficiency. Researchers have found that blood levels of haemoglobin and running performance are very similar between non-vegetarian

Table 15.2	THE IRON CONTENT OF VARIOUS PLANT FOODS
Food	**Amount of Iron (mg)**
5 heaped tbsp (250 g) cooked quinoa (75 g dry weight)	5.9
4 heaped tbsp (200 g) boiled red lentils (75 g dry weight)	4.8
5 heaped tbsp (250 g) cooked wholegrain pasta (75 g dry weight)	3.5
4 heaped tbsp (200 g) tinned chickpeas	3.0
100 g tofu	2.7
1 small handful (25 g) pumpkin seeds	2.5
3 tbsp (100 g) spinach	2.1
50 g oats	2.0
2 slices wholemeal bread (80 g)	1.9
4 ready-to-eat dried apricots (50 g)	1.7
3 tbsp (100 g) broccoli	1.7
1 level tbsp (15 g) tahini (sesame seed paste)	1.6
1 small handful (25 g) cashews	1.6

and vegetarian female runners (Snyder, 1989; Seiler, 1989).

Eating vitamin C-rich food (e.g. fruit and vegetables) at the same time as iron-rich foods greatly

Should plant-based athletes take iron supplements?

You should only take iron supplements if you have been diagnosed with iron deficiency. The usual recommended dose is 60–100 mg iron per day taken in the form of iron sulphate for 3 months, although doses depend on gender, weight and iron level. However, if you are not deficient then you shouldn't take supplements – they won't benefit your performance and may do more harm than good. Supplements containing more than 50–60 mg of iron may cause constipation and stomach discomfort.

improves iron absorption. Citric acid (found naturally in fruit and vegetables) and amino acids also promote iron absorption. Good sources of iron for vegetarians include whole grains, wholemeal bread, nuts, beans, lentils, chickpeas, peas, leafy green vegetables (broccoli, watercress and spinach), fortified cereals, seeds and dried fruit. Table 15.2 shows the iron content of various plant-based foods.

The absorption of iron from plant foods can be reduced by phytates. This rarely presents a problem since phytates are destroyed during cooking or canning, so provided you eat beans, lentils and grains cooked rather than raw, your body will be able to absorb the iron it needs.

The UK recommended intake is 8.7 mg/day for men; 14.8 mg/day for women aged 19 to

Table 15.3	THE OMEGA-3 CONTENT OF VARIOUS PLANT-BASED FOODS		
Good sources	**g per 100 g**	**Portion**	**g per portion**
Flaxseed oil	57 g	1 tbsp (14 g)	8.0 g
Flaxseeds (ground)	16 g	1 tbsp (24 g)	3.8 g
Rapeseed oil	9.6 g	1 tbsp (14 g)	1.3 g
Walnuts	7.5 g	1 tbsp (28 g)	2.6 g
Walnut oil	11.5 g	1 tbsp (14 g)	1.6 g
Sweet potatoes	0.03 g	Medium (130 g)	1.3 g
Peanuts	0.4 g	Handful (50 g)	0.2 g
Broccoli	0.1 g	3 tbsp (125 g)	1.3 g
Pumpkin seeds	8.5 g	2 tbsp (25 g)	2.1 g
Omega-3 enriched eggs	0.8 g	1 egg	0.4 g

50; and 8.7 mg/day for women over 50. There is no official recommendation for athletes or for vegetarians but the requirement for iron is thought to be 30–70% higher (DellaValle, 2013).

Omega-3s

Omega-3s are vital for heart health and brain function but can also help reduce inflammation and promote recovery after intense exercise. Oily fish are rich in the long chain omega-3 fatty acids, eicosapentaenoic acid (EPA), docosahexaenoic acid (DHA), so vegetarians and vegans who don't eat fish are at risk of deficiency. However, these long chain fatty acids can be made in the body from the conversion of alpha-linolenic acid (ALA) into EPA and DHA. ALA is found in rapeseed oil, pumpkin, flax, chia and hemp seeds, walnuts, dark green leafy vegetables and flaxseed oil (*see* Table 15.3 on p. 271, which gives the omega-3 fatty acid content of various foods).

The European Food Safety Authority recommends 2–3 g ALA a day and 250 mg EPA and DHA (EFSA, 2009). A tablespoon of flaxseed oil should provide enough of the parent omega-3 fatty acid to ensure enough EPA and DHA are formed by the body (conversion rates are around 5–10% for EPA and 2–5% for DHA). Include some of the foods listed in Table 15.4 in your daily diet.

You should also aim to consume the right balance of omega-3 and omega-6 fatty acids as a high intake of omega-6s interferes with the conversion process of ALA to EPA and DHA (*see* p. 89). Replace fat high in omega-6 oils (such as sunflower or corn oil) with fats higher in mono-unsaturated oils (such as olive oil and nuts), which do not disrupt the formation of EPA and DHA.

It's a good idea to take vegan omega-3 supplements if you don't get food sources of omega-3s

Table 15.4	THE OMEGA-3 CONTENT OF VARIOUS PLANT FOODS
Food	**Omega-3 content**
I tbsp flaxseed oil	7.2 g
I tbsp ground flaxseed	1.6 g
I tbsp hemp seeds	0.9 g
I tbsp rapeseed oil	1.3 g
25 g walnuts	2.5 g

regularly. Opt for supplements made from algae oil – these are better options than those made from flaxseed oil as they contain high levels of both the omega-3 fatty acids DHA and EPA instead of ALA.

Calcium

Calcium is needed for strong, healthy bones and teeth. It also helps with blood clotting and nerve and muscle function. Low intakes over time may result in weak bones and increase the risk of stress fractures and brittle bones (osteoporosis). Obtaining sufficient amounts of calcium can be more difficult for those who don't consume milk or dairy foods as these foods are rich in calcium.

Vegan sources include calcium-fortified non-dairy milk alternatives, calcium-set tofu, beans, lentils, peas, green leafy vegetables (spring greens, kale, broccoli and pak choi), okra, chia seeds, sesame seeds, tahini (sesame seed paste), dried figs and almonds. Table 15.5 shows the calcium content and Table 15.6 shows the absorbability of calcium from various plant foods.

The recommended intake for adults is 700 mg daily. You can get one-third of this amount from

Table 15.5   THE CALCIUM CONTENT OF VARIOUS PLANT FOODS

Food	Amount of calcium (mg)
100 g calcium-set tofu	400
1 cup (200 ml) calcium-fortified plant milk alternative	240
150 ml calcium-fortified plant yoghurt alternative (plain, Greek or sweetened)	180
2 ready-to-eat dried figs (50 g)	115
4 heaped tbsp (200 g) cooked red kidney beans (75 g dry weight)	140
3 tbsp (100 g) kale	130
1 level tbsp (15 g) tahini (sesame seed paste)	102
4 tbsp (200 g) tinned chickpeas	86
1 tbsp chia seeds	72
1 small handful (25 g) almonds	60
2–3 florets (80 g) broccoli	56
3 tbsp (100 g) pak choi	54

Table 15.6   CALCIUM ABSORPTION OF PLANT FOODS

Absorbability	Plant food
Good	Calcium-fortified plant milk and yoghurt alternatives, calcium-set tofu, kale, broccoli, pak choi, Brussels sprouts, cauliflower, watercress
Fair	Red beans, white beans, pinto beans
Poor	Sesame seeds, rhubarb, spinach

200 ml calcium-fortified plant milk or yoghurt alternative or about 60 g calcium-set tofu. Spinach is not a good calcium source as it contains oxalate, which reduces calcium absorption.

Vitamin B_{12}

Vitamin B_{12} is needed for making red blood cells and keeping the nervous system healthy. It also acts with folic acid and vitamin B_6 to control homocysteine levels, high levels of which are associated with an increased risk of heart disease. Although symptoms usually take at least 5 years to develop, a lack of B_{12} can result in nerve damage and anaemia (abnormal red blood cell

Table 15.7	THE VITAMIN B12 CONTENT OF VARIOUS PLANT FOODS
Food	**Amount of Vitamin B12 (mcg)**
100 ml fortified plant milk alternative	0.38
100 g fortified plant yoghurt alternative	0.38
2 tsp (8 g) fortified yeast extract (e.g. Marmite)	1.90
1 tbsp (5 g) fortified nutritional yeast flakes	2.20
30 g fortified bran flakes	0.63
30 g fortified instant porridge	0.63

development and shortness of breath) and impact adversely on endurance performance. If you notice persistent fatigue, ask your doctor for a blood test to check for B_{12} deficiency.

Deficiency of vitamin B_{12} is a particular risk for vegans, as it is not found naturally in any plant sources. Vegetarians can get their daily quota from eggs and dairy products but vegans will need to take a supplement or include vitamin B_{12}-fortified foods such as non-dairy milk alternatives, non-dairy yoghurt alternatives, yeast extract, nutritional yeast or certain breakfast cereals.

The Nutrient Reference Value (NRV) for vitamin B_{12} is 1.5 mcg, which can be obtained from 160 ml milk or 400 ml fortified non-dairy milk alternative. However, the Vegan Society recommends a daily intake of 3 mcg and advises eating fortified foods two or three times a day as it is absorbed more efficiently in small frequent doses. Table 15.7 gives the vitamin B_{12} content of various plant foods. Alternatively, you can take a vitamin B_{12} supplement either as part of a multivitamin or as a single supplement. The Vegan Society recommends either a daily supplement providing at least 10 mcg of vitamin B_{12}, or a weekly B_{12} supplement providing at least 2000 mcg.

Iodine

Iodine is a mineral that is needed to make thyroid hormones, T3 (triiodothyronine) and T4 (thyroxine), which help regulate the metabolic rate, growth and development. It is especially important during pregnancy for normal brain development in the foetus, and for growth in young children. Having low levels can lead to a lower metabolic rate and weight gain, and in pregnant women is linked to lower IQ and reading scores in their children.

There are very few plant sources of iodine, so vegans will need to take a supplement or use a non-dairy milk alternative fortified with iodine. Although seaweed and kelp contain iodine, they are not reliable alternatives because iodine levels can sometimes be extremely high, which carries a risk of excessive intakes. Excessive iodine can result in thyroid problems. The safe upper limit is approximately 600 mcg per day for adults.

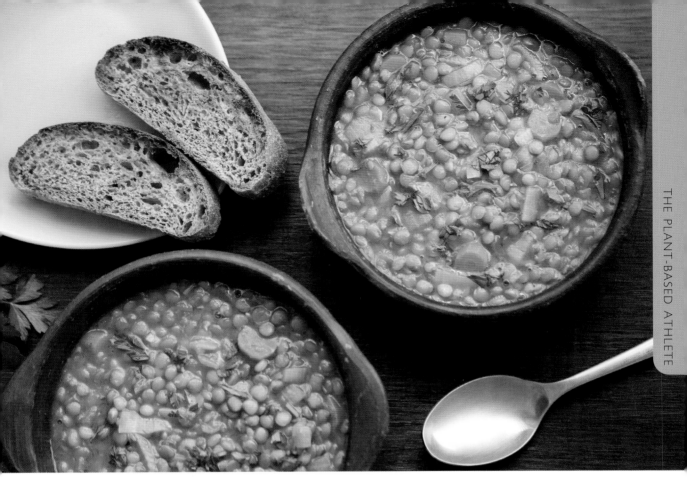

Zinc

Zinc is needed for growth and also plays a role in the proper functioning of the immune system, hormone production and fertility. A deficiency may impair your performance. The recommended daily amount is 7 mg for women and 9.5 mg for men. It is found in whole grains, beans, lentils, chickpeas, nuts, seeds and quinoa. Table 15.8 on p. 275 gives the zinc content of various foods. As with iron, the phytates found in beans, lentils and the bran layer of whole grains may reduce the amount of zinc that can be absorbed from food. Phytates are removed during soaking or cooking so, in practice, are unlikely to present a problem.

Summary of key points

- Overall, vegetarians and vegans have higher intakes of fruit and vegetables, fibre, antioxidant nutrients and phytonutrients, and lower intakes of saturated fat compared with omnivores.
- Large-scale population studies show that those following plant-based diets are less likely to suffer from chronic diseases, such as heart disease, hypertension, obesity, type 2 diabetes and certain cancers than omnivores.
- The nutritional needs of athletes can be fully met through a well-planned plant-based diet.
- Studies have shown that well-planned plant-based diets don't hinder athletic potential and can support athletic performance.

Table 15.8	THE ZINC CONTENT OF VARIOUS PLANT FOODS
Food	**Amount of zinc (mg)**
2 tbsp (30 g) chia seeds	1.4
2 tbsp (30 g) pumpkin seeds	2.0
100 g tofu	1.6
2 slices (80 g) wholemeal bread	1.3
4 heaped tbsp (200 g) cooked lentils (75 g dry weight)	2.0
4 heaped tbsp (200 g) tinned red kidney beans	1.4
5 heaped tbsp (250 g) cooked quinoa (75 g dry weight)	2.5
4 tbsp (200 g) tinned chickpeas	1.6
3 tbsp (45 g) oats	1.0

- There are no significant differences in performance, physical fitness (aerobic or anaerobic capacities) and strength between plant-based and omnivorous athletes.
- The health and performance benefits of plant-based diets may be via their positive effect on the gut microbiota. Increasing the diversity of gut micororganisms increases immunity, reduces oxidative stress and inflammation, all of which are key factors necessary for optimal performance and recovery.
- Plant-based diets are typically lower in protein than omnivorous diets but, nevertheless, athletes can meet their protein requirement from a plant-based diet as long as a variety of protein-rich foods are consumed and energy intakes are adequate.
- Plant proteins are as effective as animal proteins for increasing strength and muscle mass, provided they are consumed in sufficient amounts.

- The lower anabolic potential of plant-based diets can be overcome by consuming larger amounts of protein, including leucine-rich foods and eating a variety of plant proteins.
- Protein supplements can be a convenient option for plant-based athletes who find it difficult to meet their protein requirement from food alone.
- Plant-based athletes are likely to gain greater performance benefits from creatine supplementation than omnivores, due to their initially lower muscle creatine levels.
- A poorly planned plant-based diet may result in low energy availability, low intakes of iron, omega-3 fatty acids, vitamin B_{12}, calcium, zinc, iodine and vitamin D. These can be avoided by including plant sources of 'at risk' nutrients in the diet, fortified foods and supplementation where necessary.

The Masters //Athlete

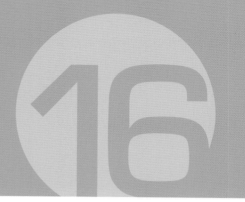

Now, more than ever, many people in their 50s, 60s and beyond want to improve their health, retain a high level of fitness, and remain competitive and at the top of their game. However, the ageing process is accompanied by many physiological changes that affect your exercise capacity, muscle mass and strength. Typically, most athletes start to see a drop in their peak performance after their 30s.

Fortunately, a combination of better training, recovery and nutrition practices can help prevent or reduce age-related declines in muscle mass, strength and physiological functioning. By 'training smarter, not harder' athletes can make gains, reap great health benefits and maintain a high level of fitness over the age of 40. This chapter explains how you can adjust your diet and training so you will continue to perform to your potential in sport as you get older.

HOW DOES AGEING AFFECT PERFORMANCE?

For most athletes, peak performance begins to drop some time in their 20s or 30s, depending on the sport and activity. The rate of decline gradually increases to about 0.7% per year throughout their 40s, 50s and 60s, with progressively steeper increases thereafter (Tanaka and Seals, 2008).

The physiological reasons for this decline are varied and not very well understood. What is known is that the natural ageing process is associated with a gradual reduction in cardiovascular and respiratory functioning, muscle mass, strength and bone mass. Women are more likely to suffer from these physical changes than men. Many of these changes are underpinned by a decline in growth hormone (GH), testosterone and oestrogen. GH is important for maintaining a favourable body composition, and thus a decrease will lead to a reduction in muscle mass and increase in subcutaneous and visceral fat. The major age-related changes that may affect nutritional requirements are summarised in Table 16.1.

Power and strength, however, decline much more quickly unless you include resistance exercise in your training programme.

Body composition

Inactive adults typically experience an increase in body fat and loss of muscle with age. This is mainly due to reduced physical activity without a concomitant reduction in energy intake. However, active adults and athletes also experience body composition changes due to hormonal changes that occur with age. We typically lose

Table 16.1	THE MAIN AGE-RELATED CHANGES THAT MAY INFLUENCE NUTRITIONAL REQUIREMENTS
Age-related change	**Nutritional implication**
Reduced aerobic capacity	Reduced energy requirements
Reduced muscle mass	Reduced energy requirements
Reduced bone mass	Increased requirement for calcium and vitamin D
Reduced skin capacity for vitamin D synthesis	Increased requirement for vitamin D
Reduced gastric acid	Increased requirement for B_{12}, folic acid, calcium, iron and zinc
Reduced absorption of calcium	Increased requirement for calcium and vitamin D
Reduced thirst perception	Increased requirement for fluid
Reduced kidney function	Increased requirement for fluid

around 3–8% of our muscle mass per decade from our 30s onwards (Westcott, 2012, Janssen *et al.*, 2000), increasing to about 15% per decade after our 70s (Mitchell *et al.*, 2012). After the age of 50, strength declines by 3% per year (Bell *et al.*, 2016). Most of the loss of muscle fibres is accounted for by loss of type 2 (fast-twitch) fibres, which are the large fibres used primarily for power and strength. The type 1 (slow-twitch) fibres, the endurance fibres, show practically no change. This age-related loss of muscle mass and strength, called sarcopenia, can dramatically reduce mobility, quality of life and ability to perform everyday activities. It also increases the risk of falls and fractures, and contributes to the development of chronic metabolic diseases such as type 2 diabetes.

This age-related muscle atropy also includes a reduction in heart muscle mass, which accounts for the drop in cardiovascular and respiratory function observed with ageing.

Cardiovascular and respiratory fitness – in sedentary people, resting stroke volume, maximum heart rate and the maximal ability to utilise oxygen (VO_2max) decline at a rate of approximately 10% per decade from the mid-20s (Downes, 2002). From middle age onwards, the drop in endurance performance is due mainly to a reduction in VO_2max, whereas from young adulthood to middle age it is mainly due to a reduction in lactate threshold (Tanaka and Seals, 2008). The reason VO_2max declines with age is that maximal heart rate decreases. This reduces both cardiac output and oxygen delivery to the muscles, which translates to a lower VO_2max and thus to lower endurance performance as we age.

Bone mass – this also declines from the mid 30s and one in three women over the age of 50 will experience fractures as a result of osteopososis (thinning of the bones), as will one in five men. All of these physiological changes inevitably result in a drop in endurance, strength and physical performance.

Flexibility – this tends to decrease due to accumulated wear and tear. Recovery from hard workouts and healing after injury take longer, and chronic overuse injuries become more common, accounting for as many as 70% of injuries in athletes over 60 years of age. To reduce your injury risk, you may need to reduce the amount of repetitive impact exercise you do and focus instead on low-impact activities, as well as building extra recovery and sleep into your programme.

Recovery – this can take longer and, as they age, many athletes find that their ability to recover from hard sessions diminishes. This can affect the intensity and volume of training of all sports. In many sports, recovering from injuries and their cumulative effects becomes the limiting factor in continuing to play at the highest level. For masters athletes, experiencing more training-associated injuries leads to reduced training intensity and volume, and thus poorer performance come race day.

Are there performance differences between men and women?

In men, performance starts to decline markedly around the age of 70–75 years while in women, it starts earlier, around the age of 55–60 years. This difference is explained by the hormonal changes in women that take place around the perimenopause and menopause.

Perimenopause is the transition period leading up to the menopause when hormone production decreases and menopause symptoms (such as hot flushes and mood swings) may be experienced. For many women this starts around the age of 45. The menopause is a specific point in time marking the cessation of menstruation, and is defined as not having had a period for 1 year. The average age is 51 years with a range from 45 to 55 years. During this time, levels of oestrogen and progesterone levels fall markedly, and this results in body composition changes, namely a decrease in muscle mass (Abildgaard *et al.*, 2013) and an increase in subcutaneous fat and visceral fat (Santosa *et al.*, 2013). Additionally, there are changes in body fat distribution, as fat shifts to the midsection (Davis *et al.*, 2012), which carries an increased risk of chronic diseases, such as heart disease, certain cancers and type

What is sarcopenia?

Sarcopenia is the gradual loss of muscle mass, strength and mobility that occurs with age. It can begin in your 30s and typically accelerates in your 60s onwards unless specific measures are taken to prevent it. Losses are typically 0.5–1.2% per year; most people in their 70s have only 60–80% of the muscle mass they had in their 30s. This age-related muscle loss is the result of a chronic disruption in the balance between protein synthesis and breakdown (Koopman, 2011) and is caused by lack of exercise as well as poor nutrition (particularly insufficient protein intake), a drop in hormone (growth hormone and testosterone) levels, chronic inflammation and DNA damage.

2 diabetes. Low levels of oestrogen also result in accelerated bone loss, reduced sensitivity to anabolic stimuli (exercise and protein intake), and decreased muscle protein synthesis (MPS). It also leads to a reduction in cardiovascular fitness – particularly during the 3–4 years prior to menopause (Mercuro *et al.*, 2006). Metabolic changes include decreased insulin sensitivity (raising the risk of type 2 diabetes), decreased glycogen storage and increased muscle breakdown. All of these changes result in increased risk after the menopause of osteoporosis, cardiovascular disease and stroke, together with other vasomotor symptoms and mood changes.

Does menopause cause weight gain in women?

While menopause itself doesn't cause weight gain, it can change the way fat is stored and distributed in our bodies, with it more likely to be stored around the middle than the hips (Toth *et al.*, 2000). Additionally, many of the symptoms of the perimenopause and menopause lead to weight gain, for example, fatigue and lack of sleep can result in less healthy dietary choices, and loss of motivation to exercise. In addition to providing much-needed relief from menopause symptoms, hormone replacement therapy (HRT) may have beneficial effects on body fat distribution once women reach the menopause (Yüksel *et al.*, 2009). It won't stop you gaining weight (if you consume more calories than you need) but it can minimise the shift in fat to your middle (Reubinoff *et al.*, 1995). In a Danish study, those women who took HRT gained less fat over 5 years than those who didn't (Kristensen *et al.*, 1999). They were also less likely to store this fat around their middles. In the Women's Health Initiative study, HRT helped women maintain lean body mass and prevented a shift towards 'apple-shaped' fat distribution (Chen *et al.*, 2005).

Can the age-related decline in body composition and performance be prevented?

The good news is that many of the detrimental effects of ageing can be offset by making a number of changes to your exercise programme and diet, including your warm-up and recovery. Older athletes will benefit from a longer, dynamic warm-up with controlled moblisation and muscle activation as this will help prevent injury.

Muscle mass – sarcopenia isn't inevitable. With regular weight-bearing exercise and resistance training performed at least twice a week, you can prevent and reverse sarcopenia and even gain lean body mass (Booth and Zwetsloot, 2010; Peterson *et al.*, 2011). Resistance training increases the size of the type 2 fibres, which are mostly dramatically affected by the ageing process, and the ability of motor nerves to recruit those fibres. It also increases the ability of the type 2 fibres to repair themselves, thus reaching higher levels of hypertrophy.

On the biochemical side, resistance training increases levels of testosterone and growth hormone. What's more, it increases blood glucose utilisation and ATP production.

Programmes based on low reps (1–6) and heavier weights produce greater increases in strength, power, metabolic efficiency, joint strength and stability, BMD and immunity than traditional resistance programmes.

For post-menopausal women, resistance training improves vasodilation, body composition (greater lean mass and decreased visceral and total body fat), muscle strength and endurance, bone density, vasomotor symptoms, and metabolic and glucose control.

For older men, it increases muscle size and mass, strength and power, metabolic rate and efficiency, joint strength and stability, and BMD.

A study by researchers at Top Institute Food and Nutrition, the Netherlands, of 24 women and 29 men aged 70–71 years showed that 6 months of resistance training resulted in a 10% increase in leg muscle mass and a 42% increase in leg strength (Leenders *et al.*, 2013).

Aerobic power (VO$_2$max) – high-intensity exercise and high-intensity interval training (HIIT) are more effective for reversing the decrease in VO$_2$max than traditional low- or moderate-intensity aerobic training. HIIT is the most effective and efficient form of cardiovascular training for old and young alike. It also improves blood glucose control, insulin sensitivity, blood vessel function and other markers of cardiovascular health. A 2:1 work/rest ratio, composed of 20 seconds work and 10 seconds of recovery, is thought to be the most efficient ratio to improve the cardiovascular system. However, including a variety of work-recovery cycles is best. A study of 40 post-menopausal women showed that an 8-week HIIT programme resulted in a significant reduction in body fat, and an increase in lean mass and aerobic fitness (Boutcher *et al.*, 2019).

However, this doesn't mean that you shouldn't do any moderate- or low-intensity training as it can also maintain cardiovascular health. A study

Fitness measurements explained

- **Maximal oxygen consumption (VO$_2$max)** – the maximal volume of oxygen that the body can deliver to the working muscles per minute. It is a good measure of an athlete's cardiovascular fitness and aerobic endurance.
- **Lactate threshold (LT)** – the exercise intensity at which blood lactate concentrations increase significantly above baseline. Lactate is the by-product of glucose breakdown by muscle cells. Having a high LT means you can work at a higher intensity for longer.

at the Mayo Clinic College of Medicine, found that older people (59–76 years of age) who did at least 1 hour of endurance exercise a day had a higher aerobic capacity, less body fat and greater insulin sensitivity (and therefore less risk of developing metabolic syndrome) than those who were sedentary (Lanza *et al.*, 2008). There was little difference in mitochondria function between older and younger active people in the group, which suggests that regular endurance exercise largely prevented the decline in aerobic capacity that normally occurs with age. According to the researchers at the University of Missouri, maintaining a life-long habit of regular aerobic exercise delays the onset of decline in aerobic capacity by 30 years (Booth and Zwetsloot, 2010). An active 80-year-old may have a higher level of fitness than a sedentary 50-year-old, especially when it comes to measures of VO$_2$max, muscle strength and endurance.

Recovery – older athletes should allow longer for recovery, particularly following resistance training and high-intensity or HIIT training, so workout planning needs to change. Benefits may also be gained by changing the periodisation of training from the traditional cycle of 3 weeks training followed by 1 week of recovery to a shorter cycle comprising 2 weeks training and 1 week of recovery.

Cross-training, such as weightlifting and yoga, can help to maintain muscle mass and flexibility, and reduce overuse injuries in endurance athletes. An emphasis on 'active recovery' strategies (e.g. an easy run or swim on your rest days) and improved sleeping habits are important for athletes of all ages, but become essential for older athletes.

How do energy requirements change with age?

Daily energy needs typically decrease with age, partly due to the decrease in lean body mass, resulting in an overall drop in resting metabolic rate (RMR), and partly due to a reduction in physical activity levels. However, this muscle loss can be prevented by incorporating resistance training in your training programme and maintaining training volume. This is explained more fully in the following section.

Your RMR is an estimate of how many calories you would burn if you were to do nothing but rest for 24 hours. It represents the minimum amount of energy needed to keep your body functioning, including breathing and keeping your heart beating. It can be estimated using the Mifflin-St Jeor equation, which utilises age as well as weight and height to take account of age-related muscle loss. However, it does not account for exercise or make any adjustment for body composition.

For example, the RMR for a 60-year-old male athlete who measures 1.78m and weighs 70 kg is 1518 kcal, whereas the RMR for a 30-year-old of the same height and weight is 1668 kcal. In other words, an average 60-year-old man expends 150 fewer calories per day at rest compared with an average 30-year-old. However, this is based on the assumption that the 60-year-old has less muscle mass than the 30-year-old.

The daily energy expenditure will also be correspondingly less. This can be calculated by multiplying RMR by the physical activity level (PAL) and then adding estimated exercise energy expenditure (*see* p. 306). For example, for a 60-year-old who is mostly sedentary (PAL 1.4) and expends an average 500 calories per day during exercise:

- Daily energy expenditure = 1518 x 1.4 + 500 = 2625 kcal

By comparison, a 30-year-old would expend 2835 kcal per day, a difference of 210 calories.

The Mifflin-St Jeor equation for estimating RMR

Men

10 × weight (kg) + 6.25 × height (cm) –5 × age (y) + 5

Women

10 × weight (kg) + 6.25 × height (cm) –5 × age (y) – 161

(Mifflin et al., 1990)

This equates to two chocolate biscuits or a pint of beer! Clearly, you can compensate for the age-related drop in calorie expenditure by consuming fewer calories, increasing energy exercise expenditure or avoiding muscle loss in the first place by including resistance training in your programme.

Calorie intake should come from nutrient-dense foods that promote maximum performance, enhance recovery from workouts and reduce the risk of chronic diseases such as cardiovascular disease, type 2 diabetes, cancer and osteoporosis and other debilitating diseases of ageing.

How do protein requirements change with age?

Both protein ingestion and resistance training are powerful anabolic stimuli, triggering muscle protein synthesis (MPS). However, as you get older, the muscles become less able to respond to the anabolic effects of dietary protein and exercise on muscle protein synthesis (MPS), and develop an 'anabolic resistance' (Burd *et al.*, 2013; Rennie, 2009). The exact mechanisms are unclear but it is thought that the absorption of amino acids from the gut is reduced as well as the uptake of amino acids by the muscles. In essence, this means that, without regular resistance exercise, MPS declines and many people experience an age-related loss of muscle.

HOW MUCH PROTEIN?

Studies suggest that older people (both inactive and active) may require a higher protein intake than previously thought to offset protein loss and maintain muscle mass, strength and physiological functioning (Moore *et al.*, 2015; Gray-Donald *et al.*, 2014; Deutz *et al.*, 2014; Bauer *et al.*, 2013).

For healthy non-active adults aged over 65, the European Society for Clinical Nutrition and Metabolism recommend 1.0–1.2 g/kg BW/day to prevent sarcopenia and maintain muscle mass (Deutz *et al.*, 2014), which is more than the amount recommended for younger adults (0.75 g/kg BW/day). For those who do regular exercise, researchers recommend a daily protein intake of 1.2–1.5 g/kg BW/day to help preserve muscle mass and strength (Witard *et al.*, 2016, Bauer *et al.*, 2013). This equates to 84 g–105 g per day for a 70 kg person. Both protein consumption and resistance exercise independently stimulate MPS, but when protein is consumed near resistance exercise, MPS is increased to a greater extent than either stimuli alone (Breen and Phillips, 2013).

It is more practical, however, to express protein intake recommendations per meal, rather than per day. The optimal protein dose for stimulating maximal muscle protein synthesis (MPS) is believed to be in the region of 40 g or 0.4 g/kg BW per meal, which is considerably higher than the recommendation for younger athletes (20 g or 0.25 g/kg BW/day) (Moore *et al.*, 2015; Witard *et al.*, 2016).

In one study of older men (average age 71), those who consumed a drink containing 40 g whey protein after resistance exercise showed significantly greater MPS than those who consumed 20 g (Yang *et al.*, 2012(b)).

IS PROTEIN TIMING IMPORTANT?

As well as quantity, the timing of protein intake is also important when it comes to stimulating maximal MPS in older athletes. Studies have found that consuming protein either during or immediately after exercise improves the anabolic response and allows more of the dietary protein to be used to build new muscle proteins (Pennings *et al.*, 2011). This not only helps to prevent protein breakdown during exercise but also helps to compensate for the anabolic resistance that occurs with age, and builds new muscle.

Since the anabolic effect of exercise is now known to extend at least 24 hours after exercise, there are further muscle-building benefits to be gained by consuming protein throughout the day, not only in the post-workout meal. A study at the University of Texas Medical Branch, found that 24-hour MPS was significantly greater when volunteers consumed 90 g protein as 3 x 30 g meals evenly spaced, compared with a skewed meal pattern that biased protein intake towards the evening meal (Mamerow *et al.*, 2014). In practice, this means including similar quantities of foods such as milk, eggs, meat, fish, poultry, tofu, beans and lentils at every meal, including breakfast. Suitable high-protein snack options include yoghurt, nuts and nut butter.

WHICH TYPE OF PROTEIN IS BEST?

Ideally, you should include high-quality proteins that provide all nine essential amino acids, including the amino acid leucine. Leucine not only provides a substrate for building new muscle proteins but also acts as an important anabolic signal for MPS by activating enzymes within the mammalian target of rapamycin complex 1 (mTORC1) signalling pathway (*see* p. 73). These can be found in animal protein sources such as milk and dairy products, whey protein supplements, eggs and meat, as well as plant sources, namely soya (e.g. soya milk alternative, soya yoghurt alternative, tofu, tempeh and miso), quinoa, buckwheat, amaranth, chia and hemp seeds. Vegans should include a mixture of plant proteins (such as beans and grains) in order to get the full complement of EAAs.

SHOULD I CONSUME PROTEIN BEFORE SLEEP?

Studies have also shown that consuming protein before sleep can result in greater MPS in younger athletes (*see* p. 266). However, this is also advantageous for older athletes. In a study involving 16 healthy older men (average age 74) at the Maastricht Medical Centre in the Netherlands, those who were given an infusion of 40 g casein protein overnight had significantly greater MPS and whole-body protein synthesis compared with those who received a placebo (Groen *et al.*, 2012). While consuming protein overnight is not a practical strategy for most people, having a high-protein snack or drink before bed could help maximise the effects of resistance exercise and help you gain more muscle. Suitable options include:

- 300 ml milk or hot chocolate (10 g protein)
- 300 ml milk blended with 20 g casein protein, a banana or a handful of berries (30 g protein)
- 250 g strained plain Greek yoghurt mixed with berries, honey or granola (20 g protein)

How do carbohydrate requirements change with age?

As we get older, we retain the ability to store carbohydrate as glycogen in the liver and muscles; to use glycogen as a source of fuel during exercise; and to recover muscle glycogen levels following exercise. So, the carbohydrate needs of older athletes are no different from those of younger athletes. However, as mentioned previously, if daily energy expenditure typically drops then your daily carbohydrate requirement may become smaller too.

HOW MUCH CARBOHYDRATE?

Your carbohydrate intake should match the fuel needs of your training programme. Thus, the guidelines for carbohydrate requirements in Table 3.1 (*see* p. 35) apply equally to older athletes. These are based on body weight and exercise load, so the greater your body weight (a proxy for muscle mass) and exercise volume, the higher your carbohydrate requirement.

Muscles become more susceptible to the damage caused by eccentric exercise (where the muscle lengthens as it contracts, such as during the lowering phase of resistance training exercises, plyometric training or downhill running) and are not able to repair this damage as quickly between workouts.

To promote recovery after exercise, especially if you plan to train within 8 hours, you should consume 1.0–1.2 g carbohydrate/kg BW/hour for the first 4 hours. Adding protein to your post-exercise meal or snack will enhance muscle repair, glycogen storage and MPS.

CAN A LOW-CARBOHYDRATE DIET HELP WEIGHT LOSS IN MASTERS ATHLETES?

Many masters athletes find that weight loss or prevention of weight gain become harder

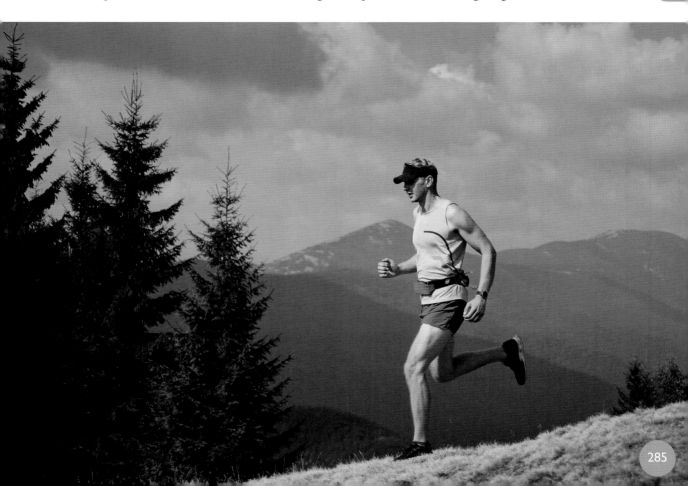

with age. Consequently, they turn to novel diet approaches, such as low-carbohydrate and very low-carbohydrate diets (including ketogenic) diets and fasted training as a means of overcoming weight loss plateaus (see p. 184). The thinking behind such regimes is that restricting carbohydrate intake will force the muscle to burn more fat and less carbohydrate during exercise. Indeed, studies have shown that carbohydrate restriction before and during exercise can increase fat oxidation. However, restricting carbohydrate also reduces exercise economy at moderate and high training intensities (64–90% VO_2max) and reduces performance in high-intensity endurance events (Burke et al., 2017; Burke et al., 2020). To date, there is no clear evidence that following a low-carbohydrate diet long term provides any performance advantage for those exercising above 64% VO_2max or participating in races that involve sprints or high-intensity efforts. However, it may suit those engaged in low- to moderate-intensity exercise, those with type 2 diabetes or those with insulin resistance (when your cells are less sensitive to insulin so cannot process carbohydrate into fuel efficiently).

In terms of weight loss, the consensus of evidence suggests that low-carbohydrate diets are no more effective than other types of diets (Kirkpatrick et al., 2019; Pagoto and Appelhans, 2013; Hu et al., 2012, Johnston et al., 2006). What matters most when it comes to weight loss is achieving a calorie deficit and then being able to sustain the diet long term.

It is important to note that the majority of studies on low-carbohydrate diets have been done with obese, diabetic men; very few have been done with athletes and even fewer on female athletes. Studies with female athletes have failed to demonstrate any performance gain. Women are already able to exercise at their maximal fat oxidation capacity and any attempt to increase this by restricting carbohydrate has no benefit.

Carbohydrate periodisation, whereby you do certain (low-intensity) workouts with low carbohydrate availability and high-intensity sessions with high carbohydrate availability, may be a better option if you are competing at elite level. The idea is to match your carbohydrate intake to the demands of your training sessions so you get the dual benefits of 'training low' (fat adaptation) as well as the performance benefits of high-intensity training.

Fluid

As we get older, our perception of thirst decreases and sweat rate decreases. You may notice that you sweat less and begin sweating later during exercise compared with younger athletes. Kidney function is also reduced, which means the ability of your kidneys to concentrate urine is reduced. Kenney and Chiu, 2001; Miescher et al., 1989; Phillips et al., 1984).

All of this means that as you age you are more susceptible to hypohydration (p.147), so make sure you begin training sessions well hydrated. Achieve this by drinking plenty of fluid in the 24 hours prior to training and approximately 5–10 ml/kg BW in the 2–4 hours before exercise. This promotes hydration and allows enough time for the excretion of excess water (Thomas et al., 2016). During exercise, you may prefer to drink to a planned schedule rather than relying totally on thirst, since thirst becomes less pronounced as we get older and is therefore a less reliable indicator of the body's fluid needs.

As a rule of thumb, an intake of 400–800 ml/hour prevents hypohydration as well as overhydration (Sawka *et al.,* 2007; Thomas *et al.,* 2016). You can work out how much fluid you lose through sweating by weighing yourself before and after a typical workout, then aim to drink sufficient to ensure a weight loss of no more than about 2% (*see* p. 153). After each session, you should drink an additional 1.2–1.5 litres of fluid for each 1 kg lost during exercise (IAAF, 2007; Shirreffs *et al.,* 2004; Shirreffs *et al.,* 1996).

Which supplements may be beneficial for masters athletes?

OMEGA-3S

Omega-3 supplements may help counter inflammation associated with sarcopenia and potentially reduce muscle loss. Chronic inflammation is believed to be a key factor in sarcopenia and the development of many chronic diseases, including heart disease. Studies have suggested that omega-3s may make muscles more sensitive to the anabolic effects of resistance exercise and protein feeding. In one study, 8 weeks of omega-3 supplementation increased the anabolic effect of protein and augment MPS in older adults (Smith *et al.,* 2011 (b)).

The UK government recommends a minimum of 450–900 mg omega-3 fatty acids per day, and advises people to eat at least two portions of fish a week, one of which should be oily fish. The best sources of omega-3s include oily fish, such as mackerel and salmon, flaxseeds, pumpkin seeds, walnuts, chia seeds and their oils.

CREATINE

Creatine supplementation may augment the benefits of resistance training (Candow *et al.,* 2014). A meta-analysis of studies with older adults (average age 64 years) showed that when combined with resistance training for an average of 12 weeks, creatine supplementation leads to greater increases in strength, power, muscle mass and functional performance compared with resistance training alone (Devries and Phillips, 2014). In one study, daily supplementation of low doses (5 g) of creatine for 12 weeks resulted in significant increase in muscle mass (Pinto *et al.,* 2016). It works by increasing PC energy stores and/or speeding PC resynthesis (*see* pp. 126–9) and reducing muscle damage, which would enhance the ability to perform short, intense exercise bouts such as resistance training and also speed recovery. There are several forms of creatine, but creatine monohydrate is the most effective and well-researched variety.

VITAMIN D

Vitamin D plays an important role in healthy bones and teeth, muscle function, supporting our immune system, lung function, cardiovascular health and the brain and nervous system. Low levels may reduce muscle function and strength, bone mineral density and impair performance (Hamilton, 2011; Larson-Meyer and Willis, 2010; Halliday *et al.,* 2011). Getting adequate levels of vitamin D – whether from sun exposure or diet – is, therefore, important for optimal performance.

Low blood levels of vitamin D are common across all age groups but this is particularly problematic as we get older as the skin's capacity to produce vitamin D from UV light diminishes.

Data from the UK National Diet and Nutrition Survey (NDNS) showed that 17% of men aged 65 or older and 24% of women had vitamin D deficiency (Bates *et al.*, 2014). A study of male cyclists found that the majority had low levels of vitamin D (below 90 nmol/litre), putting them at greater risk of injury and respiratory infection (Keay *et al.*, 2018).

There are relatively few foods that contain significant amounts of vitamin D – eggs, liver oily fish, fortified spreads, non-dairy milks and breakfast cereals – making it difficult to ensure you get enough vitamin D. For this reason, Public Health England advise taking a daily supplement containing 10 mcg of vitamin D during the autumn and winter. Those over 65 year are considered at greater risk of deficiency and are advised to take a supplement year round. However, optimising vitamin D levels may improve performance if you are deficient (i.e. with blood levels of 25(OH)D below 75 nmol/litre), in which case a supplement containing 50–100 ug or 2000–4000 IU) is recommended (Owens *et al.*, 2018).

Summary of key points

- Aerobic capacity, muscle mass and bone density gradually decline with age.
- Muscle mass starts to decline in our 30s at a rate of 3–8% per decade, increasing to about 15% per decade after our 70s.
- In female athletes, a drop in oestrogen and progesterone levels during the perimenopause and menopause results in a decrease in muscle mass, bone mineral density and cardiovascular fitness, and an increase in body fat.
- Changes in body composition in both male and female athletes can be offset by regular resistance training, especially low reps and heavier weights.
- Loss of cardiovascular fitness can be offset most effectively by high-intensity endurance training and HIIT.
- A longer dynamic warm-up and longer recovery period may reduce injury risk.
- Energy needs may decrease due to loss of muscle mass (and the resultant drop in RMR), and reduced physical activity levels.
- Muscles are less responsive to the anabolic effects of dietary protein and exercise.
- An increased daily protein intake (1.2–1.5 g/kg BW/day) can help offset protein loss and maintain muscle mass and strength.
- To maximise MPS, an intake of 0.4 g protein/kg BW per meal is recommended.
- Including proteins rich in leucine as well as consuming protein post-exercise may also help increase MPS.
- Adjust your carbohydrate intake to the fuel needs of your training programme.
- Thirst becomes less pronounced with age and is therefore a less reliable indicator of your body's fluid needs.
- Omega-3s supplements may help reduce chronic inflammation and muscle loss.
- Creatine supplementation combined with resistance training may increase muscle mass, strength and performance more than resistance training alone.
- The skin's capacity to produce vitamin D from UV light diminishes so dietary sources or supplementation become more important.

Competition // Nutrition

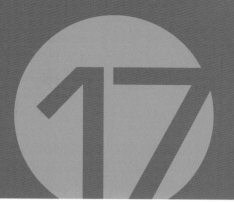

Your diet before and during a competition will have a big impact on your performance and could provide you with that winning edge. In addition, what you eat and drink on the day of the event can affect your ability to recover between heats or matches and your performance in subsequent events.

Each sport and event will have different nutritional challenges, depending on the intensity and duration of the event, and the temperature and humidity of the environment. This means that different nutrition strategies are required for different sports and types of event. For example, your fuel requirements in a marathon will be different from those in a 5k, therefore a different fuel strategy will be needed before and during the event. Additionally, your fluid requirement in hot, humid conditions will be greater than that in cool conditions, so a planned drinking schedule may be more appropriate than drinking to thirst. Every competition nutrition strategy will also need to take account of how many opportunities you will have to eat and drink and ease of access. For example, in a football match there are limited opportunities to eat and drink so you will need to ensure you consume sufficient carbohydrate and fluid after warm-up

and during the half-time break. By contrast, in a tennis match there are more frequent opportunities to eat and drink between games, so you may consume smaller amounts of carbohydrate and fluid during each break.

This chapter provides nutrition strategies for three main types of events: 1) marathon running and endurance events >90 minutes; 2) soccer and other team sports; and 3) making weight for weight-category sports. Unfortunately, it is outside the scope of this book to provide nutrition strategies for every type of event.

Marathon running and endurance events >90 minutes

If you are competing in an endurance event lasting longer than 90 minutes then you may benefit from carbohydrate loading. This is a technique originally devised in the 1960s to increase the muscles' glycogen stores above normal levels ('supercompensation'). With more glycogen available, you may be able to exercise longer before fatigue sets in. This is potentially advantageous in endurance events lasting longer than 90 minutes (e.g. marathon running or road cycling) during which glycogen depletion is a limiting factor to performance. It is unlikely to benefit you if your event lasts less than 90 minutes because muscle glycogen depletion would not be a limiting factor to your performance. Carbohydrate loading increases time to exhaustion by about 20% and improves performance by about 2–3% (Hawley et al.,1997). It can also reduce the chances of glycogen depletion, or 'hitting the wall' during the latter stages of long races, such as marathons, typically around the 20-mile mark. This is characterised by overwhelming fatigue, loss of power, weakness, nausea and disorientation. Good pacing and fuelling during the event will also help prevent glycogen depletion.

WHAT IS CARBOHYDRATE LOADING?

The classical 6-day carbohydrate loading regimen involved two bouts of glycogen-depleting exercise separated by 3 days of low carbohydrate intake and followed by 3 days of high carbohydrate intake (>70% carbohydrate, 8–10 g/kg BW/day) and minimal exercise (Ahlborg et al., 1967; Karlsson and Saltin, 1971). The theory behind this two-phase regimen is that glycogen depletion stimulates the activity of glycogen synthase, the key enzyme involved in glycogen storage, resulting in above-normal levels of muscle glycogen ('supercompensation').

However, this regimen had a number of drawbacks. In studies, not only did it interfere with exercise tapering, but the low-carbohydrate diet left athletes weak, irritable and tired. Worse, many failed to achieve high glycogen levels even after 3 days of high carbohydrate intake.

Researchers at Ohio State University, US developed a 6-day carbohydrate loading regimen that resulted in similar increases in glycogen levels but without the disadvantages described (Sherman et al., 1981). This required tapering training on 6 consecutive days while following a normal diet during the first 3 days followed by a carbohydrate-rich diet during the next 3 days.

Twenty years after this study was carried out, researchers at the University of Western Australia found that above-normal levels of glycogen can be achieved within only 24 hours after performing a short bout of high-intensity exercise followed by a high carbohydrate intake (10–12 g of carbohydrate per kilogram of body weight) (Fairchild et al., 2002; Bussau et al., 2002). In other words, a depletion phase is not necessary. The current thinking is that eating a high-carbohydrate diet for 2 days prior to competition while reducing glycogen use (tapering exercise) is sufficient to elevate muscle glycogen levels. Bear in mind, though, that glycogen storage is associated with approximately 3 g of water for each 1 g of glycogen, so carbohydrate loading can produce a weight increase of 1–2 kg. This may affect your performance in weight-sensitive sports, such as running.

24–48 HOURS BEFORE THE EVENT

For elite athletes, researchers currently recommend consuming 10–12 g/kg BW/day during the 36–48 hours prior to the event (Burke et al., 2011; Thomas et al., 2016). Table 17.4 on p. 296 gives two sample eating plans providing 500 and 700 g of carbohydrate, which you may use as a basis for developing your own plan. However, for non-elite athletes, a carbohydrate intake of 5–7 g/kg BW/day may be more appropriate since energy expenditure is reduced. In practice, your total calorie intake should remain about the same as usual while carbohydrate loading, but the proportions of carbohydrate, fat and protein will change. You will need to eat larger amounts of carbohydrate-rich foods and drinks, and smaller amounts of fats and proteins.

Distribute your carbohydrate intake evenly across your meals, include a portion of oats, rice, potatoes, sweet potatoes or bread with each meal; and add two or three high-carbohydrate snacks, such as bananas, cereal bars or toast. Eating little and often can be an easier strategy than eating big meals the day before the event so you don't over-burden your stomach. Avoid overeating or eating a large meal late in the evening so you don't go to bed feeling uncomfortable.

As a rule, stick to familiar and simple foods, avoid fatty, spicy or oily foods and avoid alcohol, as it is a diuretic. Suitable pre-competition meals and snacks are given on p. 293. Avoid any new or untried foods or food combinations during the pre-competition week in case they upset your stomach. If you are prone to bloating or other GI problems then you may wish to limit your intake of fibre (e.g. whole grains, beans, lentils and vegetables) during the day or two before competition. You may also find that avoiding FODMAP foods or simply cutting fructose and lactose may also help to avoid GI problems during an event (see pp. 237–8). On the other hand, if you're normally fine with these foods, there's no need to avoid them.

If you will be travelling or staying away from home, be prepared to take food with you. Try to find out beforehand what type of food will be available at the event venue and predict any nutritional shortfalls.

Rehearse your pre-competition and competition day eating and drinking strategy during train-

What should I eat when I am anxious before competition?

Most athletes get pre-competition anxiety and this can reduce your appetite or cause GI problems such as nausea, diarrhoea and stomach cramps. If you find it difficult to eat solid food during this time, try liquid meals such as meal replacement drinks, sports drinks, milkshakes and smoothies. Alternatively, opt for smooth, semi-liquid foods such as puréed fruit (e.g. apple purée, mashed banana, apple and apricot purée), yoghurt, porridge, custard and rice pudding. Bland foods such as semolina, mashed potato or a porridge made from cornmeal or ground rice may agree with your digestive system better. To reduce gastrointestinal problems, avoid high-fibre foods such as bran cereals, dried fruit and pulses. You may wish to avoid vegetables that cause flatulence such as the brassica vegetables (cabbage, cauliflower, Brussels sprouts, broccoli). Caffeine can exacerbate anxiety and cause problems such as diarrhoea so you may wish to avoid it on the day and the day before your competition. In essence, avoid anything that is new or unfamiliar. The golden rule with pre-competition eating is stick with tried and tested foods, which you know agree with you.

ing to find out the timing and amounts of food and fluid that work best for you. Simulate race-day conditions as far as possible, using the same strategy you anticipate during the race. Never try a new regime before an important competition. You may need to try carbohydrate loading in training more than once, adjusting the types and amounts of foods you eat.

Ensure you stay hydrated by drinking at frequent intervals throughout the day. You can check your hydration status by monitoring urine colour, thirst and, if available, urine osmolality or specific gravity (see p. 151).

ON THE DAY

On the day of your competition, your aims are to top up liver glycogen stores following the overnight fast, maintain blood sugar levels, keep hunger at bay and maintain hydration.

Carbohydrate intake in the 1–4 hours before exercise helps increase liver and muscle glycogen levels and enhances your subsequent performance (Thomas et al., 2016; Hargreaves et al., 2004). Plan to have your main pre-competition meal 2–4 hours before the event. For example, if your event is at 10 a.m., have your breakfast at 7 a.m. However, the exact timing of your pre-exercise meal will depend on your schedule. You will need to leave enough time to digest the food and for your stomach to settle so that you feel comfortable by the start of the event, not too full and not too hungry. Eating a meal too close to exercise may result in stomach discomfort and indigestion, as the blood supply is diverted away from the digestive system to your muscles. Anxiety can slow down your digestion rate, so if you have pre-competition nerves you may need to leave a little longer than usual between eating and competing.

If you are competing in the morning, you may need to get up a little earlier to eat your pre-competition breakfast. Some athletes skip break-fast, preferring to feel 'light' when they compete. However, it is not a good strategy to compete on an empty stomach if your event lasts longer than 90 minutes. Low liver glycogen and blood sugar levels may reduce your endurance and result in early fatigue. As explained in Chapter 3, liver glycogen is important for maintaining blood sugar levels and supplying fuel to the exercising muscles when muscle glycogen is depleted.

If you are competing in the afternoon, schedule lunch approximately 2–4 hours before the competition. If you are competing in the evening, eat your meals at 3-hourly intervals during the day, again scheduling your last meal to occur approximately 2–4 hours before competition.

Your pre-competition meal should be high in carbohydrate, relatively low in fat, low or moderate in protein, low in fibre, not too filling, not salty or spicy, enjoyable, familiar and easy to digest. Most athletes find that low-GI foods avoid any risk of hypoglycaemia at the start of the competition, so include a small amount of protein or fat (e.g. avocado, eggs or chicken) as well as carbohydrate (e.g. oats, bread or pasta). Suitable types of meals are given on p. 293. The ACSM advise consuming 1–4 g carbohydrate/kg BW (Thomas et al., 2016). The longer the interval you have between eating and competing, the more carbohydrate you may consume, e.g. 4 g/kg BW may be consumed 4 hours before competition, 3 g/kg BW consumed 3 hours before competition, 2 g/kg BW 2 hours before competition and so on. However, in practice you will need to experiment in training to find the amount that suits you best without causing stomach discomfort or gastrointestinal symptoms. If you really do not feel like eating, have a liquid meal or semi-liquid foods (see p. p. 291).

Make sure that you have rehearsed your eating strategy plenty of times during training before the event. Do not try anything new on the day of competition. The timing is fairly individual, so experiment in training first!

If you feel hungry when you arrive at the start of the event, have a carbohydrate-rich snack about 30–60 minutes before the race. A sports drink, banana, some dried fruit, a gel or a fruit and nut bar are good options. This isn't essential but if you had breakfast some hours ago then a small amount of carbohydrate beforehand may maintain blood glucose and stave off hunger.

Hydration is a fine balance. As a rule, the ASCM advise 5–10 ml of water/kg BW in the 2–4 hours before the race – or 350–700 ml for a 70 kg athlete (Thomas *et al.*, 2016). To avoid an early pitstop during the event, avoid drinking large amounts during the 60 minutes before the event; sip just enough to satisfy your thirst.

DURING THE EVENT

Consuming carbohydrate during events >90 minutes will help maintain blood glucose, delay fatigue and maintain performance, particularly in the latter stages. Depending on your exercise intensity and duration, aim to consume 30–60 g carbohydrate per hour. In events >2½ hours, up to 90 g carbohydrate/hour from a mixture of glucose/maltodextrin and fructose (e.g. sports drinks, gels or bananas) may be optimal.

Begin fuelling early in the event before glycogen stores become depleted. Many athletes prefer to consume fuel after approximately 30 minutes and then at 20–30 minute intervals, depending on exercise intensity. It takes 15–30 minutes for the carbohydrate you have consumed to reach your muscles, so do not wait until you are completely fatigued before you begin fuelling.

Any carbohydrate with a high or moderate GI would be suitable, but you may find liquids easier to consume than solids. Table 17.1 on p. 294 gives quantities of foods and drinks providing 30 g or 60 g carbohydrate. Isotonic sports drinks or energy drinks are popular because they serve to replenish fluid losses and prevent hypohydration (p. 147) as well as supplying carbohydrate. Recommended quantities of isotonic drinks for different types of events are given in Table 17.2.

Pre-competition meals

(2–4 hrs before event)
- Porridge or overnight oats with bananas
- Muesli or granola
- Avocado or egg on toast
- Sandwiches, wraps or rolls with falafel, avocado or chicken
- Pasta with a tomato-based sauce
- Rice with chicken, beans or peas
- Baked potato with hummus or tuna

Pre-competition snacks

(30–60 minutes before event)
- Banana
- Smoothie
- Fruit and nut, cereal or granola bar
- Dried fruit
- Energy bar
- Gel
- Rice cakes
- Mini pancakes
- Toast or bread with jam or honey

Table 17.1	SUITABLE FOODS AND DRINKS TO CONSUME DURING EVENTS	
Food or drink	Portion size providing 30 g carbohydrate	Portion size providing 60 g carbohydrate
Isotonic sports drink (6 g/100 ml)	500 ml	1000 ml
Banana	1 large (150 g)	2 large (300 g)
Energy bar	1 bar (45 g)	2 bars (90 g)
Diluted fruit juice (1:1)	500 ml	1000 ml
Raisins	40 g	80 g
Medjool dates	2 dates (40 g)	4 dates (80 g)
Fruit and nut bar	2 × 35 g bars	4 × 35 g bars
Energy gel	1 gel (45–55 g)	2 gels (90–110 ml)
Energy chews	4 chews (40 g)	8 chews (80 g)

Table 17.2	RECOMMENDED QUANTITY OF A 6% ISOTONIC DRINK DURING EXERCISE (60 G GLUCOSE/SUCROSE/GLUCOSE POLYMER DISSOLVED IN 1 LITRE WATER)	
Moderate intensity (30 g carbohydrate/h)	Moderate–high intensity (45 g carbohydrate/h)	High-intensity (60 g carbohydrate/h)
500 ml/h	750 ml/h	1000 ml/h

Whether you consume whole foods (e.g. fruit and nut bars, cereal bars, bananas, flapjacks and dried fruit) or energy products (e.g. gels, chews and energy bars) is down to personal preference. Many athletes prefer consuming whole foods nearer the start as it allows time to digest, then consume energy products nearer the end as they are digested faster. You can use caffeine before or during the event if you've used it successfully in training (*see* pp. 118–21).

Gut problems, such as bloating, nausea, cramping and diarrhoea, during endurance events >90 minutes are common, especially in sports that involve running. Nutritional strategies to alleviate symptoms are given in Chapter 12.

Depending on your sweat rate and anticipated fluid losses, you may opt either to drink to thirst (if fluid losses are likely to be <2% BW) or follow a planned drinking strategy you used in training. However, you should be prepared to adjust your strategy according to the temperature and humidity on event day. Your aim is to avoid under-drinking (hypohydration) as well as over-drinking (hyperhydration, which can lead to hyponatraemia). Aim for approximately 400–800 ml/h. Drinks containing electrolytes are recommended during events longer than 2 hours or when total sweat losses are more than 2–3 litres, or if you're a salty sweater (look for white marks on your kit or even on your skin after exercise).

AFTER THE EVENT

To promote recovery, aim to consume at least 1 g carbohydrate/kg BW/hour during the 4-hour post-exercise period since muscle glycogen replenishment is faster during this time. If you don't feel hungry immediately after the event then you may prefer liquid meals such as sports drinks, smoothies and milk-based drinks. These will help replace both glycogen and fluid. If you are able to eat solid food, choose carbohydrates with a high GI that you find easy to digest and that are not too filling. Suitable foods are listed in Table 17.5 p. 299. Take these with you in your kit bag and begin refuelling in the changing room or whenever practical. Drink fluid immediately after the event and continue drinking at regular intervals to replace fluid losses. To optimise muscle protein synthesis for repair and adaptation, you should also aim to include 20–25 g protein in meals at 3–4 hourly intervals (*see* pp. 75–6).

Football and other team sports

Energy requirements during a football match can be high, with elite outfield players typically burning 1300–1600 kcal. Add in the warm-up and warm-down, and total match day energy

Table 17.3	RECOMMENDED CARBOHYDRATE INTAKE FOR ATHLETES OF DIFFERENT BODY WEIGHTS	
Body weight (kg)	**Daily carbohydrate intake equivalent to 10–12 g/kg body weight**
50	500–600 g
55	550–660 g
60	600–720 g
65	650–780 g
70	700–840 g
75	750–900 g
80	800–960 g
85	850–1020 g

demands are likely to be close to 3500 kcal (Anderson *et al.*, 2017). The main focus of your match day nutrition strategy is ensuring sufficient carbohydrate intake and hydration.

THE DAY BEFORE THE MATCH

As carbohydrate is the main fuel used during a match, you should aim to start the match with full glycogen stores. Depletion of glycogen will result in early fatigue and reduced physical and cognitive performance. The UEFA expert consensus statement on nutrition in elite football recommends consuming at least 6–8 g carbohydrate/kg BW on the day before the match (Collins *et al.*, 2021). To maximise muscle glycogen replenishment, you should do only very light training or

Table 17.4	PRE-COMPETITION SAMPLE EATING PLAN	
	Providing 500 g carbohydrate	**Providing 700 g carbohydrate**
Breakfast	50 g porridge oats	75 g porridge oats
	300 ml milk	450 ml milk
	50 g raisins	70 g raisins
	1 large banana	2 large bananas
Morning snack	2 slices bread	3 slices bread
	30 g honey	45 g honey
Lunch	250 g jacket potato	350 g jacket potato
	100 g sweetcorn and 1 tbsp (50 g) tuna or hummus	150 g sweetcorn and 1 tbsp (50 g) tuna or hummus
	Beetroot and spinach salad	Beetroot and spinach salad
	150 g fresh fruit	150 g fresh fruit
Snack	2 x 35 g cereal bars	3 x 35 g cereal bars
	500 ml sports drink or smoothie	500 ml sports drink or smoothie
Dinner	75 g rice (uncooked weight)	125 g rice (uncooked weight)
	125 g stir-fried vegetables	125 g stir-fried vegetables
	60 g stir-fried chicken or tofu	60 g stir-fried chicken or tofu
	150 g banana	150 g banana
	100 g Ice cream	150 g Ice cream
Snack	50 g granola	75 g granola
	150 g low-fat yoghurt	150 g low-fat yoghurt

rest completely. Table 17.4 gives a sample eating plan providing 500 g and 700 g carbohydrate, which you may use as a basis for developing your own plan.

You will need to eat larger amounts of carbohydrate-rich foods and drinks than usual, and include potatoes, pasta, oats, rice, bread or bananas with each meal. You may need to add two or three high-carbohydrate snacks, such as bananas, cereal bars or toast. Eating little and often can be an easier strategy than eating a big meal the evening before the match event. You may need to compensate for the additional calories by consuming smaller amounts of fat and possibly protein.

As a rule, stick to familiar and simple foods, avoid fatty or oily foods and avoid alcohol, as it is a diuretic. Suitable pre-competition meals and snacks are given on p. 293. Avoid any new or untried foods or food combinations during the pre-competition week in case they upset your stomach. If you are prone to bloating or other GI problems, you may wish to limit your intake of fibre (e.g. whole grains, beans, lentils and vegetables) during the day or two before competition. Avoiding FODMAP foods or simply cutting out fructose and lactose may also help to avoid GI problems during an event in those who are susceptible to GI symptoms (see pp. 237–8). On the other hand, if you're normally fine with these foods, there's no need to avoid them.

If you will be travelling or staying away from home, be prepared to take food with you. Try to find out beforehand what type of food will be available at the event venue and predict any nutritional shortfalls. Ensure you stay hydrated by drinking at frequent intervals throughout the day. You can check your hydration status by monitoring urine colour, thirst and, if available, urine osmolality or specific gravity (see p. 151).

ON MATCH DAY

On match day, your aims are to top up liver glycogen stores following the overnight fast, maintain blood sugar levels, keep hunger at bay and maintain hydration. Carbohydrate intake in the 1–4 hours before exercise helps increase liver and muscle glycogen levels and enhances your subsequent performance (Thomas et al., 2016; Hargreaves et al., 2004).

The UEFA expert consensus statement on nutrition in elite football recommends consuming 1–3 g carbohydrate/kg BW 3–4 hours before kick-off, which equates to 70–210 g for a 70 kg player (Collins et al., 2021). For example, for a 3 p.m. kick-off, schedule your pre-match meal between 11 a.m. and midday. For later kick-off times, schedule your pre-match meal 3–4 hours beforehand, then work backwards so you eat your meals at roughly 3-hourly intervals during the day. You will need to leave enough time to digest the food and for your stomach to settle so that you feel comfortable by the start of the match, not too full and not too hungry. Eating a meal too close to the match may result in stomach discomfort and indigestion, as the blood supply is diverted away from the digestive system to your muscles.

Your pre-competition meal should be high in carbohydrate, low in fat, low or moderate in protein, low in fibre, not too filling, not salty or spicy, enjoyable, familiar and easy to digest. Suitable types of meals are given on p. 293. Most players find that low-GI foods avoid any risk of hypoglycaemia at the start of the competition. However, make sure that you have rehearsed your eating strategy plenty of times during training or

acute weight loss during the pre-competition week. However, this should not be achieved at the expense of performance or health. Severe calorie and carbohydrate restriction and rapid weight loss may result in loss of muscle mass and strength. Restricting carbohydrate may result in depleted glycogen stores and, if there is not sufficient time to replenish glycogen between the weigh-in and competition then you may suffer early fatigue and performance below par. Rapid dehydration before weigh-in is a common practice in many weight-class sports. However, restricting fluid intake or using methods to induce sweating such as saunas, sweat-suits or diuretics prior to the weigh-in can result in hypohydration and electrolyte imbalances, which can be detrimental to performance and health if you do not fully rehydrate before competition. Rapid last-minute loss can also have a negative

psychological impact since it may increase anger, fatigue, tension and anxiety (Sundgot-Borgon and Garthe, 2011). Extreme weight-cutting in MMA athletes has been shown to result in signs of relative energy deficiency (RED-S) (*see* Chapter 11), including a drop in RMR, reduced performance and altered hormone levels (Kasper et al, 2019).

Ideally, you should seek professional guidance from a registered sports nutrition practitioner who will be able to advise on safe weight loss (*see* p. 406 'Online resources').

8–12 WEEKS BEFORE COMPETITION

The principles for making weight for competition are similar to those for weight loss (*see* pp. 189–99). In summary:

1. Set a realistic and achievable goal and allow enough time to achieve this. This is crucial to your strategy and cannot be over-emphasised. You must plan to begin 'making weight' many weeks before your event and *not* at the last minute. For example, bodybuilders traditionally follow a 2–4 month pre-competition diet (Helms *et al.*, 2014(b)).
2. Set your calorie intake at a level that results in approximately 0.5–1% body weight loss per week (Helms *et al.*, 2014(b)). Weight loss >1 kg/week has been shown to result in 5% decrease in bench press strength and 30% drop in testosterone levels (Mero *et al.*, 2010). Also, the greater the calorie deficit, the greater the amount of lean tissue that will be lost (Garthe *et al.*, 2011).
3. Monitor your weight and body composition – skinfold thickness measurements and girth measurements are the most practical (*see* pp. 173–4).

Endurance events lasting less than 90 minutes; or multiple heats

If your event lasts less than 90 minutes, or if your competition schedule includes multiple heats in 1 day, your muscle glycogen stores can become depleted and result in early fatigue and reduced performance. Examples of events with multiple heats include swimming, track cycling and track and field athletics. Carbohydrate loading is unlikely to be beneficial; instead, ensure you start the event with full glycogen stores by tapering your training during the final week and maintaining or increasing your carbohydrate intake to about 6–8 g/kg BW/day during the 24–48 hours prior to your competition.

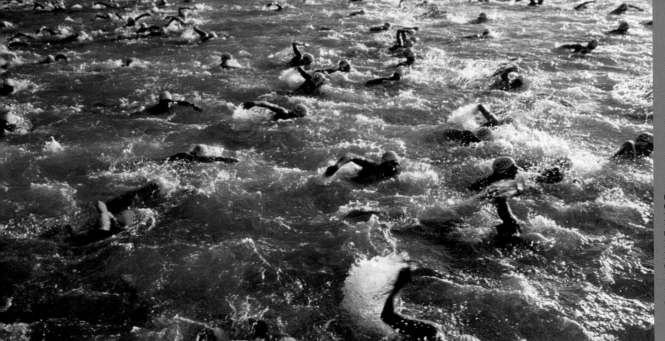

4. Reduce your calorie intake by 10–20% (Garthe *et al.*, 2011) and never eat less than your resting metabolic rate (*see* pp. 5–6). A step-wise calorie reduction may be a better strategy than consuming the same calories throughout the weight loss period, since the leaner you become, the greater the likelihood of lean mass loss (Forbes, 2000).

5. Increasing the amount and frequency of aerobic training may help achieve a calorie deficit and mean a less severe reduction in calorie intake will be required.

6. Adjust your carbohydrate intake according to your training load, eating less on days when you perform lower-intensity or shorter workouts. Restricting carbohydrate too severely during the final weeks before competition may result in losses in muscle mass, lowered RMR and hormone levels (Mäestu *et al.*, 2010). Once you are close to your desired level of leanness, increase your carbohydrate intake by 25–50 g/day to maintain performance and minimise muscle loss (Helms *et al.*, 2014(a)).

7. Adjust fat intake to 15–30% of total calories to achieve your calorie deficit. Minimise saturated fats.

8. Minimise muscle loss by consuming approximately 1.8–2.7 g protein/kg BW/day and at least 0.4 g protein/kg BW/meal (Phillips and Van Loon, 2011). However, an intake of 2.3–3.1 g/kg BW/day may be more appropriate for bodybuilding (Helms *et al.*, 2014(b)).

9. Aim to be at or within 2–3% your weight category at least 24–48 hours before the weigh-in.

24–48 HOURS BEFORE COMPETITION

If you still have further weight to lose, it may be possible to lose 2–3% body weight through acute strategies such as reducing carbohydrate, fibre, salt and/or fluid in the final 24–48 hours before weigh-in, without compromising performance in competition. Provided you have at least 24 hours between weigh-in and competition, restoration of glycogen and fluid can usually be achieved safely (Langan-Evans *et al.*, 2011).

A registered practitioner will be able to help you make weight safely by monitoring your food intake and weight. Acute calorie restriction or dehydration just before your competition can be dangerous without professional guidance, and may result in depleted glycogen stores, fatigue, electrolyte disturbances, cramp and heartbeat irregularities. In other words, the negative effects of rapid weight loss may outweigh any potential performance advantages. Following weigh-in, you will need to refuel and rehydrate as fully as possible before your competition. If you find it very difficult to make weight without resorting to dangerous weight loss methods or compromising your health and performance then you may need to consider competing in the next weight category.

Summary of key points

- If you are competing in an endurance event lasting longer than 90 minutes then you may benefit from carbohydrate loading. It is not advantageous for shorter events.
- Carbohydrate loading is a dietary protocol to increase the muscles' glycogen stores above normal levels. It may be achieved by performing a short bout of high-intensity exercise followed by a high-carbohydrate intake (10–12 g/kg BW/day) for 36–48 hours prior to the event.
- Practical carbohydrate loading recommendations include spreading carbohydrate intake evenly across meals, avoiding any unfamiliar foods, limiting fibre if prone to GI problems,

and rehearsing your eating and drinking strategy during training.
- It is recommended to consume 1–4 g carbohydrate/kg BW between 1 and 4 hours prior to endurance events >90 minutes and 5–10 ml of water/kg BW in the 2–4 hours beforehand. Aim to consume 30–60 g carbohydrate/h, or 90 g/h for events >2½ hours.
- For football and other team sports, it is recommended to consume >6–8 g carbohydrate/kg BW on the day before the match.
- On match day, it is recommended to consume 1–3 g carbohydrate/kg BW 3–4 hours before kick-off, and 5–7 ml fluid/kg BW in the 2–4 hours beforehand. Aim to consume 30–60 g carbohydrate after warm-up and again at half-time.
- After the match, consuming 1 g carbohydrate/kg BW/hour during the 4-hour post-exercise period will promote rapid recovery.
- To make weight for weight-class sports, you should allow enough time to achieve your weight loss goal.
- Set your calorie intake at a level that results in approximately 0.5–1% body weight loss per week, ideally 10–20% less than your usual intake in order to minimise muscle mass loss.
- Minimise muscle loss by consuming approximately 1.8–2.7 g protein/kg BW/day and at least 0.4 g protein/kg BW/meal.
- Weight loss of 2–3% body weight may be achieved through acute strategies such as reducing carbohydrate, fibre, salt and/or fluid in the final 24–48 hours before weigh-in, without compromising performance in competition, but should be undertaken with the guidance of a registered sports nutrition practitioner.

Your Personal Nutrition Plan

Sports organisations have provided general guidelines for the amounts of nutrients athletes should consume to optimise their performance. Tailoring this information to suit your specific goals is the next critical step. Your nutritional requirements depend on many factors, including your body weight, your body composition, the energy demands of your training programme, your daily activity levels, your health status and your individual metabolism.

This chapter provides a summary of the macronutrient recommendations for athletes and gives a step-by-step guide to calculating your individual calorie, carbohydrate, protein and fat needs. Some of the calculations have been detailed previously in other chapters but are amalgamated here to help you devise your personal nutrition plan.

To help guide you through, sample calculations are shown for a 30-year-old male athlete, who measures 1.78 m, weighs 70 kg, and has a moderately active lifestyle.

1: ESTIMATE YOUR DAILY CALORIE NEEDS

Your daily calorie needs will depend on your genetic make-up, age, weight, body composition, your daily activity and your training programme.

You can estimate how many calories you need to consume each day from your total daily energy expenditure (TDEE). TDEE is an estimate of how many calories you burn each day. It is calculated by first estimating your Basal Metabolic Rate (BMR), then multiplying that value by an activity multiplier, a Physical Activity Level (PAL).

a. Estimate your resting metabolic rate (RMR)

Your RMR is an estimate of how many calories you would burn if you were to do nothing but rest for 24 hours. It represents the minimum amount of energy needed to keep your body functioning, including breathing and keeping your heart beating. The simplest way to calculate your RMR is using an online calculator. Alternatively, you can use the Mifflin-St. Jeor equation (*see* p. 282) and punch in the numbers:

Men
- $(10 \times \text{weight (kg)}) + (6.25 \times \text{height (cm)}) - (5 \times \text{age (y)}) + 5$

Women
- $(10 \times \text{weight (kg)}) + (6.25 \times \text{height (cm)}) - (5 \times \text{age (y)}) - 161$

Example for a male athlete (70 kg, 178 cm, 30y):

- RMR = (10 x 70) + (6.25 x 178) – (5 x 30) + 5 = 1668 kcal

b. Multiply your RMR by your physical activity level (PAL)

PAL is the ratio of your overall daily energy expenditure to your RMR, a rough measure of your lifestyle activity. Table 18.3 on p. 306 provides a description of different PALs.

Example for a male athlete (70 kg, 178cm, moderately active):

- TDEE = RMR x PAL
- TDEE = 1668 x 1.4 = 2335 kcal

This figure gives you a rough idea of your daily calorie requirement to maintain your weight. If you eat fewer calories, you will lose weight; if you eat more then you will gain weight.

To lose body fat: reduce your calorie intake by 15% – i.e. multiply your maintenance calories by 0.85 (85%).

- Example: TDEE = 2335 × 0.85 = 1,985 kcal

To increase lean body weight: increase your calorie intake by 20% – i.e. multiply your maintenance calories by 1.2 (120%).

- Example: TDEE = 2335 x 1.2 = 2,802 kcal

2: CALCULATE YOUR CARBOHYDRATE REQUIREMENT

Calculate your carbohydrate requirement according to your activity level and body weight, using Table 18.1.

Table 18.4 shows ample calculations for weight maintenance, fat loss and muscle gain for a 70 kg male athlete.

Table 18.1	SUMMARY OF SPORTS NUTRITION MACRONUTRIENT GUIDELINES
Macronutrient	**Daily guideline**
Carbohydrate	3–5 g/kg BW for low-intensity training days 5–7 g/kg BW for moderate-intensity training days (approx. 1 h) 6–10 g/kg BW for moderate- to high-endurance training (1–3 h) 8–12 g/kg BW for high-intensity training (>4 h) or fuelling up for an endurance event
Protein	1.2–2.0 g/kg BW/day (weight maintenance) 1.2–1.4 g/kg BW/day (endurance training) 1.4–2.0 g/kg BW/day (power and resistance training) 1.8–2.7 g/kg BW/day (weight loss) 1.4–2.0 g/kg BW/day (weight gain) **Per meal:** **0.25–0.4 g/kg BW/meal (all goals)**
Fat	20–35% of daily energy

Table 18.2	SUMMARY OF FLUID INTAKE GUIDELINES
Before exercise	• Ensure you are fully hydrated. • Drink 5–10 ml/kg BW of fluid slowly in the 2–4 hours before exercise to promote hydration and allow enough time for excretion of excess water.
During exercise	• Drink according to thirst or to a plan. • For most athletes and events, an intake of 400–800 ml/hour prevents hypohydration as well as overhydration. • For most activities lasting <45 min, water is fine for replacing fluid losses. • For high-intensity exercise lasting >1 hour, a hypotonic or isotonic sports drink containing 40–80 g carbohydrate/litre may reduce fatigue and improve performance. • For high-intensity exercise lasting 1–2½ hours, consuming between 30 and 60 g carbohydrate/hour will help increase endurance. • For high-intensity exercise lasting >2½ hours, an intake of 90 g carbohydrate/hour is recommended. This should be provided by a mixture of glucose and fructose.
After exercise	• Drink 1.25–1.5 litres for every 1 kg body weight lost as sweat during exercise.

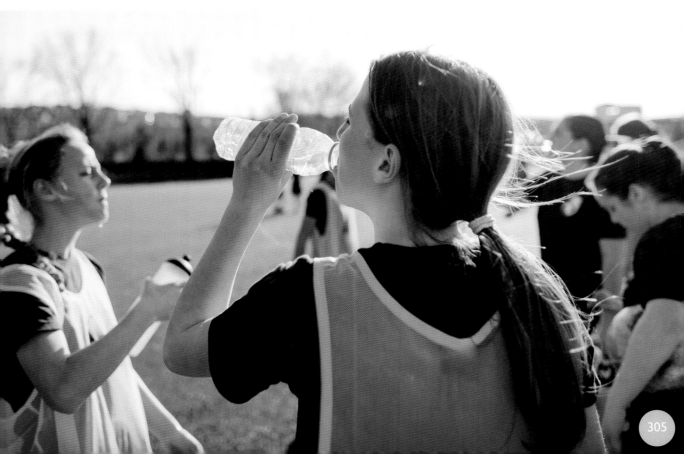

Table 18.3 — PHYSICAL ACTIVITY LEVELS

Physical Activity Level (PAL)	Multiplier	Description
Mostly inactive	1.2	Mainly sitting
Fairly active	1.3	Sitting, some walking, exercise once or twice per week
Moderately active	1.4	Regular walking, or exercise two to three times per week
Active	1.5	Exercise or sport more than three times per week
Very active	1.7	Physically active job or intense daily exercise or sport

Table 18.4 — CALORIE AND CARBOHYDRATE REQUIREMENTS FOR WEIGHT MAINTENANCE, FAT LOSS AND MUSCLE GAIN

	Weight maintenance	Weight loss	Weight gain
Calorie requirement	2335 kcal	1985 kcal	2802 kcal
Carbohydrate requirement, g/kg BW	5 g	3 g	6 g
Example: 70 kg male athlete Carbohydrate requirement, g/day	350 g	210 g	420 g

Table 18.5 — PROTEIN REQUIREMENTS FOR WEIGHT MAINTENANCE, WEIGHT LOSS AND WEIGHT GAIN

	Endurance training	Power and resistance training	Weight loss	Weight gain
Protein, g/kg BW/day	1.3 g/kg BW	1.6 g/kg BW	2.0 g/kg BW	1.6 g/kg BW
Example: 70 kg male athlete, g/day	91 g	112 g	140 g	112 g

Table 18.6	MACRONUTRIENT REQUIREMENTS FOR A 70 KG MALE ATHLETE			
		Weight maintenance	Weight loss	Weight gain
A	Total daily calorie intake	2335 kcal	1985 kcal	2803 kcal
B	Carbohydrate intake	350 g	210 g	420 g
C	Carbohydrate calories (B x 4)	1400 kcal	840 kcal	1680 kcal
D	Protein intake (endurance)	91 g	140 g	112 g
E	Protein calories (D x 4)	364 kcal	560 kcal	448 kcal
F	Fat calories (A − C − E)	571 kcal	585 kcal	675 kcal
	Fat intake (F 9)	63 g	65 g	75 g

3: CALCULATE YOUR PROTEIN INTAKE

Your protein requirement is based on the following recommendations:

- Endurance training: 1.2–1.4 g/kg BW/day
- Power and resistance training: 1.4–2.0 g/kg BW/day
- Weight loss: 1.8–2.7 g/kg BW/day
- Weight gain: 1.4–2.0 g/kg BW/day

Table 18.5 shows the calculations for estimating the protein requirements for different training and body composition goals.

4: CALCULATE YOUR FAT INTAKE

This is the balance left once you have calculated your carbohydrate and protein requirements. This should provide 20–35% of daily calorie intake. Use the following calculation:

- Carbohydrate calories = grams carbohydrate x 4
- Protein calories = grams protein x 4
- Fat calories = total daily calories – carbohydrate calories – protein calories
- Grams fat = fat calories ÷ 9

Table 18.6 shows the calculations for estimating the macronutrient requirements for different training and body composition goals for a 70 kg male athlete.

Meal plans

To help you plan your personal diet, here are two sets of daily meal plans, providing 2000 kcal, 2500 kcal, 3000 kcal, 3500 kcal, 4000 kcal, 4500 kcal and 5000 kcal for omnivores and vegetarians. Each meal plan is in line with the nutritional recommendations outlined in this chapter. Opt for the meal plan that most closely matches your calorie requirement and use it as a guide for devising your individual eating plan. Adapt the types and foods to suit your particular food preferences, and adjust portion sizes to suit your day-to-day training goals. For example, on low-intensity training or recovery days you will need fewer calories and less carbohydrate than on high-intensity training days, so adjust portion sizes accordingly. Similarly, when performing higher-intensity or longer workouts you will need to eat larger portions. For meal ideas, *see* Chapter 19, which includes more than 50 recipes for all types of diets.

The macronutrient composition of each food has been listed to show its relative contribution of calories, protein, carbohydrate and fat to your daily totals. If you wish to carry out similar calculations for other foods and construct new meal plans, you may use a reputable set of food composition tables, an online nutrition calculator or a nutritional analysis software program (*see* pp. 364–406).

Notes:

- For cooking and dressings, use oils rich in monounsaturated fats e.g. olive, rapeseed, flax, soya, walnut.
- Use spreads high in monounsaturates or polyunsaturates, containing no hydrogenated or trans fatty acids.
- Weights are for dried/uncooked foods, i.e. 50 g uncooked pasta or 75 g uncooked rice noodles, not the cooked weight.

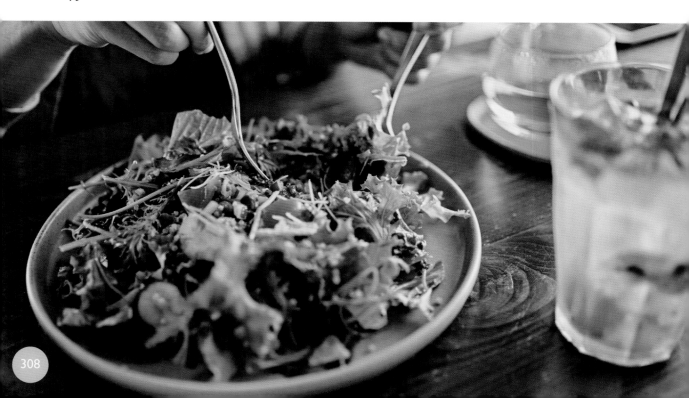

2000 KCAL MEAL PLAN

		kcal	Protein (g)	Carbohydrate (g)	Fat (g)
Breakfast	2 clementines	65	1	13	0
	1 slice (40 g) wholegrain toast	95	4	16	1
	2 tsp (10 g) olive oil spread	57	0	0	6
	2 scrambled or poached eggs	148	12	0	11
Mid-morning	100 g 0% fat plain Greek yoghurt	57	10	4	0
	100 g strawberries	30	1	6	0
Lunch	50 g pasta	179	7	35	1
	75 g tuna in brine	75	18	0	1
	100 g chopped peppers	36	1	6	0
	100 g tomatoes	20	1	2	0
	1 tbsp (11 g) oil dressing	69	0	0	7
	1 pear	69	1	14	0
Mid-afternoon	25 g mixed nuts	149	7	3	12
Workout	Water	0	0	0	0
Post-workout	25 g whey protein	174	18	26	0
Dinner	100 g grilled turkey breast	155	35	0	2
	75 g rice noodles	249	4	58	0
	100 g kale	42	3	1	2
	100 g cauliflower	39	4	3	1
	150 g mango	98	1	20	0
Total		**2037**	**122**	**256**	**51**

2500 KCAL MEAL PLAN

		Kcal	Protein (g)	Carbohydrate (g)	Fat (g)
Breakfast	75 g oats	320	10	52	7
	300 ml skimmed milk	104	10	14	1
	100 g blueberries	68	1	15	0
Mid-morning	25 g almonds	158	6	2	14
	100 g low-fat plain Greek yoghurt	98	8	9	4
Lunch	200 g baked potato	158	4	33	0
	10 g olive oil spread	57	0	0	6
	100 g tuna in brine	99	24	0	1
	Rocket salad	16	1	2	0
	15 g oil/vinegar dressing	69	0	0	7
	2 kiwi fruit	65	1	12	1
Mid-afternoon	1 flapjack	265	5	24	16
Workout	Water	0	0	0	0
Post-workout	25 g whey	100	18	2	2
	300 ml skimmed milk	104	10	14	1
Dinner	125 g grilled skinless chicken breast fillet	127	30	0	1
	75 g pasta	269	10	53	1
	1 tbsp (11 g) olive oil	99	0	0	11
	100 g broccoli	40	4	2	1
	100 g carrots	42	1	8	0
	30 g pasta sauce/tomato salsa	13	0	2	0
Evening	2 slices (80 g) wholemeal toast	190	8	32	2
	20 g peanut butter	124	5	3	10
Total		2587	157	276	87

3000 KCAL MEAL PLAN

		Kcal	Protein (g)	Carbohydrate (g)	Fat (g)
Breakfast	75 g oats	320	10	52	7
	300 ml semi-skimmed milk	140	10	13	5
	100 g blueberries	68	1	15	0
	1 slice (40 g) wholegrain toast	95	4	16	1
	10 g peanut butter	62	3	1	5
Mid-morning	25 g almonds	158	6	2	14
	100 g low-fat plain Greek yoghurt	98	8	9	4
	1 banana	99	1	22	0
Lunch	200 g baked potato or sweet potato	158	4	33	0
	10 g olive oil spread	57	0	0	6
	100 g tuna in brine	99	24	0	1
	Rocket salad	16	1	2	0
	15 g oil/vinegar dressing	69	0	0	7
	2 clementines	65	1	13	0
Mid-afternoon	1 flapjack	265	5	24	16
Workout	Water	0	0	0	0
Post-workout	25 g whey	100	18	2	2
	300 ml semi-skimmed milk	140	10	13	5
	1 banana	99	1	22	0
Dinner	125 g grilled skinless chicken breast fillet	127	30	0	1
	75 g pasta	269	10	53	1
	1 tbsp (11 g) olive oil	99	0	0	11
	100 g broccoli	40	4	2	1
	100 g carrots	42	1	8	0
	30 g pasta sauce/tomato salsa	13	0	2	0
Evening	2 slices (80 g) wholemeal toast	190	8	32	2
	20 g peanut butter	124	5	3	10
Total		**3013**	**165**	**338**	**102**

3500 KCAL MEAL PLAN

		kcal	Protein (g)	Carbohydrate (g)	Fat (g)
Breakfast	75 g oats	320	10	52	7
	300 ml semi-skimmed milk	140	10	13	5
	25 g raisins	70	1	17	1
	100 g blueberries	68	1	15	0
	1 slice (40 g) wholegrain toast	95	4	16	1
	10 g peanut butter	62	3	1	5
Mid-morning	50 g mixed nuts and raisins	252	8	15	17
	100 g low-fat plain Greek yoghurt	98	8	9	4
	1 banana	99	1	22	0
Lunch	200 g baked potato or sweet potato	158	4	33	0
	10 g olive oil spread	57	0	0	6
	100 g tuna in brine	99	24	0	1
	150 g sweetcorn	191	4	38	2
	Rocket salad	16	1	2	0
	15 g oil/vinegar dressing	69	0	0	7
	2 clementines	65	1	13	0
Mid-afternoon	1 flapjack	265	5	24	16
Workout	500 ml isotonic sports drink	130	0	33	0
Post-workout	25 g whey	100	18	2	2
	300 ml semi-skimmed milk	140	10	13	5
	1 banana	99	1	22	0
Dinner	125 g grilled skinless chicken breast fillet	127	30	0	1
	75 g pasta	269	10	53	1
	1 tbsp (11 g) olive oil	99	0	0	11
	100 g broccoli	40	4	2	1
	100 g carrots	42	1	8	0
	30 g pasta sauce/tomato salsa	13	0	2	0
Evening	2 slices (80 g) wholemeal toast	190	8	32	2
	20 g peanut butter	124	5	3	10
Total		3500	172	438	107

4000 KCAL MEAL PLAN

		kcal	Protein (g)	Carbohydrate (g)	Fat (g)
Breakfast	100 g oats	427	13	69	9
	400 ml semi-skimmed milk	187	14	18	7
	25 g raisins	70	1	17	1
	100 g blueberries	68	1	15	0
	1 slice (40 g) wholegrain toast	95	4	16	1
	2 eggs	148	12	0	11
Mid-morning	50 g mixed nuts and raisins	252	8	15	17
	100 g low-fat plain Greek yoghurt	98	8	9	4
	1 banana	99	1	22	0
Lunch	300 g baked potato or sweet potato	237	6	49	1
	20 g olive oil spread	114	0	0	13
	100 g tuna in brine	99	24	0	1
	150 g sweetcorn	191	4	38	2
	Rocket salad	16	1	2	0
	15 g oil/vinegar dressing	69	0	0	7
	2 clementines	65	1	13	0
Mid-afternoon	1 flapjack	265	5	24	16
Workout	500 ml isotonic sports drink	130	0	33	0
Post-workout	25 g whey	100	18	2	2
	300 ml semi-skimmed milk	140	10	13	5
	1 banana	99	1	22	0
Dinner	125 g grilled skinless chicken breast fillet	127	30	0	1
	75 g pasta	269	10	53	1
	1 tbsp (11 g) olive oil	99	0	0	11
	100 g broccoli	40	4	2	1
	100 g carrots	42	1	8	0
	30 g pasta sauce/tomato salsa	13	0	2	0
	150 g mango	98	1	20	0
Evening	2 slices (80 g) wholemeal toast	190	8	32	2
	20 g peanut butter	124	5	3	10
Total		**3973**	**192**	**496**	**123**

4500 KCAL MEAL PLAN

		kcal	Protein (g)	Carbohydrate (g)	Fat (g)
Breakfast	100 g oats	427	13	69	9
	400 ml semi-skimmed milk	187	14	18	7
	25 g raisins	70	1	17	1
	100 g blueberries	68	1	15	0
	2 slices (80 g) wholegrain toast	190	8	32	2
	2 eggs	148	12	0	11
Mid-morning	50 g mixed nuts and raisins	252	8	15	17
	100 g low-fat plain Greek yoghurt	98	8	9	4
	1 banana	99	1	22	0
	1 raw energy bar	173	5	13	11
Lunch	300 g baked potato or sweet potato	237	6	49	1
	20 g olive oil spread	114	0	0	13
	200 g tuna in brine	199	47	0	1
	150 g sweetcorn	191	4	38	2
	Rocket salad	16	1	2	0
	15 g oil/vinegar dressing	69	0	0	7
	2 clementines	65	1	13	0
Mid-afternoon	1 flapjack	265	5	24	16
	25 g mixed nuts	149	7	3	12
Workout	500 ml isotonic sports drink	130	0	33	0
Post-workout	25 g whey	100	18	2	2
	300 ml semi-skimmed milk	140	10	13	5
	1 banana	99	1	22	0
Dinner	125 g grilled skinless chicken breast fillet	127	30	0	1
	75 g pasta	269	10	53	1
	1 tbsp (11 g) olive oil	99	0	0	11
	150 g broccoli	59	7	3	1
	150 g carrots	63	1	11	1
	30 g pasta sauce/tomato salsa	13	0	2	0
	150 g mango	98	1	20	0
Evening	2 slices (80 g) wholemeal toast	190	8	32	2
	20 g peanut butter	124	5	3	10
Total		**4529**	**234**	**532**	**148**

5000 KCAL MEAL PLAN

		kcal	Protein (g)	Carbohydrate (g)	Fat (g)
Breakfast	100 g oats	427	13	69	9
	400 ml semi-skimmed milk	187	14	18	7
	25 g raisins	70	1	17	1
	100 g blueberries	68	1	15	0
	2 slices (80 g) wholegrain toast	190	8	32	2
	2 eggs	148	12	0	11
Mid-morning	50 g mixed nuts and raisins	252	8	15	17
	100 g low-fat plain Greek yoghurt	98	8	9	4
	1 banana	99	1	22	0
	1 energy bar	173	5	13	11
Lunch	300 g baked potato or sweet potato	237	6	49	1
	20 g olive oil spread	114	0	0	13
	200 g tuna in brine	199	47	0	1
	150 g sweetcorn	191	4	38	2
	Rocket salad	16	1	2	0
	15 g oil/vinegar dressing	69	0	0	7
	2 clementines	65	1	13	0
Mid-afternoon	2 flapjacks	530	10	47	32
	25 g mixed nuts	149	7	3	12
Workout	500 ml isotonic sports drink	130	0	33	0
Post-workout	25 g whey	100	18	2	2
	300 ml semi-skimmed milk	140	10	13	5
	1 banana	99	1	22	0
Dinner	125 g grilled skinless chicken breast fillet	127	30	0	1
	100 g pasta	359	13	71	2
	1 tbsp (11 g) olive oil	99	0	0	11
	150 g broccoli	59	7	3	1
	150 g carrots	63	1	11	1
	60 g pasta sauce/tomato salsa	27	1	5	0
	150 g mango	98	1	20	0
Evening	2 slices (80 g) wholemeal toast	190	8	32	2
	20 g peanut butter	124	5	3	10
	100 g low-fat plain Greek yoghurt	98	8	9	4
Total		**4995**	**250**	**584**	**169**

2000 KCAL VEGETARIAN MEAL PLAN

		kcal	Protein (g)	Carbohydrate (g)	Fat (g)
Breakfast	2 clementines	65	1	13	0
	1 slice (40 g) wholegrain toast	95	4	16	1
	2 tsp (10 g) olive oil spread	57	0	0	6
	2 scrambled or poached eggs	148	12	0	11
Mid-morning	100 g 0% fat plain Greek yoghurt	57	10	4	0
	100 g strawberries	30	1	6	0
Lunch	50 g pasta	179	7	35	1
	125 g mixed beans	144	11	17	3
	100 g chopped peppers	36	1	6	0
	100 g tomatoes	20	1	2	0
	1 tbsp (11 g) oil dressing	69	0	0	7
Mid-afternoon	25 g mixed nuts	149	7	3	12
Workout	Water	0	0	0	0
Post-workout	25 g whey protein	174	18	26	0
Dinner	Tofu with Noodles (recipe p. 336)	555	21	75	19
	100 g kale	42	3	1	2
	100 g cauliflower	39	4	3	1
	150 g mango	98	1	20	0
Total		**2010**	**89**	**251**	**68**

2500 KCAL VEGETARIAN MEAL PLAN

		kcal	Protein (g)	Carbohydrate (g)	Fat (g)
Breakfast	75 g oats	320	10	52	7
	300 ml skimmed milk	104	10	14	1
	100 g blueberries	68	1	15	0
Mid-morning	25 g almonds	158	6	2	14
	100 g low-fat plain Greek yoghurt	98	8	9	4
Lunch	200 g baked potato	158	4	33	0
	100 g cottage cheese or low-fat soft cheese	100	12	3	4
	Rocket salad	16	1	2	0
	15 g oil/vinegar dressing	69	0	0	7
	2 kiwi fruit	65	1	12	1
Mid-afternoon	1 flapjack	265	5	24	16
Workout	Water	0	0	0	0
Post-workout	25 g whey	100	18	2	2
	300 ml skimmed milk	104	10	14	1
Dinner	Chickpeas with Butternut Squash and Tomatoes (recipe p. 338)	342	15	48	10
	50 g pasta	179	7	35	1
	100 g broccoli	40	4	2	1
	100 g carrots	42	1	8	0
Evening	2 slices (80 g) wholemeal toast	190	8	32	2
	20 g peanut butter	124	5	3	10
Total		**2544**	**127**	**307**	**82**

3000 KCAL VEGETARIAN MEAL PLAN

		kcal	Protein (g)	Carbohydrate (g)	Fat (g)
Breakfast	75 g oats	320	10	52	7
	300 ml semi-skimmed milk	140	10	13	5
	100 g blueberries	68	1	15	0
	1 slice (40 g) wholegrain toast	95	4	16	1
	10 g peanut butter	62	3	1	5
Mid-morning	25 g almonds	158	6	2	14
	100 g low-fat plain Greek yoghurt	98	8	9	4
	1 banana	99	1	22	0
Lunch	200 g baked potato	158	4	33	0
	100 g cottage cheese or low-fat soft cheese	100	12	3	4
	Rocket salad	16	1	2	0
	15 g oil/vinegar dressing	69	0	0	7
	2 clementines	65	1	13	0
Mid-afternoon	1 flapjack	265	5	24	16
Workout	Water	0	0	0	0
Post-workout	25 g whey	100	18	2	2
	300 ml semi-skimmed milk	140	10	13	5
	1 banana	99	1	22	0
Dinner	Chickpeas with Butternut Squash and Tomatoes (recipe p. 338)	342	15	48	10
	75 g pasta	269	10	53	1
	100 g broccoli	40	4	2	1
	100 g carrots	42	1	8	0
Evening	2 slices (80 g) wholemeal toast	190	8	32	2
	20 g peanut butter	124	5	3	10
Total		**3060**	**139**	**387**	**97**

3500 KCAL VEGETARIAN MEAL PLAN

		kcal	Protein (g)	Carbohydrate (g)	Fat (g)
Breakfast	75 g oats	320	10	52	7
	300 ml semi-skimmed milk	140	10	13	5
	100 g blueberries	68	1	15	0
	25 g raisins	70	1	17	1
	1 slice (40 g) wholegrain toast	95	4	16	1
	10 g peanut butter	62	3	1	5
Mid-morning	50 g mixed nuts and raisins	252	8	15	17
	100 g low-fat plain Greek yoghurt	98	8	9	4
	1 banana	99	1	22	0
Lunch	200 g baked potato	158	4	33	0
	100 g cottage cheese or low-fat soft cheese	100	12	3	4
	150 g sweetcorn	191	4	38	2
	Rocket salad	16	1	2	0
	15 g oil/vinegar dressing	69	0	0	7
	2 clementines	65	1	13	0
Mid-afternoon	1 flapjack	265	5	24	16
Workout	500 ml isotonic sports drink	130	0	33	0
Post-workout	25 g whey	100	18	2	2
	300 ml semi-skimmed milk	140	10	13	5
	1 banana	99	1	22	0
Dinner	Chickpeas with Butternut Squash and Tomatoes (recipe p. 338)	342	15	48	10
	75 g pasta	269	10	53	1
	100 g broccoli	40	4	2	1
	100 g carrots	42	1	8	0
Evening	2 slices (80 g) wholemeal toast	190	8	32	2
	20 g peanut butter	124	5	3	10
Total		**3546**	**145**	**487**	**102**

4000 KCAL VEGETARIAN MEAL PLAN

		kcal	Protein (g)	Carbohydrate (g)	Fat (g)
Breakfast	100 g oats	427	13	69	9
	400 ml semi-skimmed milk	187	14	18	7
	100 g blueberries	68	1	15	0
	25 g raisins	70	1	17	1
	1 slice (40 g) wholegrain toast	95	4	16	1
	2 eggs	148	12	0	11
Mid-morning	50 g mixed nuts and raisins	252	8	15	17
	100 g low-fat plain Greek yoghurt	98	8	9	4
	1 banana	99	1	22	0
Lunch	300 g baked potato or sweet potato	237	6	49	1
	20 g olive oil spread	114	0	0	13
	100 g cottage cheese or low-fat soft cheese	100	12	3	4
	150 g sweetcorn	191	4	38	2
	Rocket salad	16	1	2	0
	15 g oil/vinegar dressing	69	0	0	7
	2 clementines	65	1	13	0
Mid-afternoon	1 flapjack	265	5	24	16
Workout	500 ml isotonic sports drink	130	0	33	0
Post-workout	25 g whey	100	18	2	2
	300 ml semi-skimmed milk	140	10	13	5
	1 banana	99	1	22	0
Dinner	Chickpeas with Butternut Squash and Tomatoes (recipe p. 338)	342	15	48	10
	75 g pasta	269	10	53	1
	100 g broccoli	40	4	2	1
	100 g carrots	42	1	8	0
Evening	2 slices (80 g) wholemeal toast	190	8	32	2
	20 g peanut butter	124	5	3	10
Total		**3978**	**164**	**524**	**124**

4500 KCAL VEGETARIAN MEAL PLAN

		kcal	Protein (g)	Carbohydrate (g)	Fat (g)
Breakfast	100 g oats	427	13	69	9
	400 ml semi-skimmed milk	187	14	18	7
	100 g blueberries	68	1	15	0
	25 g raisins	70	1	17	1
	2 slices (80 g) wholegrain toast	190	8	32	2
	2 eggs	148	12	0	11
Mid-morning	50 g mixed nuts and raisins	252	8	15	17
	100 g low-fat plain Greek yoghurt	98	8	9	4
	1 banana	99	1	22	0
	1 energy bar	173	5	13	11
Lunch	300 g baked potato or sweet potato	237	6	49	1
	20 g olive oil spread	114	0	0	13
	100 g cottage cheese or low-fat soft cheese	100	12	3	4
	150 g sweetcorn	191	4	38	2
	Rocket salad	16	1	2	0
	15 g oil/vinegar dressing	69	0	0	7
	2 clementines	65	1	13	0
Mid-afternoon	2 flapjacks	530	10	47	32
Workout	500 ml isotonic sports drink	130	0	33	0
Post-workout	25 g whey	100	18	2	2
	300 ml semi-skimmed milk	140	10	13	5
	1 banana	99	1	22	0
Dinner	Chickpeas with Butternut Squash and Tomatoes (recipe p. 338)	342	15	48	10
	75 g pasta	269	10	53	1
	100 g broccoli	40	4	2	1
	100 g carrots	42	1	8	0
Evening	2 slices (80 g) wholemeal toast	190	8	32	2
	20 g peanut butter	124	5	3	10
Total		**4511**	**178**	**577**	**153**

5000 KCAL VEGETARIAN MEAL PLAN

		kcal	Protein (g)	Carbohydrate (g)	Fat (g)
Breakfast	100 g oats	427	13	69	9
	400 ml semi-skimmed milk	187	14	18	7
	100 g blueberries	68	1	15	0
	25 g raisins	70	1	17	1
	2 slices (80 g) wholegrain toast	190	8	32	2
	2 eggs	148	12	0	11
Mid-morning	50 g mixed nuts and raisins	252	8	15	17
	100 g low-fat plain Greek yoghurt	98	8	9	4
	1 banana	99	1	22	0
	1 energy bar	173	5	13	11
Lunch	300 g baked potato or sweet potato	237	6	49	1
	20 g olive oil spread	114	0	0	13
	200 g cottage cheese or low-fat soft cheese	200	25	6	9
	150 g sweetcorn	191	4	38	2
	Rocket salad	16	1	2	0
	15 g oil/vinegar dressing	69	0	0	7
	2 clementines	65	1	13	0
Mid-afternoon	2 flapjacks	530	10	47	32
	25 g mixed nuts	149	7	3	12
Workout	500 ml isotonic sports drink	130	0	33	0
Post-workout	25 g whey	100	18	2	2
	300 ml semi-skimmed milk	140	10	13	5
	1 banana	99	1	22	0
Dinner	Chickpeas with Butternut Squash and Tomatoes (recipe p. 338)	342	15	48	10
	25 g Cheddar cheese	103	6	0	9
	75 g pasta	269	10	53	1
	100 g broccoli	40	4	2	1
	100 g carrots	42	1	8	0
	150 g mango	98	1	20	0
Evening	2 slices (80 g) wholemeal toast	190	8	32	2
	20 g peanut butter	124	5	3	10
	100 g low-fat plain Greek yoghurt	98	8	9	4
Total		**5059**	**212**	**611**	**182**

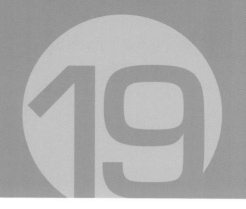

//The Recipes

Breakfasts

FRUIT MUESLI

Serves 4
175 g (6 oz) oats
300 ml (½ pint) milk
40 g (1½ oz) sultanas
40 g (1½ oz) toasted flaked almonds, chopped hazelnuts or cashews
225 g (8 oz) fresh fruit, e.g. bananas, blueberries, strawberries, raspberries
1 apple, peeled and grated
1 tbsp honey

- In a large bowl, mix together the oats, milk, sultanas and nuts. Cover and leave overnight in the fridge.
- Just before serving, stir in the fruit, grated apple and honey. Spoon into cereal bowls.

Nutritional information (per serving):
Calories = 329; protein = 11 g; carbohydrate = 52 g; fat = 10 g; fibre = 6 g

ATHLETE'S PORRIDGE

Serves 1
50 g (2 oz) porridge oats
350 ml (12 fl oz) milk
1 banana, sliced
25 g (1 oz) dried fruit e.g. raisins, dates or figs

- Mix the oats and milk in a pan. Bring to the boil and simmer for approx. 5 minutes, stirring frequently.
- Top with the banana and dried fruit.

Nutritional information (per serving):
Calories = 476; protein = 20 g; carbohydrate = 85 g; fat = 5 g; fibre = 5 g

BREAKFAST MUFFINS

Makes 8 muffins

125 g (4 oz) self-raising flour
125 g (4 oz) oatmeal
25 g (1 oz) butter or margarine
40 g (1½ oz) soft brown sugar
1 egg
150 ml (5 fl oz) milk
50 g (2 oz) chopped dates or raisins

- Preheat the oven to 220°C/425°F/Gas mark 7.
- Mix the flour and oatmeal together in a bowl.
- Add the butter, sugar, egg and milk. Mix well.
- Stir in the dried fruit.
- Spoon into a non-stick muffin tray and bake for approx. 15 minutes until golden brown.

YOGHURT WITH DRIED FRUIT COMPOTE

Serves 4

Grated zest and juice of 1 orange
2 tbsp (30 ml) acacia honey
300 ml (½ pint) water
150 ml (5 fl oz) orange juice
75 g (3 oz) ready-to-eat dried figs, halved
75 g (3 oz) ready-to-eat dried apricots
75 g (3 oz) ready-to-eat pitted prunes
450 ml (¾ pint) plain whole-milk or Greek yoghurt

- Combine the orange zest and freshly squeezed juice, honey, water and orange juice in a pan.
- Bring the mixture to the boil, stirring until the honey is dissolved, then add the dried fruit and simmer, covered, for about 15 minutes until the fruit becomes plump and soft. Allow to cool and keep covered in the fridge until you are ready to serve.
- Divide the yoghurt between 4 bowls. Top with the fruit compote.

Nutritional information (per serving):
Calories = 189; protein = 5 g;
carbohydrate = 33 g; fat = 5 g;
fibre = 2 g

Nutritional information (per serving):
Calories = 223; protein = 9 g;
carbohydrate = 41 g; fat = 4 g;
fibre = 4 g

GREEK YOGHURT WITH BANANA AND HONEY

Serves 2

2 bananas

300 g (11 oz) plain Greek yoghurt

1–2 level tbsp honey (to taste)

2 tbsp toasted flaked almonds (or walnuts, hazelnuts or pecans)

- Slice the bananas into two bowls. Spoon half the yoghurt on top of each bowl. Drizzle with honey and scatter over the toasted nuts.

Main meals

SALMON AND VEGETABLE PASTA

Serves 2

175 g (6 oz) pasta

175 g (6 oz) salmon steak

1 tbsp olive oil

1 red pepper, deseeded and chopped

1 courgette, sliced

1 garlic clove, crushed

75 g (3 oz) cherry tomatoes

A handful of rocket

- Cook the pasta according to the pack instructions, adding the salmon to the pan 6 minutes before the end of the cooking time.
- Heat the oil in a pan, and cook the pepper, courgette, garlic and cherry tomatoes for 5 minutes until they start to soften.
- When the pasta is cooked, remove the salmon, then drain the pasta. Fork the salmon into large chunks and add to the vegetables along with the pasta and rocket. Toss together, then serve.

Nutritional information (per serving):
Calories = 368; protein = 12 g; carbohydrate = 43 g; fat = 18 g; fibre = 2 g

Nutritional information (per serving):
Calories = 570; protein = 31 g; carbohydrate = 69 g; fat = 18 g; fibre = 6 g

FISH TAGINE WITH CHICKPEAS

Serves 2

1 tbsp light-in-colour olive oil
1 onion, chopped
1 garlic clove, crushed
½ tsp each of ground cumin, coriander,
    cinnamon and turmeric
2 small potatoes, peeled and cut into quarters
300 ml (10 fl oz) fish or chicken stock
75 g (3 oz) cherry tomatoes, halved
1 tbsp ground almonds
½ tin (200 g/7 oz) chickpeas, drained
300 g (10 oz) white fish, cut into chunks
125 g (4 oz) baby spinach
Squeeze of lemon juice
A handful of fresh coriander, chopped
25 g (1 oz) flaked almonds
Plain Greek yoghurt, to serve

- Heat the oil in a large pan. Add the onion and cook for a few minutes until soft. Add the garlic and spices and cook for a few minutes more.
- Add the potatoes, stock, tomatoes, ground almonds and chickpeas. Simmer for 10 minutes, then add the fish. Cover and simmer on a low heat for 2–3 minutes until just cooked. Stir in the spinach, allow to wilt for 1–2 minutes, then add a squeeze of lemon juice and the coriander and scatter with the flaked almonds.
- Serve with plain Greek yoghurt.

Nutritional information (per serving):
Calories = 598; protein = 46 g;
carbohydrate = 49 g; fat = 21 g;
fibre = 14 g

QUINOA AND CHICKEN SALAD WITH BEETROOT YOGHURT

Serves 2

125 g (4oz) quinoa
1 small cooked beetroot, finely chopped
2 tbsp plain Greek yoghurt
1 garlic clove, crushed
2 cooked skinless chicken breast fillets,
    shredded
½ red onion, chopped
½ tin (200 g/7oz) flageolet beans (or other
    variety of beans)
2 tomatoes, chopped
100 g (3½ oz) spinach, watercress and rocket
    salad leaves
Salt and freshly ground black pepper

- Cook the quinoa according to the pack instructions. Drain.
- Meanwhile, mix the beetroot, plain Greek yoghurt and garlic with a little salt and freshly ground black pepper in a small bowl.
- In a large bowl, mix the quinoa, chicken, vegetables and beans. Serve with the beetroot yoghurt.

Nutritional information (per serving):
Calories = 496; protein = 58 g;
carbohydrate = 58 g; fat = 6 g;
fibre = 9 g

CHICKEN AND BROCCOLI PASTA

Serves 2

175 g (6 oz) wholewheat pasta
150 g (5 oz) broccoli, cut into small florets
1–2 tbsp light-in-colour olive oil
2 skinless chicken breast fillets, cut into
 bite-sized chunks
1 garlic clove, crushed
150 g (5 oz) passata
1 tbsp tomato purée
75 g (3 oz) baby spinach
25 g (1 oz) flaked almonds, toasted

• Cook the pasta according to the pack instructions. Add the broccoli 3 minutes before the
 end of cooking.
• Meanwhile, fry the chicken in half the olive oil
 for 8–10 minutes or until cooked and golden.
• Heat the remaining olive oil, add the garlic
 and cook for 2 minutes, then stir in the passata
 and tomato purée. Simmer for 5 minutes.
• Drain the pasta and broccoli. Add to the pan
 with the tomato sauce then add the chicken,
 spinach and almonds. Allow the spinach to
 wilt, then serve.

CHICKEN AND VEGETABLE STIR-FRY

Serves 2

1 tbsp light-in-colour olive oil
1 small onion, chopped
1 cm (½ inch) piece of fresh ginger, finely
 chopped
1 garlic clove, crushed
2 chicken thigh fillets, thinly sliced
1 red pepper, deseeded and thinly sliced
75 g (3 oz) green or white cabbage, shredded
A handful of beansprouts
1 courgette, sliced
1 tbsp soy sauce
2 nests of dried egg noodles

• Heat the oil in a wok or frying pan and fry
 the onion for 2 minutes. Add the ginger, garlic
 and chicken and stir-fry until the chicken is
 browned all over. Add the vegetables to the
 pan and stir-fry for 2–3 minutes until starting
 to soften.
• Stir in the soy sauce and a little water.
 Continue to stir-fry over a medium–high heat
 for 3–4 minutes, or until the chicken is cooked
 through.
• Cook the noodles according to the pack
 instructions. Add to the chicken and vegetables and stir to combine.

Nutritional information (per serving):
Calories = 618; protein = 50 g;
carbohydrate = 62 g; fat = 16 g;
fibre = 14 g

Nutritional information (per serving):
Calories = 497; protein = 29 g;
carbohydrate = 47 g; fat = 20 g;
fibre = 7 g

MOROCCAN CHICKEN WITH RICE

Serves 1
1 skinless chicken breast fillet
1 garlic clove, crushed
½ red chilli, deseeded and chopped
   (use according to taste)
A pinch of paprika
A pinch of ground cumin
Juice of ½ lemon
1 tbsp chopped fresh mint leaves
75 g (3 oz) wholegrain rice
1 tbsp toasted pumpkin seeds
Cooked green vegetables, to serve

- Slash the chicken breast fillet 3 or 4 times.
- Place the garlic, chilli, paprika, cumin, lemon juice and mint in a bowl and mix well. Add the chicken and turn a few times. Leave to marinate, ideally for 30 minutes.
- Meanwhile, boil the rice according to the pack instructions, approx. 25 minutes. Drain and mix with the toasted pumpkin seeds.
- Preheat the grill. Place the chicken on a baking tray and grill for 6–7 minutes on each side, until cooked through.
- Spoon the rice on to a plate and place the chicken on top. Serve with green vegetables.

Nutritional information (per serving):
Calories = 545; protein = 48 g;
carbohydrate = 63 g; fat = 13 g;
fibre = 2 g

SALMON AND BEAN SALAD

Serves 4
150 g (5 oz) salad leaves
400 g (14 oz) tin mixed beans,
   drained and rinsed
4 tbsp French dressing
2 tbsp chopped fresh parsley
200 g (7 oz) tin wild red salmon, drained
200 g (7 oz) cherry tomatoes, halved
4 spring onions, chopped
Freshly ground black pepper

- Arrange the salad leaves on 4 plates.
- Mix the beans with the French dressing, parsley and freshly ground black pepper to taste.
- Remove the skin and bones from the salmon and lightly flake the flesh. Mix with the tomatoes, spring onions and the bean mixture. Heap on top of the salad leaves.

Nutritional information (per serving):
Calories = 219; protein = 17 g;
carbohydrate = 14 g; fat = 9 g;
fibre = 7 g

SWEET AND SOUR CHICKEN WITH MANGO

Serves 4
For the sweet and sour sauce:
4 tbsp water
2 tbsp each dry sherry, sesame oil and
  white wine vinegar
1 tbsp light soy sauce
2 tsp honey

2 tbsp sunflower oil
4 skinless chicken breast fillets, cut into 1 cm
  (½ inch) pieces
2 onions, sliced
250 g (9 oz) broccoli, divided into small florets
1 tsp grated fresh ginger
1 large mango, peeled and cubed
Boiled basmati rice, to serve

- For the sauce, combine the water, sherry, sesame oil, vinegar, soy sauce and honey.
- Heat half the sunflower oil in a wok or large frying pan, add the chicken and quickly brown on all sides for 2–3 minutes. Transfer to a warm plate.
- Heat the remaining oil, add the onions and cook until softened. Add the broccoli and ginger, followed by the sauce and the mango.
- Bring to the boil and then simmer gently for 3 minutes. Return the chicken to the wok and continue to cook for a further 2–3 minutes until thoroughly cooked. Serve with basmati rice.

Nutritional information (per serving):
Calories = 255; protein = 23 g;
carbohydrate = 9 g; fat = 14 g;
fibre = 3 g

CHICKEN AND LENTIL SALAD

Serves 4
1 tbsp olive oil
4 skinless chicken breast fillets, sliced
1 garlic clove, crushed
1 small onion, chopped
400 g (14 oz) tin lentils, drained and rinsed
3–4 tomatoes, finely chopped
2 tbsp roughly chopped fresh flat-leaf parsley

For the dressing:
1 tbsp olive oil
2 tbsp lemon juice
1 tbsp clear honey

- Heat the oil in a large frying pan over a high heat and sauté the chicken for 5–6 minutes or until cooked through.
- Add the garlic, onion, lentils and tomatoes and cook, stirring, for about 2 minutes until heated.
- For the dressing, shake together the ingredients in a bottle or screw-top jar.
- Stir the dressing and half the parsley into the lentils in the pan. Transfer to a serving dish, scatter over the remaining parsley and serve warm.

Nutritional information (per serving):
Calories = 347; protein = 45 g;
carbohydrate = 20 g; fat = 10 g;
fibre = 2 g

PILAFF WITH PLAICE

Serves 2
175 g (6 oz) raw brown rice
600 ml (1 pint) water
1 small onion, chopped
Pinch of turmeric (or mild curry powder)
1 courgette, sliced
1 small red pepper, deseeded and chopped
350 g (12 oz) plaice fillets, cut into strips
Salt and freshly ground black pepper
1 tbsp sunflower seeds (optional)

- Place the rice, water, onion and turmeric in a large pan.
- Bring to the boil, cover and simmer for 20 minutes.
- Add the courgette, red pepper and plaice and season to taste.
- Cook for a further 5 minutes or until the fish is cooked and the water absorbed.
- Scatter the sunflower seeds over before serving, if using.

NOODLES WITH PRAWNS AND GREEN BEANS

Serves 2
225 g (8 oz) frozen or fresh whole green beans
175 g (6 oz) egg noodles
1 tsp sunflower oil
175 g (6 oz) peeled rawns
1 tbsp soy sauce

- Cook the green beans in a little boiling water until just tender, then drain.
- Cook the noodles in a large pan until soft.
- Meanwhile, heat the oil in a wok or frying pan and stir-fry the prawns for 2 minutes.
- Add the beans, noodles and soy sauce, and heat through.

Nutritional information (per serving):
Calories = 530; protein = 40 g;
carbohydrate = 76 g; fat = 10 g;
fibre = 3 g

Nutritional information (per serving):
Calories = 483; protein = 32 g;
carbohydrate = 66 g; fat = 12 g;
fibre = 5 g

POTATO AND FISH PIE

Serves 2
450 g (1 lb) potatoes
200 g (7 oz) white fish fillets
   (e.g. cod or plaice)
3 tbsp skimmed milk
2 eggs
1 tbsp parsley
1 tbsp lemon juice
Cooked green vegetables, to serve

- Cut the potatoes into chunks and boil until tender.
- Drain, then mash with the flaked fish, milk, eggs, parsley and lemon juice.
- Place in a dish, then cook either in microwave at full power for 5 minutes, or in the oven at 200°C/400°F/gas mark 6 for 20 minutes.
- Serve with green vegetables.

Vegetarian main meals

BAKED EGGS WITH ROASTED MEDITERRANEAN VEGETABLES

Serves 2
½ aubergine, sliced
1 courgette, sliced
½ yellow pepper, deseeded and sliced
½ red pepper, deseeded and sliced
½ fennel bulb, cut into wedges
1 small onion, sliced
1 tbsp olive oil
1 garlic clove, crushed
A few sprigs of rosemary
A handful of black olives
2 large eggs
Crusty bread, to serve

- Preheat the oven to 200°C/400°F/gas mark 6.
- Place all the vegetables in an ovenproof dish.
- Drizzle over the olive oil, add the garlic and rosemary, then toss lightly so that the vegetables are well coated in the oil. Roast in the oven for about 20 minutes, until the vegetables are just tender.
- Mix in the black olives. Make two wells in the middle of the vegetables. Crack an egg into each indentation. Bake for a further 8–10 minutes or until the eggs are set.
- Serve with crusty bread.

Nutritional information (per serving):
Calories = 352; protein = 33 g;
carbohydrate = 39 g; fat = 8 g;
fibre = 3 g

Nutritional information (per serving):
Calories = 201; protein = 10 g;
carbohydrate = 9 g; fat = 14 g;
fibre = 4 g

STIR-FRIED VEGETABLE OMELETTE

Serves 1
For the stir-fried vegetables:
2 tsp vegetable oil
1 small onion, sliced
1 garlic clove, crushed
1 tsp chopped fresh root ginger
Vegetables, e.g. carrot, cut into strips; red
    pepper, deseeded and sliced; mangetout,
    trimmed and halved; button mushrooms
1 tbsp soy sauce
Juice of ½ lime

For the omelette:
2 large eggs
2 tsp vegetable oil
Salt and freshly ground black pepper

- Heat the oil in a wok or heavy-based pan, and then add the onion, garlic and ginger. Cook for 2 minutes then add the vegetables. Stir-fry for 3–4 minutes, until softened. Stir in the soy sauce and lime juice and set aside.
- For the omelette, beat the eggs in a small bowl and season to taste with salt and pepper.
- Heat the oil in a medium non-stick frying pan, add the eggs and cook for 2–3 minutes over a medium heat until the egg is almost set.
- Pile the stir-fried vegetables on one half of the omelette and fold the other half over the top. Slide on to a plate and serve.

Nutritional information (per serving):
Calories = 372; protein = 20 g;
carbohydrate = 16 g; fat = 26 g;
fibre = 4 g

TOFU WITH NOODLES

Serves 2
For the marinade:
2 tbsp soy sauce
2 tbsp dry sherry
1 tbsp wine vinegar

225 g (8 oz) tofu, cubed
1 tbsp olive oil
1 garlic clove, crushed
1 piece of fresh root ginger, chopped
1 red pepper, deseeded and sliced
100 g (3½ oz) mangetout
1 tsp cornflour
175 g (6 oz) noodles

- Mix the ingredients for the marinade together. Add the tofu and leave for at least 30 minutes in the fridge (or overnight).
- Heat the oil in a wok and stir-fry the garlic, ginger and vegetables for 4 minutes.
- Remove the tofu from the marinade.
- Blend the marinade with the cornflour and pour over the vegetables. Stir until the sauce has thickened. Place the vegetables and sauce in a serving dish.
- Meanwhile, cook the noodles according to the packet instructions
- Stir-fry the tofu for 2 minutes and add to the vegetables. Serve with noodles.

Nutritional information (per serving):
Calories = 533; protein = 21 g;
carbohydrate = 75 g; fat = 19 g;
fibre = 4 g

POTATO, PEA AND SPINACH FRITTATA

Serves 2

1 potato (175 g/6 oz), peeled and sliced
75 g (3 oz) frozen peas
2 tsp olive oil
1 onion, finely sliced
1 garlic clove, crushed
4 large eggs
200 g (7 oz) fresh baby leaf spinach
Salt and freshly ground black pepper
Green salad, to serve

- Cook the potato in a small pan of boiling water for 5–6 minutes, or until just tender. Add the peas during the last 3 minutes. Drain.
- Heat the oil in a frying pan, add the onion and garlic and cook until softened.
- Beat the eggs in a large bowl and season to taste with salt and freshly ground pepper.
- Add the eggs to the pan, stir in the potatoes, peas and spinach and cook over a medium heat for a few minutes until the eggs are almost set.
- Place the pan underneath a hot grill to finish cooking. The frittata should be set and golden on top.
- Slide a knife around the edge and slide the frittata on to a large plate. Serve in wedges with a green salad.

CHICKPEAS WITH BUTTERNUT SQUASH AND TOMATOES

Serves 4

2 tbsp extra virgin olive oil
2 onions, chopped
1 red pepper, deseeded and chopped
225 g (8 oz) butternut squash, peeled and chopped
400 g (14 oz) tin chopped tomatoes
250 ml (8 fl oz) vegetable stock
2 x 400 g (14 oz) tins chickpeas, drained and rinsed
225 g (8 oz) potatoes, peeled and chopped
Grated cheese, to serve

- Heat the oil in a heavy-based pan, add the onion and pepper and cook over a moderate heat for 5 minutes.
- Add the squash, tomatoes, vegetable stock, chickpeas and potatoes, stir and then bring to the boil. Lower the heat and simmer for 20 minutes, stirring occasionally.
- Serve sprinkled with a little grated cheese.

Nutritional information (per serving):
Calories = 347; protein = 23 g;
carbohydrate = 27 g; fat = 18 g;
fibre = 6 g

Nutritional information (per serving):
Calories = 331; protein = 15 g;
carbohydrate = 48 g; fat = 10 g;
fibre = 10 g

SPICY COUSCOUS

Serves 4
250 g (9 oz) couscous
400 ml (14 fl oz) hot vegetable stock or water
½ red pepper, deseeded and cut into wide strips
½ yellow pepper, deseeded and cut into wide strips
1 red onion, sliced
10–12 cherry tomatoes, halved
2 tbsp extra virgin olive oil
½ tsp cumin seeds
A small handful of fresh coriander, chopped
1 tbsp lemon juice
Salt and freshly ground black pepper

- Preheat the oven to 200°C/400°F/gas mark 6.
- Put the couscous in a large bowl and cover with the hot stock or water. Stir briefly, cover and allow to stand for 5 minutes until the stock has been absorbed. Fluff up with a fork.
- Place the pepper in a large roasting tin with the onion and cherry tomatoes, drizzle over the oil, scatter over the cumin seeds and toss so that the vegetables are well coated in oil.
- Roast in the oven for about 15 minutes until the peppers are slightly charred on the outside and tender in the middle. Allow to cool, then roughly chop the peppers.
- Add the roasted vegetables (with the cumin seeds), coriander and lemon juice to the couscous. Season to taste, stir well and serve.

Nutritional information (per serving):
Calories = 224; protein = 5 g;
carbohydrate = 39 g; fat = 7 g;
fibre = 2 g

ROASTED VEGETABLES WITH MARINATED TOFU

Serves 2
1 small red onion, roughly sliced
½ red pepper, deseeded and cut into strips
½ yellow pepper, deseeded and cut into strips
½ orange pepper, deseeded and cut into strips
1 small courgette, trimmed and thickly sliced
¼ aubergine, cut into 2 cm (¾ inch) cubes
2 garlic cloves, crushed
2 tbsp extra virgin olive oil
200 g (7 oz) marinated tofu pieces
A small handful of fresh basil, roughly torn
Freshly ground black pepper

- Preheat the oven to 200°C/400°F/gas mark 6.
- Place the prepared vegetables in a large roasting tin and scatter over the crushed garlic. Pour over the oil and toss lightly, thoroughly coating the vegetables.
- Roast in the oven for 25 minutes, turning them occasionally. Scatter the tofu pieces over and continue roasting for 5 minutes until the vegetables are slightly charred on the outside and tender in the middle.
- Remove from the oven and spoon on to a serving dish. Grind over black pepper to taste and sprinkle with the torn basil.

Nutritional information (per serving):
Calories = 245; protein = 11 g;
carbohydrate = 14 g; fat = 16 g;
fibre = 4 g

VEGETABLE RISOTTO WITH CASHEW NUTS

Serves 2

2 tbsp olive oil
1 onion, chopped
1 red pepper, deseeded and chopped
1 garlic clove, crushed
1 bay leaf
150 g (5 oz) wholegrain rice
500 ml (18 fl oz) hot vegetable stock
75 g (3 oz) green beans, cut into 2 cm
   (¾ inch) lengths
125 g (4 oz) sugar snap peas
2 tomatoes, deseeded and chopped
50 g (2 oz) baby spinach leaves
50 g (2 oz) cashew nuts, lightly toasted
Freshly ground black pepper

- Heat the oil in a large heavy-based pan and cook the onion with the pepper, garlic and bay leaf over a moderate heat, stirring frequently, until softened.
- Stir in the rice and cook for 1–2 minutes, stirring constantly until the grains are coated with oil and translucent.
- Add half the hot vegetable stock and bring to the boil. Reduce the heat and simmer gently until the liquid is absorbed. Stir in the remaining stock, a ladleful at a time, and continue to simmer until the rice is almost tender (about 25–30 minutes).
- Add the green beans, peas and tomatoes and continue cooking for a further 5 minutes. As a guide, the total cooking time should be around 35 minutes.
- Add the spinach leaves to the hot risotto. Stir until the leaves have wilted. Remove the pan from the heat.
- Season to taste with freshly ground black pepper, then scatter over the cashew nuts.

Nutritional information (per serving):
Calories = 652; protein = 16 g;
carbohydrate = 84 g; fat = 29 g;
fibre = 9 g

PASTA WITH CHICKPEAS AND SPINACH

Serves 4

400 g (14 oz) tin chickpeas, drained and rinsed
350 g (12 oz) tub fresh tomato pasta sauce
400 g (14 oz) fresh penne pasta
200 g (7 oz) fresh spinach
25 g (1 oz) Parmesan cheese shavings
Olive oil, to drizzle
Freshly ground black pepper

- Place the chickpeas in a medium pan with the tomato sauce and 100 ml (3½ fl oz) cold water. Bring to the boil over a low heat. Turn off the heat and cover.
- Meanwhile, bring a large pan of water to the boil. Add the pasta and return to the boil for 5 minutes or until the pasta is just tender. Drain thoroughly. Stir in the spinach and allow to wilt.
- Place the pasta in a serving dish and pour the hot pasta sauce and chickpea mixture over the top, then toss together and season to taste with black pepper. Top each serving with Parmesan cheese shavings and a drizzle of olive oil.

VEGETABLE STIR-FRY WITH SESAME NOODLES

Serves 4

1 tsp clear honey
Juice of 1 large orange
3 tbsp soy sauce
2 tbsp oil
1 onion, sliced
1 large carrot, peeled and cut into thin strips
225 g (8 oz) pak choi or spring cabbage, shredded
2.5 cm (1 inch) piece of root ginger, peeled and grated
1 garlic clove, crushed
225 g (8 oz) ready-cooked egg noodles
3 tbsp sesame seeds, toasted

- In a small bowl, mix together the honey, orange juice and soy sauce and set aside.
- Heat the oil in a wok or large frying pan.
- Add the onion and carrot and stir-fry for 2–3 minutes. Add the pak choi or cabbage, ginger and garlic and stir-fry for a further 2–3 minutes.
- Add the ready-cooked egg noodles to the wok and pour in the sauce mix. Toss everything together and cook for a further 2–3 minutes, or until piping hot. Scatter with the toasted sesame seeds and serve.

Nutritional information (per serving):
Calories = 434; protein = 20 g;
carbohydrate = 76 g; fat = 8 g;
fibre = 7 g

Nutritional information (per serving):
Calories = 330; protein = 9 g;
carbohydrate = 44 g; fat = 14 g;
fibre = 4 g

RICE, BEAN AND VEGETABLE STIR-FRY

Serves 2
175 g (6 oz) raw brown rice
1 tbsp olive oil
1 onion, chopped
2 garlic cloves, crushed
1 piece of fresh root ginger, chopped
125 g (4 oz) large mushrooms, sliced
2 celery stalks, chopped
125 g (4 oz) peas
½ tin (200 g/7 oz) red kidney beans, rinsed
   and drained

- Cover the rice with plenty of boiling water. Bring to the boil and simmer for 25–30 minutes.
- Meanwhile, heat the oil in a wok over a high heat. Add the onion, and stir-fry for 1 minute.
- Add the garlic, ginger, mushrooms, celery and peas and stir-fry for 3 minutes.
- Tip in the red kidney beans and cooked rice. Cook for a further 2 minutes, until all the ingredients are thoroughly heated through.

VEGETARIAN CHILLI

Serves 2
1 garlic clove, crushed
1 onion, chopped
1 green or red pepper, deseeded and chopped
½ tsp chilli powder (or to taste)
225 g (8 oz) tinned tomatoes
50 g (2 oz) red lentils
175 g (6 oz) raw rice
300 ml (½ pint) water
½ tin (200 g/7 oz) red kidney beans, rinsed
   and drained
Salt and freshly ground black pepper
Cooked broccoli or green salad, to serve

- Place the garlic, onion, pepper, chilli powder, tomatoes, lentils, rice and water in a large pan.
- Bring to the boil and simmer for 20 minutes.
- Add the kidney beans and cook for a further 5 minutes.
- Season to taste. Serve with broccoli or green salad.

Nutritional information (per serving):
Calories = 526; protein = 18 g;
carbohydrate = 94 g; fat = 11 g;
fibre = 11 g

Nutritional information (per serving):
Calories = 550; protein = 21 g;
carbohydrate = 119 g; fat = 2 g;
fibre = 10 g

MIXED BEAN HOTPOT

Serves 2

400 g (14 oz) tin beans (e.g. red kidney beans, chickpeas or haricot beans), rinsed and drained
125 g (4 oz) green beans
225 g (8 oz) tinned tomatoes
1 tbsp tomato purée
1 tsp mixed herbs
450 g (1 lb) potatoes, boiled and cooled
Cooked green vegetables or salad, to serve

- Place the beans in a large casserole dish and mix in the green beans, tomatoes, tomato purée and herbs.
- Thinly slice the potatoes and arrange on top.
- Bake at 170°C/325°F/gas mark 3 for 30 minutes until the potatoes are cooked, or microwave on full for 8 minutes.
- Serve with green vegetables or salad.

Nutritional information (per serving):
Calories = 346; protein = 17 g;
carbohydrate = 71 g; fat = 2 g;
fibre = 14 g

LENTIL AND VEGETABLE LASAGNE

Serves 2
6 sheets ready-cooked lasagna

For the lentil and vegetable sauce:
100 g (4 oz) red lentils
1 onion, chopped
400 g (14 oz) tin tomatoes
2 carrots, chopped
1 tsp oregano
150 ml (¼ pint) water

For the topping:
2 eggs
125 g (4 oz) fromage frais
1 tbsp freshly grated Parmesan cheese
Mixed salad, to serve

- For the lentil and vegetable sauce, place all the ingredients in a pan and bring to the boil.
- Simmer for 20 minutes or cook in a pressure cooker for 3 minutes (release the steam slowly).
- Place half of the sauce in a dish, with 3 lasagne sheets on top. Spread over the rest of the sauce, followed by the remaining lasagne sheets.
- For the topping, beat the eggs with the fromage frais, then spoon the mixture on top of the lasagne. Sprinkle with the Parmesan cheese.
- Bake at 200°C/400°F/gas mark 6 for 40 minutes, until the topping is golden. Serve with a large mixed salad.

Nutritional information (per serving):
Calories = 513; protein = 33 g;
carbohydrate = 75 g; fat = 11 g; fibre = 6 g

BEAN BURGERS

Serves 2

2 tsp oil, plus extra if frying the burgers
1 small onion, finely chopped
1 garlic clove, crushed
400 g (14 oz) tin red kidney beans, rinsed
    and drained
1 tbsp parsley
1 tbsp lemon juice
Flour (optional)
Oats, for coating
Wholemeal bap or pitta and salad, to serve

- Put the oil in a pan, add the onion and garlic and cook until softened.
- Mash the onion and garlic with a fork or blend in a food processor with the other ingredients, except the oats, until a coarse purée is formed. Add a little flour if necessary for a firmer texture.
- Place the oats in a dish. Using your hands, form the mixture into 4 large burgers, coating them with oats. Preheat a grill, if using.
- Grill for about 2 minutes on each side, fry in a small amount of hot oil, or barbecue.
- Serve in a wholemeal bap or pitta with lots of salad.

Desserts

BANANA PANCAKES

Makes 8 pancakes

100 g (3½ oz) wholemeal flour, or fine
    oatmeal
300 ml (½ pint) milk
2 eggs
1 tsp oil
3 ripe bananas
Low-fat plain yoghurt, to serve

- Blend the flour, milk and eggs in a liquidiser for 30 seconds.
- Heat a non-stick frying pan and add the oil.
- Pour in 1 tbsp of the batter, tilting the pan to coat it evenly.
- Cook until the underside of the pancake is brown.
- Turn, and cook for a further 10 seconds until the other side is brown. Transfer to an oven-proof plate and keep warm in the oven on a very low heat. Repeat the cooking process until the batter is used up.
- Mix one mashed banana with two sliced bananas.
- Place a spoonful on each pancake and fold into quarters.
- Serve with plain yoghurt.

Nutritional information (per serving):
Calories = 234; protein = 12 g;
carbohydrate = 34 g; fat = 7 g;
fibre = 10 g

Nutritional information (per serving):
Calories = 103; protein = 5 g;
carbohydrate = 17 g; fat = 2 g;
fibre = 2 g

BAKED APPLES

Serves 1

1 large cooking apple
1 tbsp raisins or sultanas
1 tsp honey
1 tsp toasted, chopped hazelnuts (optional)
Yoghurt, low-fat custard or fromage frais,
  to serve

- Remove the core from the apple.
- Score the skin lightly around the middle. Place the apple in a small ovenproof dish.
- Mix together the raisins or sultanas, honey and nuts and use to fill the centre of the apple.
- Cover loosely with foil and bake at 180°C/ 350°F/gas mark 4 for 45–60 minutes or cover with another dish and microwave on medium power for 5–7 minutes (depending on the size of the apple), until tender.
- Serve with yoghurt, low-fat custard or fromage frais.

Nutritional information (per serving):
Calories = 144; protein = 1 g;
carbohydrate = 33 g; fat = 2 g;
fibre = 1 g

WHOLEMEAL BREAD AND BUTTER PUDDING

Serves 4

8 slices wholemeal bread
40 g (1½ oz) butter or olive oil spread
75 g (3 oz) sultanas
1 tbsp brown sugar
3 eggs
600 ml (1 pint) milk
Freshly ground nutmeg

- Spread the bread with the butter or spread.
- Cut each slice into 4 squares and layer in a 1 litre (2 pint) dish, scattering sultanas between each layer.
- Beat together the sugar, eggs and milk and pour over the bread.
- Sprinkle with a little grated nutmeg.
- Leave to soak for 30 minutes, if time allows.
- Bake at 350°F/180°C/gas mark 4 for 30–40 minutes, until the top is golden.

Nutritional information (per serving):
Calories = 345; protein = 17 g;
carbohydrate = 49 g; fat = 11 g;
fibre = 4 g

OAT APPLE CRUMBLE

Serves 6
700 g (1½ lb) cooking apples, peeled
    and sliced
75 g (3 oz) clear honey
½ tsp cinnamon
4 tbsp water

For the topping:
125 g (4 oz) plain flour
75 g (3 oz) butter or olive oil spread
50 g (2 oz) oats
50 g (2 oz) brown sugar

- Preheat the oven to 190°C/375°C/gas mark 5.
- Place the apples, honey and cinnamon in a deep baking dish. Combine well and pour the water over.
- For the topping, put the flour in a bowl and rub in the margarine until the mixture resembles coarse breadcrumbs. Mix in the oats and sugar. Alternatively, mix in a food mixer or processor.
- Sprinkle the crumble mixture over the fruit.
- Bake for 40–45 minutes, until the topping is golden and the fruit is tender.

SPICED FRUIT SKEWERS

Serves 4
50 g (2 oz) clear honey
1 tbsp lemon juice
Juice of 1 orange
8 cardamom pods, lightly crushed
1 cinnamon stick, halved
8 Medjool dates, pitted
8 apricots, halved and stoned
4 plums, halved and stoned

- Place the honey, lemon juice, orange juice, cardamom pods and cinnamon stick in a shallow dish. Add the dates, apricots and plums. Marinate for at least 30 minutes.
- Drain the fruits, reserving the honey syrup, and thread on to 4 long wooden skewers. Cook under a preheated grill (or over a prepared barbecue) for 10–15 minutes, or until beginning to colour.
- Remove the cardamom pods and cinnamon sticks from the honey syrup. Serve the fruit skewers drizzled with the syrup.

Nutritional information (per serving):
Calories = 311; protein = 3 g;
carbohydrate = 52 g; fat = 11 g;
fibre = 3 g

Nutritional information (per serving):
Calories = 147; protein = 2 g;
carbohydrate = 37 g; fat = 1 g;
fibre = 3 g

EXOTIC FRUIT WITH LIME

Serves 4
2 tbsp clear honey
100 ml (3½ fl oz) hot water
Grated zest of 1 lime
20 g (⅔ oz) pack fresh mint leaves
1 pineapple, skin removed, quartered
  and cored
3 kiwi fruit, peeled and cut into chunks
1 mango, peeled and sliced
Plain yoghurt, to serve

- Place the honey, water, lime zest and half the mint in a jug. Allow to infuse for 1 hour, then strain.
- Cut the pineapple into small wedges and toss gently in a large bowl with the kiwi fruit and mango pieces. Pour the cooled syrup over and combine well.
- Divide the fruit between 4 bowls, decorate with the remaining mint and serve with plain yoghurt.

ROASTED PEACHES AND PLUMS WITH YOGHURT

Serves 4
4 ripe peaches
4 ripe plums
1 cinnamon stick, broken in half
Grated zest and juice of 2 oranges
400 g (14 oz) plain Greek yoghurt
2 tbsp clear honey

- Preheat the oven to 200°C/400°F/gas mark 6.
- Halve and stone the peaches and plums and arrange, cut sides up, in a shallow dish large enough to hold them all in one layer.
- Put the cinnamon stick, orange zest and juice and honey in a small pan. Heat gently until the honey has melted. Pour evenly over the fruit. Roast in the oven for 25–30 minutes, basting halfway through the cooking time, until the fruit is tender.
- Cool for 10 minutes, then divide between serving plates. Place a dessertspoonful of yoghurt into the cavity of each fruit and drizzle some of the honey syrup over. Serve the rest of the yoghurt separately.

Nutritional information (per serving):
Calories = 124; protein = 1 g;
carbohydrate = 30 g; fat = 1 g;
fibre = 4 g

Nutritional information (per serving):
Calories = 179; protein = 6 g;
carbohydrate = 26 g; fat = 6 g;
fibre = 3 g

Snacks

FRUIT SCOTCH PANCAKES

Serves 2–4

100 g (3½ oz) plain flour
1 tbsp sugar
1 tsp baking powder
2 medium eggs
150 ml (5 fl oz) semi-skimmed milk
50 g (2 oz) raisins
50 g (2 oz) ready-to-eat dried apricots, chopped
Oil, for brushing
Fresh fruit and honey, to serve

- Mix together the dry ingredients in a bowl.
- Add the eggs and a splash of milk and whisk until smooth, then add the remaining milk and whisk to a smooth batter. Stir in the raisins and apricots.
- Heat a large griddle or heavy-based non-stick frying pan and brush it lightly with oil. Drop small spoonfuls of the batter on to the griddle to make 8–10 cm (3–4 inch) rounds and cook for about 2 minutes or until air bubbles start to form on the surface.
- Turn and cook the other side for 1–2 minutes or until golden. You may need to cook in 2 batches.
- Serve with fresh fruit and honey.

Nutritional information (per serving):
For 2 servings: Calories = 423;
protein = 25 g; carbohydrate = 76 g;
fat = 9 g; fibre = 4 g
For 4 servings: Calories = 212;
protein = 8 g; carbohydrate = 38 g;
fat = 5 g; fibre = 2 g

HUMMUS WITH PINE NUTS

Serves 4

400 g (14 oz) tin chickpeas or 125 g (4 oz) dried chickpeas, soaked overnight and then boiled for 45 minutes
1–2 garlic cloves, crushed
2 tbsp extra virgin olive oil
1 tbsp tahini (sesame seed paste)
Juice of ½ lemon
2–4 tbsp water
1–2 tbsp pine nuts
Salt and freshly ground black pepper

- Drain and rinse the chickpeas. Reserve 1–2 tbsp of the chickpeas and put the remainder in a food processor or blender with the garlic, oil, tahini, lemon juice and 2 tbsp water. Whizz until smooth, add a little salt and freshly ground black pepper and process again. Taste to check the seasoning. Add extra water if necessary to give the desired consistency.
- Meanwhile, lightly toast the pine nuts under a hot grill or in a frying pan for 3–4 minutes until they are lightly coloured but not brown (watch carefully because they colour quickly).
- Stir the reserved whole chickpeas into the hummus. Spoon into a shallow dish. Scatter over the pine nuts and drizzle over a few drops of olive oil. Chill in the fridge for at least 2 hours before serving.

Nutritional information (per serving):
Calories = 193; protein = 7 g;
carbohydrate = 12 g; fat = 13 g;
fibre = 4 g

BANANA MUFFINS

Makes 10 muffins
50 g (2 oz) butter
75 g (3 oz) brown sugar
1 egg
225 g (8 oz) flour (wholemeal or half
   wholemeal, half white)
2 mashed bananas
Pinch of salt
1 tsp baking powder
1 tsp vanilla essence
5 tbsp milk

- Preheat the oven to 190°C/375°F/gas mark 5.
- Combine all the ingredients in a large bowl until just mixed.
- Spoon into 10 non-stick bun tins (or paper cases).
- Bake for approx. 20 minutes, until well risen and golden.

Variations:
- Add 50 g (2 oz) chocolate chips to the mixture (recommended!).
- Substitute 225 g (8 oz) fresh blueberries or 75 g (3 oz) dried blueberries for the bananas.
- Substitute 225 g (8 oz) fresh cranberries or 75 g (3 oz) dried cranberries for the bananas.
- Substitute 100 g (3½ oz) chopped dried apricots for the bananas.
- Add the grated zest of 1 lemon instead of the vanilla essence.
- Add 50 g (2 oz) chopped walnuts.

Nutritional information (per serving):
Calories = 164; protein = 4 g;
carbohydrate = 27 g; fat = 5 g;
fibre = 2 g

RAISIN BREAD

Makes 1 loaf (10 slices)
225 g (8 oz) strong flour (half wholemeal,
   half white)
½ tsp salt
1½ tbsp sugar
1 sachet (7 g) easy-blend yeast
1 tbsp melted butter
180 ml (6fl oz) warm water
100 g (3½ oz) raisins

- Mix together the flour, salt, sugar, yeast and butter.
- Add the warm water and mix to form a dough.
- Turn out on to a floured surface and knead for 5–10 minutes until smooth and silky.
- Knead in the raisins.
- Place in a bowl, cover and leave in a warm place or at room temperature to rise until doubled in size (approx. 1 hour).
- Preheat the oven to 220°C/425°F/gas mark 7.
- Knead the dough for a few minutes then shape into a round loaf.
- Place on an oiled baking tray, leave to rise for approximately 60 – 90 minutes, and bake for 20 minutes or until the bread sounds hollow when tapped underneath.

Variations:
- Add 2 tsp cinnamon to the flour mixture.
- Substitute 100 g (3½ oz) chopped dried apricots for the raisins.

Nutritional information (per serving):
Calories = 120; protein = 3 g;
carbohydrate = 25 g; fat = 2 g;
fibre = 2 g

APPLE AND CINNAMON OAT BARS

Makes 12 bars
2 apples, sliced and cooked, or 175 g (6 oz)
   no-added-sugar apple purée
175 g (6 oz) oats
2 tsp cinnamon
4 egg whites
1 tbsp honey
50 g (2 oz) raisins
6 tbsp skimmed milk

- Preheat the oven to 200°C/400°F/gas mark 6.
- Mix all the ingredients together in a bowl.
- Transfer to a non-stick baking tin 23 cm x 15 cm (approx. 9 inches x 6 inches).
- Bake for 15 minutes until golden and set.
- When cool, cut into squares.

SULTANA FLAPJACKS

Makes 12 slices
200 g (7 oz) butter or margarine
200 g (7 oz) sugar
200 g (7 oz) honey or golden syrup
400 g (14 oz) porridge oats
75 g (3 oz) sultanas

- Preheat the oven to 180°C/350°F/gas mark 4.
- Butter a 20 cm x 30 cm cake tin.
- Put the butter, sugar and honey in a pan and heat, stirring occasionally, until the butter has melted and the sugar has dissolved. Add the oats and sultanas and mix well.
- Transfer the oat mixture to the prepared tin and spread to about 2 cm (¾ inch) thick. Smooth the surface with the back of a spoon.
- Bake in the oven for 15–20 minutes, until lightly golden around the edges, but still slightly soft in the middle.
- Leave to cool in the tin, then turn out and cut into 12 slices.

Nutritional information (per serving):
Calories = 87; protein = 3 g;
carbohydrate = 17 g; fat = 1 g;
fibre = 1 g

Nutritional information (per serving):
Calories = 389; protein = 5 g;
carbohydrate = 59 g; fat = 17 g;
fibre = 2 g

BANANA AND WALNUT LOAF

Makes 10 slices or 12 muffins
2 medium bananas
125 g (4 oz) butter
125 g (4 oz) dark brown sugar
2 eggs
1 tsp vanilla essence
1 tsp ground cinnamon
250 g (9 oz) plain flour
1 tsp baking powder
3 tbsp milk
125 g (4 oz) walnuts

- Preheat the oven to 180°C/350°F/gas mark 4.
- Butter a 1 kg (2 lb) loaf tin or use 12 large muffin cases.
- Mash the bananas. Cream the butter and sugar until smooth and then beat in the mashed bananas. Add the eggs, vanilla essence and cinnamon and mix well.
- Add the flour, baking powder and milk, and mix until smooth. Fold in the walnuts.
- Spoon the mixture into the tin and bake for about 50 minutes, until the loaf is crusty on the top and a skewer inserted into the middle comes out clean.
- Cool in the tin, then turn out on to a cooling rack. For muffins, cook for 20–25 minutes.

Nutritional information (per serving):
Calories = 348; protein = 6 g;
carbohydrate = 37 g; fat = 217 g;
fibre = 1 g

BLUEBERRY MUFFINS

Makes 18
250 g (9 oz) plain flour
1 tsp baking powder
100 g (3½ oz) caster sugar
2 eggs
50 g (2 oz) melted butter
200 ml (7 fl oz) buttermilk or plain yoghurt
125 g (4 oz) blueberries

- Preheat the oven to 200°C/400°F/gas mark 6.
- Line 2 x 12-hole muffin trays with paper cases.
- Sift the flour and baking powder into a large bowl then stir in the sugar.
- In another bowl, whisk together the eggs, melted butter and buttermilk or yoghurt. Fold this mixture into the flour and stir the blueberries through. Do not overmix.
- Spoon into paper cases and bake for 20–25 minutes or until cooked and golden.

Nutritional information (per serving):
Calories = 164; protein = 4 g;
carbohydrate = 26 g; fat = 6 g;
fibre = 1 g

RASPBERRY MUFFINS

Makes 10
4 tbsp sunflower oil
5 tbsp milk
1 large egg
150 g (5 oz) self-raising flour
100 g (4 oz) caster sugar
175 g (6 oz) fresh or thawed frozen
   raspberries

For the icing:
4 tbsp icing sugar, sifted
2 tsp lemon juice

- Preheat the oven to 200°C/400°F/gas mark 6.
- Line a 12-hole deep muffin tray with paper cases.
- Mix the oil, milk and egg together.
- Sift the flour and sugar into a bowl. Add the liquid and half the raspberries to the flour and briefly mix until just coming together.
- Spoon into the muffin cases and scatter over the remaining raspberries.
- Bake for 25–30 minutes or until cooked and golden. Cool on a wire rack.
- For the icing, sift the icing sugar into a bowl and stir in the lemon juice to make a runny icing.
- Drizzle the icing over the muffins and leave to set.

Nutritional information (per serving):
Calories = 131; protein = 3 g;
carbohydrate = 19 g; fat = 5 g;
fibre = 1 g

CHERRY, ALMOND AND OAT COOKIES

Makes 15
125 g (4 oz) butter or margarine
125 g (4 oz) granulated or caster sugar
1 tbsp golden syrup
½ tsp vanilla essence
150 g (5 oz) plain flour
100 g (3½ oz) rolled oats
100 g (3½ oz) ground almonds
100 g (3½ oz) glacé cherries, chopped
Oil, for greasing

- Preheat the oven to 170°C/350°F/gas mark 3.
- Oil two baking sheets (or use baking parchment).
- Cream together the butter or margarine and the sugar in a large bowl until light and smooth. Beat in the golden syrup and vanilla essence.
- Add the flour, oats and almonds to the mixture, mixing well. Stir in the cherries.
- Place spoonfuls on to the baking sheets, about 2.5 cm (1 inch) apart, then flatten with your hand.
- Bake for 10–12 minutes or until light golden.

Nutritional information (per serving):
Calories = 216; protein = 3 g;
carbohydrate = 27 g; fat = 11 g;
fibre = 1 g

Vitamin	Function(s)	Sources	RNI and SUL*
A	Essential for normal colour vision and for the cells in the eye that enable us to see in dim light; promotes healthy skin and mucous membranes lining the mouth, nose, digestive system, etc.	Liver, meat, eggs, whole milk, cheese, oily fish, butter, margarine	Men: 700 mcg/day Women: 600 mcg/day SUL: 1500 mcg/day (800 mcg for pregnant women)
Beta-carotene	Converted into vitamin A (6 mcg produces 1 μg vitamin A): a powerful antioxidant and ROS scavenger	Brightly coloured fruit and vegetables (e.g. carrots, spinach, apricots, tomatoes)	No official carotene RNI. 15 mg is suggested intake SUL: 7 mg
B (Thiamin)	Forms a co-enzyme essential for the conversion of carbohydrates into energy; used for the normal functioning of nerves, brain and muscles	Wholemeal bread and cereals, liver, kidneys, red meat, pulses (beans, lentils, peas)	Men: 1.0 mg Women: 0.8 mg No SUL. FSA recommends 100 mg
B2 (Riboflavin)	Required for the conversion of carbohydrates to energy; promotes healthy skin and eyes and normal nerve functions	Liver, kidneys, red meat, chicken, milk, yoghurt, cheese, eggs	Men: 1.3 mg/day Women: 1.1 mg/day No SUL. FSA recommends 40 mg

*RNI = Reference Nutrient Intake for males and females aged 19–64

Sources: Department of Health, Dietary Reference Values for Food Energy and Nutrients for the United Kingdom, HMSO. SACN Vitamin D and Health, 20161991)

**NV = no value published.

SUL = Safe upper limit recommended by the Expert Group on Vitamins and Minerals, an independent advisory committee to the Food Standards Agency (Food Standards Agency, 2003)

Claim(s) of supplements	The evidence	Possible dangers of high doses
Maintains normal vision, healthy skin, hair and mucous membranes; may help to treat skin problems such as acne and boils; may affect protein manufacture	Not involved in energy production; little evidence to suggest it can improve sporting performance	Liver toxicity from taking supplements: symptoms include liver and bone damage; abdominal pain; dry skin; double vision; vomiting; hair loss; headaches. May also cause birth defects. Pregnant women should avoid liver. Never exceed 9000 mcg/day (men), 7500 mcg/day (women)
Reduces risk of heart disease, cancer and muscle soreness	As an antioxidant, may help prevent certain cancers. Other carotenoids in food may also be important	Orange tinge to the skin – probably harmless and reversible
May optimise energy production and performance; is usually present within a B-complex or multivitamin	Involved in energy (ATP) production, so the higher the energy expenditure, the higher the thiamin requirement; increased needs can normally be met in the diet; there is no evidence to suggest that high intakes enhance performance; supplements are probably unnecessary	Cannot be stored – excess is excreted, therefore unlikely to be toxic; toxic symptoms (rare) may include insomnia, rapid pulse, weakness and headaches. Avoid taking more than 3 g/day
Sportspeople may need more B2 because they have higher energy needs – supplements may optimise energy production; usually present within a B-complex or multivitamin	Forms part of the enzymes involved in energy production, so exercise may increase the body's requirements; however, these can usually be met by a balanced diet; there is no evidence that supplements improve performance; if you take the contraceptive pill you may need extra B2	Rarely toxic as it cannot be stored; any excess is excreted in the urine (a bright yellow colour)

Vitamin	Function(s)	Sources	RNI and SUL*
Niacin	Helps to convert carbohydrates into energy; promotes healthy skin, normal nerve functions and digestion	Liver, kidneys, red meat, chicken, turkey, nuts, milk, yoghurt and cheese, eggs, bread, cereals	Men: 6.6 mg/1000 calories Women: 6.6 mg/1000 calories UL: 17 mg
B6 (Pyridoxine)	Involved in the metabolism of fats, proteins and carbohydrates; promotes healthy skin, hair and normal red blood cell formation; is actively used in many chemical reactions of amino acids and proteins	Liver, nuts, pulses, eggs, bread, cereals, fish, bananas	Men: 1.4 mg/day Women: 1.2 mg/day UL: 80 mg
Pantothenic acid (B vitamin)	Involved in the metabolism of fats, proteins and carbohydrates; promotes healthy skin, hair and normal growth; helps in the manufacture of hormones and antibodies, which fight infection; helps energy release from food	Liver, wholemeal bread, brown rice, nuts, pulses, eggs, vegetables	No RNI in the UK No SUL
Folic acid (B vitamin)	Essential in the formation of DNA; necessary for red blood cell manufacture	Liver and offal, green vegetables, yeast extract, wheatgerm, pulses	Men: 200 mcg/day Women: 200 mcg/day UL: 1000 mcg (1 mg)
B12	Needed for red blood cell manufacture and to prevent some forms of anaemia; used in fat, protein and carbohydrate metabolism; promotes cell growth and development; needed for normal nerve functions	Meat, fish, offal, milk, cheese, yoghurt; vegan sources (fortified foods) are soya protein and milk, yeast extract, breakfast cereals	Men: 1.5 mcg/day Women: 1.5 mcg/day UL: 2 mg

Claim(s) of supplements	The evidence	Possible dangers of high doses
Sportspeople need more niacin since it is involved in metabolism; higher doses may help to reduce blood cholesterol levels	Not enough evidence to prove that high doses can help to improve performance; requirements can be met by a balanced diet	Excess is excreted in the urine; doses of more than 200 mg of niacin may cause dilation of the blood vessels near the skin's surface (hot flushes)
Sportspeople may need higher doses to meet their increased energy requirements	Requirements are related to protein intake, so sportspeople on high-protein diets may need extra B6; endurance work may cause greater than normal losses; there is no evidence to suggest that high doses improve performance; extra doses may help to alleviate PMS (premenstrual syndrome)	Excess is excreted in the urine; very high doses (over 2 g/day) over months or years may cause numbness and unsteadiness
Since it is involved in protein, fat and carbohydrate metabolism, sportspeople may need higher doses; usually present within a B-complex or multivitamin – for overall well-being	No evidence to suggest that high doses improve performance	Excess is excreted in the urine
Supplements help overall well-being, and also prevent folic acid deficiency and anaemia; these would, in theory, hinder aerobic performance	No studies have been carried out on athletic performance and folic acid	Dangers of toxicity are very small, though high doses may reduce zinc absorption and disguise a deficiency of vitamin B12
Since it is involved in the development of red blood cells, the implication is that B12 can improve the body's oxygen carrying capacity (and therefore its aerobic performance); athletes have been known to use injections of vitamin B12 before competition in the hope that it will improve their endurance; usually present within a B-complex or multivitamin	Extra vitamin B12 has no effect on endurance or strength; there is no benefit to be gained from taking supplements (deficiencies are very rare)	Excess is excreted in the urine

Vitamin	Function(s)	Sources	RNI and SUL*
Biotin	Involved in the manufacture of fatty acids and glycogen, and in protein metabolism; needed for normal growth and development	Egg yolk, liver and offal, nuts, whole grains, oats	No RNI in the UK; 10–200 mcg/day is thought to be a safe and adequate range UL: 900 mcg
C	Growth and repair of body cells; collagen formation (in connective tissue) and tissue repair; promotes healthy blood vessels, gums and teeth; haemoglobin and red blood cell production; manufacture of adrenalin; powerful antioxidant	Fresh fruit (especially citrus), berries and currants, vegetables (especially dark green, leafy vegetables, tomatoes, peppers)	Men: 40 mg/day Women: 40 mg/day UL: 1000 mg
D	Controls absorption of calcium from the intestine and helps to regulate calcium metabolism; prevents rickets in children and osteomalacia in adults; helps to regulate bone formation	Sunlight (UV light striking the skin), fresh oils, oily fish, eggs, vitamin-D-fortified cereals, margarines and some yoghurts	10 mcg SUL: 25 mcg
E	As an antioxidant, it protects tissues against ROS damage; promotes normal growth and development; helps in normal red blood cell formation	Pure vegetable oils, wheatgerm, wholemeal bread and cereals, egg yolk, nuts, sunflower seeds, avocado	No RNI in the UK; FSA suggests 4 mg (men) 3 mg (women) (10 mg in EU) SUL: 540 mg

Claim(s) of supplements	The evidence	Possible dangers of high doses
Although biotin was once known among bodybuilders as the 'dynamite vitamin', no specific role for this vitamin in sporting performance has been claimed; it is usually present within a B-complex or multivitamin	The body can make its own biotin, so supplements are unnecessary	There are no known cases of biotin toxicity
Vitamin C may help to increase oxygen uptake and aerobic energy production; exercise causes an increased loss so extra may be needed; intense exercise tends to cause greater ROS damage, so sportspeople need higher doses	A deficiency reduces physical performance; exercise may increase requirements to approximately 80 mg/day – these can be met by including five portions of fresh fruit and vegetables in the diet each day; intakes of 100–150 mg may help prevent heart disease and cancer	Excess is excreted, so toxic symptoms are unlikely; high doses may lead to diarrhoea and increase the risk of kidney stones in people who are prone to them
No specific claims for athletic performance	So far not shown to be beneficial to performance	Fat-soluble and can be stored in the body; toxicity is rare but symptoms may include high blood pressure, nausea, and irregular heart beat and thirst
Since it is an antioxidant, it may improve oxygen utilisation in the muscle cells; it may also help to protect the cells from the damaging effects of intense exercise; may help to protect against heart disease and cancer	Supplements may have a beneficial effect on performance at high altitudes, and may help reduce heart disease, cancer risk, and post-exercise muscle soreness; requirements are related to intake of polyunsaturated fatty acids	Although it cannot be excreted, toxicity is extremely rare

Mineral	Function(s)	Sources	RNI and SUL*	
Calcium	Important for bone and teeth structure; helps with blood clotting; acts to transmit nerve impulses; helps with muscle contraction	Milk, cheese, yoghurt, soft bones of small fish, seafood, green leafy vegetables, fortified white flour and bread, pulses	700 mg SUL: 1500 mg	
Sodium	Helps to control body fluid balance; involved in muscle and nerve functions	Table salt, tinned vegetables, fish, meat, ready-made sauces and condiments, processed meats, bread, cheese	Men: 1.6 g/day (= 4 g salt) Women: 1.6 g/day (= 4 g salt) FSA recommends a maximum intake of 2.5 g/day (= 6 g salt)	
Potassium	Works with sodium to control fluid balance and muscle and nerve functions	Vegetables, fruit and fruit juices, unprocessed cereals	Men: 3.5 g/day Women: 3.5 g/day SUL: 3.7 g	
Iron	Involved in red blood cell formation and oxygen transport and utilisation	Red meat, liver, offal, fortified breakfast cereals, shellfish, wholegrain bread, pasta and cereals, pulses, green leafy vegetables	Men: 6.7 mg/day Women: 16.4 mg/day SUL: 17 mg	

Claim(s) of supplements	The evidence	Possible dangers of high doses
May help to prevent calcium deficiency and, in some cases, osteoporosis (brittle bone disease)	There is no evidence that extra calcium prevents osteoporosis; exercise (with adequate calcium intake) prevents bone loss, so supplements would seem to be unnecessary; sportspeople who eat few or no dairy products may find calcium supplements useful for meeting basic dietary requirements; extra calcium may help to reduce the risk of stress fractures in sportswomen with menstrual irregularities	The balance of calcium in the bones and blood is finely controlled by hormones – calcium toxicity is thus virtually unknown. Very high intakes may interfere with the absorption of iron and with kidney function
It has been claimed that extra salt is needed if you sweat a lot or exercise in hot, humid conditions; advocated for treating cramp	Excessive sweating during exercise may cause a marked loss of sodium, but as salt is present in most foods, supplements are usually unnecessary; extra salt is more likely to cause, rather than prevent, cramp – hypohydration is normally the cause of cramp (together possibly with a shortage of potassium)	High salt intakes may increase blood pressure, risk of stroke, fluid retention and upset the electrolyte balance of the body
May help to reduce blood pressure and encourage sodium excretion	Extra potassium is not known to enhance performance; may help to prevent cramp	Excess is excreted, therefore toxicity is very rare
Extra iron can improve the oxygen-carrying capacity of red blood cells, and therefore improve aerobic performance; can prevent or treat anaemia	Iron-deficiency anaemia can impair performance, especially in aerobic activity; exercise destroys red blood cells and haemoglobin and increases loss of iron, therefore iron requirements of sportspeople may be slightly higher than those of sedentary people; iron is lost through menstruation, so supplements may be sensible for sportswomen	High doses may cause constipation and stomach discomfort; they may also interact with zinc, reducing its absorption

Mineral	Function(s)	Sources	RNI and SUL*
Zinc	A component of many enzymes involved in the metabolism of proteins, carbohydrates and fats; helps to heal wounds; assists the immune system; needed for building cells	Meat, eggs, wholegrain cereals, milk and dairy products	Men: 9.5 mg/day Women: 7 mg/day SUL: 25 mg
Magnesium	Involved in the formation of new cells, in muscle contraction and nerve functions; assists with energy production; helps to regulate calcium metabolism; forms part of the mineral structure of bones	Cereals, vegetables, fruit, potatoes, milk	Men: 300 mg/day Women: 270 mg/day SUL: 400 mg
Phosphorus	Assists in bone and teeth formation; involved in energy metabolism as a component of ATP	Cereals, meat, fish, milk and dairy products, green vegetables	550 mg/day SUL: 250 mg from supplements

Claim(s) of supplements	The evidence	Possible dangers of high doses
Suggest a possible role in high-intensity and strength exercises; may help to boost the immune system	Studies have failed to show that extra zinc is of any benefit to performance; sportspeople with a zinc deficiency may have an impaired immune system, so an adequate intake is important	High doses may cause nausea and vomiting; daily doses of more than 50 mg also interfere with the absorption of iron and other minerals, leading to iron deficiency anaemia
Magnesium status may be related to aerobic capacity	Studies have failed to show that magnesium supplements are beneficial to performance	May cause diarrhoea
It has been claimed that phosphate loading enhances aerobic performance and delays fatigue	The consensus is that phosphate loading is of little benefit to performance	High intakes over a long period of time may lower blood calcium levels

LIST OF ABBREVIATIONS

ACSM	American College of Sports Medicine
ADP	adenosine diphosphate
ALA	alpha-linolenic acid
ATP	adenosine triphosphate
BCAA	branched-chain amino acids
BMI	Body Mass Index
BMR	basal metabolic rate
BV	Biological Value
EAA	essential amino acid
DHA	docosahexaenoic acid
DHEA	dehydroepiandrosterone
DoH	Department of Health
DRV	Dietary Reference Value
EFA	essential fatty acid
EPA	eicosapentaenoic acid
FT	fast-twitch (type II) muscle fibres
GI	glycaemic index
GL	glycaemic load
HDL	high density lipoprotein
HMB	beta-hydroxy beta-methylbutyrate
IGF-I	insulin-like growth factor-I
IOC	International Olympic Committee
LDL	low density lipoprotein
MRP	meal replacement product
NEAA	non-essential amino acid
PC	phosphocreatine
NRV	Nutrient Reference Value (on supplement labels)
RMR	resting metabolic rate
RNI	Reference Nutrient Intake
ST	slow-twitch (type I) muscle fibres
SUL	safe upper limit
VO_2max	maximal aerobic capacity

SYMBOLS USED AND CONVERSIONS

SYMBOLS USED

g	gram
h	hour
kcal	kilocalorie
kJ	kilojoule
m	metre
min	minute
mcg	microgram
mg	milligram (1000 g = 1 g)
ml	millilitre
mmol	millimole
mph	miles per hour
sec	seconds
tbsp	tablespoon
tsp	teaspoon
dl	decilitre (10 dl = 1 l)
mcg	microgram (1000 mcg = 1 mg)
<	less than
>	greater than
°C	degree Celsius

CONVERSIONS

1 kcal	=	4.2 kJ
25 g	=	1 oz
450 g	=	1 lb
1 kg	=	2.2 lb
5 ml	=	1 tsp
15 ml	=	1 tbsp
25 ml	=	1 fl oz
600 ml	=	1 pint

FURTHER READING

Bean, Anita (2021) *The Vegan Athlete's Cookbook*, Bloomsbury Publishing Plc

Bean, Anita (2019) *Vegetarian Meals in 30 Minutes*, Bloomsbury Publishing Plc

Bean, Anita (2017) *The Runner's Cookbook*, Bloomsbury Publishing Plc

Bean, Anita (2016) *The Vegetarian Athlete's Cookbook*, Bloomsbury Publishing Plc

Bubbs, D. M. (2019), *Peak: The New Science of Athletic Performance That Is Revolutionizing Sports*, 1st ed., White River Junction, Vermont: Chelsea Green Publishing Co.

Burke, L. (2007), *Practical Sports Nutrition*, Human Kinetics.

Burke, L. and Deakin, V. (2015), *Clinical Sports Nutrition*, McGraw-Hill Medical.

Food Standards Agency (2002), *McCance and Widdowson's The Composition of Foods*, 6th summary ed., Royal Society of Chemistry.

Hutchinson, A. (2019), *Endure: Mind, Body and the Curiously Elastic Limits of Human Performance*, HarperCollins.

Institute of Food Research and Department of Health (2014), *McCance and Widdowson's The Composition of Foods: Seventh Summary Edition*, 7th ed., Cambridge: Royal Society of Chemistry.

Jeukendrup, A. and Glesson, M. (2018), *Sport Nutrition*, 3rd ed., Human Kinetics.

Larson-Meyer, D. E. and Ruscigno, M. (2019), *Plant-Based Sports Nutrition: Expert fueling strategies for training, recovery, and performance*, Illustrated ed., Champaign, IL: Human Kinetics.

McArdle, W. D., Katch, F. I. and Katch, V. L. (2015), *Essentials of Exercise Physiology*, 5th North American ed., Philadelphia: Lippincott Williams and Wilkins.

Wilson, P. (2020), *The Athlete's Gut: The Inside science of Digestion, Nutrition, and Stomach Distress*, VeloPress.

REFERENCES

Abildgaard, J. *et al.* (2013), 'Menopause is associated with decreased whole body fat oxidation during exercise', *American Journal of Physiology. Endocrinology and Metabolism*, 304(11), pp. E1227-1236. doi: 10.1152/ajpendo.00492.2012.

Aceto, C. (1997), *Everything You Need to Know about Fat Loss*, (Adamsville TN: Fundco).

Acheson, K. J. *et al.* (1988), 'Glycogen storage capacity and de novo lipogenesis during massive carbohydrate overfeeding in man', *The American Journal of Clinical Nutrition*, 48(2), pp. 240–247. doi: 10.1093/ajcn/48.2.240.

Achten J. *et al.* (2004), 'Higher dietary carbohydrate content during intensified running training results in better maintenance of performance and mood state', *J. Appl. Physiol.*, vol. 96(4), pp. 1331–40.

Ackerman, K. E. *et al.* (2019), 'Low energy availability surrogates correlate with health and performance consequences of Relative Energy Deficiency in Sport', *British Journal of Sports Medicine*, 53(10), pp. 628–633. doi: 10.1136/bjsports-2017-098958.

Ackland T. *et al.* (2012), 'Current Assessment of Body Composition in Sport'. *Sports Med.*, vol. 42(3): 227–49.

ACSM (1982), 'American College of Sports Medicine Position Statement on: The Use of Alcohol in Sports', *Medicine & Science in Sports & Exercise*, 14(6), p. ix.

ACSM (1996), 'Position stand on exercise and fluid replacement', *Med. Sci. Sports and Ex.*, vol. 28, pp. i–vii.

ACSM (2007), Armstrong, L. E., Casa, D. J. *et al.*, 'American College of Sports Medicine position stand on:. Exertional heat illness during training and competition', *Med. Sci. Sports and Ex.*, vol. 39(3): 556–72.

Adams, R. B., Egbo, K. N., and Demmig-Adams, B. (2014), 'High-dose vitamin C supplements diminish the benefits of exercise in athletic training and disease prevention', *Nutrition & Food Science*, vol. 44(2), pp. 95–101

Ahlborg, B. *et al.* (1967), 'Human muscle glycogen content and capacity for prolonged exercise after different diets', *Forsvarsmedicin*, vol. 3, pp. 85–99.

Ahnen, R. T., Jonnalagadda, S. S. and Slavin, J. L. (2019), 'Role of plant protein in nutrition, wellness, and health', *Nutrition Reviews*, 77(11), pp. 735–747. doi: 10.1093/nutrit/nuz028.

Aird, T. P., Davies, R. W. and Carson, B. P. (2018), 'Effects of fasted vs fed-state exercise on performance and post-exercise metabolism: A systematic review and meta-analysis', *Scandinavian Journal of Medicine & Science in Sports*, 28(5), pp. 1476–1493. doi: 10.1111/sms.13054.

Alexander, D. D. *et al.* (2016), 'Dairy consumption and CVD: a systematic review and meta-analysis', *The British Journal of Nutrition*, 115(4), pp. 737–750. doi: 10.1017/S0007114515005000.

Alexander, D., Ball, M. J. and Mann, J. (1994), 'Nutrient intake and hematological status of vegetarians and age-sex matched omnivores', *Eur. J. Clin. Nutr.*, vol. 48, pp. 538–46.

Alghannam, A. F. *et al.* (2016), 'Impact of muscle glycogen availability on the capacity for repeated exercise in man', *Med. Sci. Sports and Ex.*, vol. 48(1), pp. 123–31.

Alghannam, A. F., Gonzalez, J. T. and Betts, J. A. (2018), 'Restoration of Muscle Glycogen and Functional Capacity: Role of Post-Exercise Carbohydrate and Protein Co-Ingestion', *Nutrients*, 10(2). doi: 10.3390/nu10020253.

Alghannam, A. F., Gonzalez, J. T. and Betts, J. A. (2018), 'Restoration of Muscle Glycogen and Functional Capacity: Role of Post-Exercise Carbohydrate and Protein Co-Ingestion', *Nutrients*, 10(2), p. E253. doi: 10.3390/nu10020253.

Allaway, H. C. M., Southmayd, E. A. and Souza, M. J. D. (2016), 'The physiology of functional hypothalamic amenorrhea associated with energy deficiency in exercising women and in women with anorexia nervosa', *Hormone Molecular Biology and Clinical Investigation*, 25(2), pp. 91–119. doi: 10.1515/hmbci-2015-0053.

Allen, J. M. *et al.* (2018), 'Exercise Alters Gut Microbiota Composition and Function in Lean and Obese Humans', *Medicine and Science in Sports and Exercise*, 50(4), pp. 747–757. doi: 10.1249/MSS.0000000000001495.

Alvares, T. S. *et al.* (2012), 'Acute L-Arginine supplementation does not increase nitric oxide production in healthy subjects', *Nutrition & Metabolism*, 9(1), p. 54. doi: 10.1186/1743-7075-9-54.

Anderson, L. *et al.* (2017), 'Energy Intake and Expenditure of Professional Soccer Players of the English Premier League: Evidence of Carbohydrate Periodization', *International Journal of Sport Nutrition and Exercise Metabolism*, 27(3), pp. 228–238. doi: 10.1123/ijsnem.2016-0259.

Anthony, J. C. *et al.* (2001), 'Signaling pathways involved in translational control of protein synthesis in skeletal muscle by leucine', *J. Nutr.*, vol. 131(3), pp. 856S–860S.

Antoni, R. *et al.* (2018), 'A pilot feasibility study exploring the effects of a moderate time-restricted feeding intervention on energy intake, adiposity and metabolic physiology in free-living human subjects', *Journal of Nutritional Science*, 7. doi: 10.1017/jns.2018.13.

Antonio, J. and Street, C. (1999), 'Glutamine: a potentially useful supplement for athletes', *Can. J. Appl. Physiol.*, vol. 24(1): S69–77.

Appleby, P. N. *et al.* (1999), 'The Oxford Vegetarian Study: an overview', *Am. J. Clin. Nutr.*, vol. 70 (3 Suppl), pp. 525S–31S.

Aragon, A. A. *et al.* (2017), 'International society of sports nutrition position stand: diets and body composition', *Journal of the International Society of Sports Nutrition*, 14(1), p. 16. doi: 10.1186/s12970-017-0174-y.

Areces, F. *et al.* (2014), 'A 7-day oral supplementation with branched-chain amino acids was ineffective to prevent muscle damage during a marathon', *Amino Acids*, 46(5), pp. 1169–1176. doi: 10.1007/s00726-014-1677-3.

Areta J. L. *et al.* (2013), 'Timing and distribution of protein ingestion during prolonged recovery from resistance exercise alters myofibrillar protein synthesis', *J. Physiol.*, vol. 591(9), pp. 2319–31.

Armento, A. *et al.* (2021), 'Presence and Perceptions of Menstrual Dysfunction and Associated Quality of Life Measures Among High School Female Athletes', *Journal of Athletic Training*. doi: 10.4085/624-20.

Armstrong, L. E. (2002), 'Caffeine, body fluid-electrolyte balance and exercise performance', *Int. J. Sport Nutr.*, vol. 12, pp. 189–206.

Armstrong, L. E. *et al.* (1985), 'Influence of diuretic induced dehydration on competitive running performance', *Med. Sci. Sports Ex.*, vol. 17, pp. 456–61.

Armstrong, L. E. *et al.* (1998), 'Urinary indices during dehydration, exercise and rehydration', *Int. J. Sport Nutr.*, vol. 8, pp. 345–55.

Armstrong, L. E. *et al.* (2005), 'Fluid, electrolyte and renal indices of hydration during 11 days of controlled caffeine consumption', *Int. J. Sport Nutr. Exerc. Metab.*, vol. 15, pp. 252–65.

Ashtary-Larky, D. *et al.* (2021), 'Ketogenic diets, physical activity, and body composition: A review', *The British Journal of Nutrition*, pp. 1–68. doi: 10.1017/S0007114521002609.

Ashwell, M. *et al.* (2011), 'Waist-to-height ratio is a better screening tool than waist circumference and BMI for adult cardiometabolic risk factors: systematic review and meta-analysis'. *Obes. Rev.* vol 13(3), pp. 275–86.

Asnicar, F. *et al.* (2021), 'Microbiome connections with host metabolism and habitual diet from 1,098 deeply phenotyped individuals', *Nature Medicine*, 27(2), pp. 321–332. doi: 10.1038/s41591-020-01183-8.

Astrup, A. *et al.* (2019), 'WHO draft guidelines on dietary saturated and trans fatty acids: time for a new approach?', *BMJ*, 366, p. l4137. doi: 10.1136/bmj.l4137.

Astrup, A., *et al.* (2010), 'The role of reducing intakes of saturated fat in the prevention of cardiovascular disease: where does the evidence stand in 2010?', *Am. J. Clin. Nutr.*, vol. 93, pp. 684–8.

Aykan, N. F. (2015), 'Red Meat and Colorectal Cancer', *Oncology Reviews*, 9(1), p. 288. doi: 10.4081/oncol.2015.288.

Bacon, L. *et al.* (2005), 'Size acceptance and intuitive eating improve health for obese, female chronic dieters', *J. Am. Diet. Assoc.*, vol. 105 (6), pp. 929–36.

Barnes, M. J. (2014), 'Alcohol: impact on sports performance and recovery in male athletes', *Sports Medicine (Auckland, N.Z.)*, 44(7), pp. 909–919. doi: 10.1007/s40279-014-0192-8.

Barr, S. I. and Costill, D. L. (1989), 'Water. Can the endurance athlete get too much of a good thing?', *J. Am. Diet. Assoc.*, vol. 89, pp. 1629–32.

Barr, S. I. and Rideout, C. A. (2004), 'Nutritional considerations for vegetarian athletes', *Nutrition*, vol. 20 (7–8), pp. 696–703.

Barrett, E. C., McBurney, M. I. and Ciappio, E. D. (2014), 'ω-3 fatty acid supplementation as a potential therapeutic aid for the recovery from mild traumatic brain injury/concussion', *Advances in Nutrition (Bethesda, Md.)*, 5(3), pp. 268–277. doi: 10.3945/an.113.005280.

Bartlett, J. D. *et al.* (2013), 'Reduced carbohydrate availability enhances exercise-induced p53 signaling in human skeletal muscle: implications for mitochondrial biogenesis', *American Journal of Physiology. Regulatory, Integrative and Comparative Physiology*, 304(6), pp. R450-458. doi: 10.1152/ajpregu.00498.2012.

Bartlett, J. D. *et al.* (2015), 'Carbohydrate availability and exercise training adaptation: too much of a good thing?', *Eur. J. Sport Sci.*, vol. 15(1), pp. 3–12.

Barton, W. *et al.* (2018), 'The microbiome of professional athletes differs from that of more sedentary subjects in composition and particularly at the functional metabolic level', *Gut*, 67(4), pp. 625–633. doi: 10.1136/gutjnl-2016-313627.

Bates *et al.* (2014), National Diet and Nutrition Survey. Headline results from years 1, 2, 3, 4 of the Rolling Programme (2208/9–2011/12) (Public Health England, London).

Bauer, J. *et al.* (2013), 'Evidence-based recommendations for optimal dietary protein intake in older people: a position paper from the PROT-AGE Study Group', *Journal of the American Medical Directors Association*, 14(8), pp. 542–559. doi: 10.1016/j.jamda.2013.05.021.

Bazzare, T. L. *et al.* (1986), 'Incidence of poor nutritional status among triathletes, endurance athletes and controls', *Med. Sci. Sports Ex.*, vol. 18, p. 590.

BDA, *Vegetarian, vegan and plant-based diet*. Available at: https://www.bda.uk.com/resource/vegetarian-vegan-plant-based-diet.html (Accessed: 6 May 2021).

Beals, K. A. and Hill, A. K. (2006), 'The prevalence of disordered eating, menstrual dysfunction and low bone mineral density among US collegiate athletes', *Int. J. Sports Nutr. Exerc. Metab.*, vol. 16, pp. 1–23.

Beelen, M. *et al.* (2008), 'Protein coingestion stimulates muscle protein synthesis during resistance type exercise', *Am. J. Physiol. Endocrinol Metab.*, vol. 295, pp. E70–7.

Beelen, M. *et al.* (2010), 'Nutritional strategies to promote postexercise recovery', *Int. J. Sport Nutr. Exerc. Metab.*, vol. 20, pp. S15–32.

Beis, L. Y. *et al.* (2011), 'Food and macronutrient intake of elite Ethiopian distance runners', *J. Int. Soc. Sports Nutr.*, vol. 8 pp. 7–11.

Bell, K. E. *et al.* (2016), 'Muscle Disuse as a Pivotal Problem in Sarcopenia-related Muscle Loss and Dysfunction', *The Journal of Frailty & Aging*, 5(1), pp. 33–41. doi: 10.14283/jfa.2016.78.

Bell, P. G. *et al.* (2015), 'Recovery facilitation with Montmorency cherries following high-intensity, metabolically challenging exercise', *Appl. Physiol. Nutr. Metab.*, vol. 40, pp. 414–23.

Below, P. R. *et al.* (1995), 'Fluid and carbohydrate ingestion independently improve performance during one hour of intense exercise', *Med. Sci. Sports Exerc.*, vol. 27, pp. 200–10.

Belza, A., Ritz, C., Sørensen, M. Q. *et al.* (2013), 'Contribution of gastroenteropancreatic appetite hormones to protein-induced satiety', *Am. J. Clin. Nutr.*, vol. 97(5), pp. 980–9.

Bennell K. L. *et al.* (1995), 'Risk factors for stress fractures in female track and field athletes: a retrospective anaysis'. *Clin. J. Sports Med.*, vol. 5, pp. 229–35.

Beradi, J. M. *et al.* (2008), 'Recovery from a cycling time trial is enhanced with carbohydrate-protein supplementation vs. isoenergetic carbohydrate supplementation', *J. Int. Soc. Sports Nutr.* 2008, vol. 5, p. 24.

Berg, A. and Keul, J. (1988), 'Biomechanical changes during exercise in children',. *Young athletes: Biological, psychological and educational perspectives,* ed. R. M. Malina (Champaign, IL, Human Kinetics), pp. 61–77.

Bergstrom, J. *et al.* (1967), 'Diet, muscle glycogen and physical performance', *Acta. Physiol. Scand.*, vol. 71, pp. 140–50.

Berkulo, M. A. R. *et al.* (2016), 'Ad-libitum drinking and performance during a 40-km cycling time trial in the heat', *European Journal of Sport Science*, 16(2), pp. 213–220. doi: 10.1080/17461391.2015.1009495.

Bermon, S. *et al.* (2017), 'Consensus Statement Immunonutrition and Exercise', *Exercise Immunology Review*, 23, pp. 8–50.

Berrazaga, Insaf, et al.*et al.* (2019), '"The Role of the Anabolic Properties of Plant- versus Animal-Based Protein Sources in Supporting Muscle Mass Maintenance: A Critical Review."', *Nutrients*, vol. 11, no. 8, Aug. 2019. PubMed Central, doi:10.3390/nu11081825.

Berry, D. J. *et al.* (2011), 'Vitamin D status has a linear association with seasonal infections and lung function in British adults', *British Journal of Nutrition*, 106(9), pp. 1433–1440. doi: 10.1017/S0007114511001991.

Bescos, R. *et al.* (2012), 'The effect of nitric oxide related supplements on human performance', *Sports Med.*, vol. 42(2), pp. 99–117.

Betts, J. A. and Williams, C. (2010), 'Short-term recovery from prolonged exercise: exploring the potential for protein ingestion to accentuate the benefits of carbohydrate supplements', *Sports Medicine (Auckland, N.Z.)*, 40(11), pp. 941–959. doi: 10.2165/11536900-000000000-00000.

Betts, J. A. *et al.* (2016), 'Is breakfast the most important meal of the day?', *The Proceedings of the Nutrition Society*, 75(4), pp. 464–474. doi: 10.1017/S0029665116000318.

Betts, J. *et al.* (2007), 'The influence of carbohydrate and protein ingestion during recovery from prolonged exercise on subsequent endurance performance', *J. Sports Sci.*, vol. 25(13), pp. 1449–60.

Betts, J. *et al.* (2014), 'The causal role of breakfast in energy balance and health: a randomized controlled trial in lean adults', *Am. J. Clin. Nutr.*, vol. 100(2), pp. 539–47.

Biolo, G. *et al.* (2008), 'Positive energy balance is associated with accelerated muscle atrophy and increased erythrocyte glutathione turnover during 5 wk of bed rest', *The American Journal of Clinical Nutrition*, 88(4), pp. 950–958. doi: 10.1093/ajcn/88.4.950.

Biolo, G., K. D. Tipton, S. Klein, and R. R. Wolfe (1997), 'An abundant supply of amino acids enhances the metabolic effect of exercise on muscle protein', *Am. J. Physiol.* 273: E122-E129.

Bishop, N. C. *et al.* (2001), 'Pre-exercise carbohydrate status and immune responses to prolonged cycling: I. Effect on neutrophil degranulation', *International Journal of Sport Nutrition and Exercise Metabolism*, 11(4), pp. 490–502. doi: 10.1123/ijsnem.11.4.490.

Bishop, N. C. *et al.* (2002), 'Influence of carbohydrate supplementation on plasma cytokine and neutrophil degranulation responses to high intensity intermittent exercise', *Int. J. Sport Nutr.*, vol. 12, pp. 145–56.

Bloomer, R. J. *et al.* (2000), 'Effects of meal form and composition on plasma testosterone, cortisol and insulin following resistance exercise', *Int. J. Sport Nutr.*, vol. 10, pp. 415–24.

Bodine, S. C. *et al.* (2001), 'Akt/mTOR pathway is a crucial regulator of skeletal muscle hypertrophy and can prevent muscle atrophy in vivo', *Nature Cell Biology*, 3(11), pp. 1014–1019. doi: 10.1038/ncb1101-1014.

Boirie, Y. *et al.* (1997), 'Slow and fast dietary proteins differently modulate postprandial protein accretion', *Proc. Nat. Acad. Sci. USA.*, vol. 94(26), pp. 14930–5.

Bonn-Miller, M. O. *et al.* (2017), 'Labeling Accuracy of Cannabidiol Extracts Sold Online', *JAMA*, 318(17), p. 1708. doi: 10.1001/jama.2017.11909.

Booth, F. and Zwetsloot, K. (2010), 'Basic concepts about genes, inactivity and aging', *Scand. J. Med. Sci. Sports*, vol. 20, pp. 1–4.

Borsheim E *et al.* (2004), 'Effect of an amino acid, protein, and carbohydrate mixture on net muscle protein balance after resistance training', *Int. J. Sport. Nutr. Exerc. Metab.*, vol. 14, pp. 255–71.

Bosch, A. N. *et al.* (1994), 'Influence of carbohydrate ingestion on fuel substrate turnover and oxidation during prolonged exercise', *J. Appl. Physiol.*, vol. 76, pp. 2364–72.

Bounous, G. and Gold, P. (1991), 'The biological activity of un-denatured whey proteins: role of glutathione', *Clin. Invest. Med.*, vol. 4, pp. 296–309.

Boutcher, Y. N. *et al.* (2019), 'The Effect of Sprint Interval Training on Body Composition of Postmenopausal Women', *Medicine & Science in Sports & Exercise*, 51(7), pp. 1413–1419. doi: 10.1249/MSS.0000000000001919.

Bouvard, V. *et al.* (2015), 'Carcinogenicity of consumption of red and processed meat', *The Lancet Oncology*, Oct. 26 2015.

Bowtell, J. and Kelly, V. (2019), 'Fruit-Derived Polyphenol Supplementation for Athlete Recovery and Performance', *Sports Medicine*, 49(1), pp. 3–23. doi: 10.1007/s40279-018-0998-x.

Bowtell, J. L., Sumners, D. P., Dyer, A. *et al.* (2011), 'Montmorency cherry juice reduces muscle damage caused by intensive strength exercise', *Medicine and Science in Sports Exercise*, vol. 43(8), pp. 1544–51.

Brand-Miller, J. *et al.* (2003), 'Low GI diet in the management of diabetes'. *Diabetes Care*, vol. 26, pp. 2261–7.

Brand-Miller, J., Foster-Powell, K. and McMillan Price J. (2005), *The Low GI Diet*. (Hodder Mobius).

Breen, L. and Phillips, S. M. (2013), 'Interactions between exercise and nutrition to prevent muscle waste during ageing', *British Journal of Clinical Pharmacology*, 75(3), pp. 708–715. doi: 10.1111/j.1365-2125.2012.04456.x.

Brilla, L. R. and Conte, V. (2000), 'Effects of a novel zinc-magnesium formulation on hormones and strength', *J. Exerc. Physiol. Online*, vol. 3(4), pp. 1–15.

Brinkworth, G. D. and Buckley, J. D. (2003), 'Concentrated bovine colostrum protein supplementation reduces the incidence of self-reported symptoms of upper respiratory tract infection in adult males', *Eur. J. Nutr.*, vol. 42, pp. 228–32.

Brinkworth, G. D. *et al.* (2004), 'Effect of bovine colostrum supplementation on the composition of resistance trained and untrained limbs in healthy young men', *Eur. J. Appl. Physiol.*, vol. 91, pp. 53–60.

Broeder, C. E. *et al.* (2000), 'The Andro Project', *Arch. Intern. Med.*, vol. 160(20), pp. 3093–104.

Brouns, F. *et al.* (1998), 'The effect of different rehydration drinks on post-exercise electrolyte excretion in trained athletes', *Int. J. Sports Med.*, vol. 19, pp. 56–60.

Brown, E. C. *et al.* (2004), 'Soya versus whey protein bars: Effects of exercise training impact on lean body mass and antioxidant status', *J. Nutr.*, vol. 3, pp. 22–7.

Brown, G. A. *et al.* (2000), 'Effects of anabolic precursors on serum testosterone concentrations and adaptations to resistance training in young men', *Int. J. Sport Nutr.*, vol. 10, pp. 340–59.

Brown, M. A., Stevenson, E. J. and Howatson, G. (2019), 'Montmorency tart cherry (*Prunus cerasus L.*) supplementation accelerates recovery from exercise-induced muscle damage in females', *European Journal of Sport Science*, 19(1), pp. 95–102. doi: 10.1080/17461391.2018.1502360.

Brown, R. C. and Cox, C. M. (1998), 'Effects of high fat versus high carbohydrate diets on plasma lipids and lipoproteins in endurance athletes', *Medicine & Science in Sports & Exercise*, 30(12), pp. 1677–1683.

Brownlie, T., *et al.* (2004), 'Tissue iron deficiency without anemia impairs adaptation in endurance capacity after aerobic training in previously untrained women', *Am. J. Clin. Nutr.*, vol. 79(3), pp. 437–43.

Bryer S. C. and Goldfarb, A. H. (2006), 'Effect of high dose vitamin C supplementation on muscle soreness, damage, function and oxidative stress to eccentric exercise', *Int. J. Sport Nutr. Exerc. Metab.*, vol. 16, pp. 270–80.

Buckley, J. D. *et al.* (2003), 'Effect of bovine colostrum on anaerobic exercise performance and plasma insulin-like growth factor', *J. Sports Sci.*, vol. 21, pp. 577–88.

Buford, T. W., *et al.* (2007), 'International Society of Sports Nutrition position stand: creatine supplementation and exercise', *J. Int. Soc. Sports Nutr.*, vol. 4, p. 6.

Burd, N. A. *et al.* (2009), 'Exercise training and protein metabolism: influences of contraction, protein intake, and sex-based differences', *J. Appl. Physiol.*, vol. 106(5), pp. 1692–701.

Burd, N. A. *et al.* (2011), 'Enhanced amino acid sensitivity of myofibrillar protein synthesis persists for up to 24 h after resistance exercise in young men', *J. Nutr.*, vol. 141(4), pp. 568–73.

Burd, N. A. *et al.* (2013), 'Anabolic resistance of muscle protein synthesis with aging', *Exerc. Sport Sci. Rev.*, vol. 41, pp. 169–73.

Burd, N. A. *et al.* (2015), 'Differences in postprandial protein handling after beef compared with milk ingestion during postexercise recovery: a randomized controlled trial', *The American Journal of Clinical Nutrition*, 102(4), pp. 828–836. doi: 10.3945/ajcn.114.103184.

Burd, N. A. *et al.* (2019), 'Food-First Approach to Enhance the Regulation of Post-exercise Skeletal Muscle Protein Synthesis and Remodeling', *Sports Medicine (Auckland, N.z.)*, 49(Suppl 1), pp. 59–68. doi: 10.1007/s40279-018-1009-y.

Burke L. M. *et al.* (2011), 'Carbohydrates for training and competition', *J. Sports Sci.*, vol. 29, Suppl. 1, pp. S17–27.

Burke, D. G. *et al.* (1993), 'Muscle glycogen storage after prolonged exercise: effect of glycaemic index of carbohydrate feedings', *J. Appl. Physiol.*, vol. 75, pp. 1019–23.

Burke, D. G. *et al.* (2000), 'The effect of continuous low dose creatine supplementation on force, power and total work', *Int. J. Sport Nutr.*, vol. 10, pp. 235–44.

Burke, L. M. (2010), 'Fueling strategies to optimize performance: training high or training low?', *Scand. J. Med. Sci. Sports,* vol. 20, Suppl. 2, pp. 48–58.

Burke, L. M. (2021), 'Ketogenic low-CHO, high-fat diet: the future of elite endurance sport?', *The Journal of Physiology*, 599(3), pp. 819–843. doi: 10.1113/JP278928.

Burke, L. M. and Kiens, B. (2006), '"Fat adaptation" for athletic performance: the nail in the coffin?', *Journal of Applied Physiology (Bethesda, Md.: 1985)*, 100(1), pp. 7–8. doi: 10.1152/japplphysiol.01238.2005.

Burke, L. M. and Kiens, B. (2006), '"Fat adaptation" for athletic performance: the nail in the coffin?', *Journal of Applied Physiology (Bethesda, Md.: 1985)*, 100(1), pp. 7–8. doi: 10.1152/japplphysiol.01238.2005.

Burke, L. M. *et al.* (2003), 'Effect of alcohol intake on muscle glycogen storage after prolonged exercise', *Journal of Applied Physiology (Bethesda, Md.: 1985)*, 95(3), pp. 983–990. doi: 10.1152/japplphysiol.00115.2003.

Burke, L. M. *et al.* (2004), 'Carbohydrates and fat for training and recovery', *J. Sports Sci.*, vol. 22(1), pp. 15–30.

Burke, L. M. *et al.* (2012), 'Effect of intake of different dietary protein sources on plasma amino acid profiles at rest and after exercise', *Int. J. Sport Nutr. and Exerc. Metab.*, vol. 22, pp. 452–62.

Burke, L. M. *et al.* (2017), 'Low carbohydrate, high fat diet impairs exercise economy and negates the performance benefit from intensified training in elite race walkers', *The Journal of Physiology*, 595(9), pp. 2785–2807. doi: 10.1113/JP273230.

Burke, L. M. *et al.* (2018), 'Relative Energy Deficiency in Sport in Male Athletes: A Commentary on Its Presentation Among Selected Groups of Male Athletes', *International Journal of Sport Nutrition and Exercise Metabolism*, 28(4), pp. 364–374. doi: 10.1123/ijsnem.2018-0182.

Burke, L. M. *et al.* (2019), 'International Association of Athletics Federations Consensus Statement 2019: Nutrition for Athletics', *International Journal of Sport Nutrition and Exercise Metabolism*, 29(2), pp. 73–84. doi: 10.1123/ijsnem.2019-0065.

Burke, L. M. *et al.* (2020), 'Crisis of confidence averted: Impairment of exercise economy and performance in elite race walkers by ketogenic low carbohydrate, high fat (LCHF) diet is reproducible', *PloS One*, 15(6), p. e0234027. doi: 10.1371/journal.pone.0234027.

Bussau, V. A. *et al.* (2002), 'Carbohydrate loading in human muscle: an improved 1-day protocol', *Eur. J. Appl. Physiol.*, vol. 87, pp. 290–5.

Butterfield G. E. (1996), 'Ergogenic Aids: Evaluating sport nutrition products', *Int. Sport Nutr.*, vol. 6, pp. 191–7.

Byrne, S. and McLean, N. (2002), 'Elite athletes: effects of the pressure to be thin', *Journal of Science and Medicine in Sport*, 5(2), pp. 80–94. doi: 10.1016/s1440-2440(02)80029-9.

Cahill, C. F. (1976), 'Starvation in Man', *J. Clin. Endocrinol. Metab.*, vol. 5, pp. 397–415.

Calder, P. C. (2013), 'n-3 fatty acids, inflammation and immunity: new mechanisms to explain old actions', *The Proceedings of the Nutrition Society*, 72(3), pp. 326–336. doi: 10.1017/S0029665113001031.

Calder, P. C. (2020), 'Nutrition, immunity and COVID-19', *BMJ nutrition, prevention & health*, 3(1), pp. 74–92. doi: 10.1136/bmjnph-2020-000085.

Cameron S. L. *et al.* (2010), 'Increased blood pH but not performance with sodium bicarbonate supplementation in elite rugby union players', *Int. J. Sport Nutr. Exerc. Metab.*, vol. 20(4), pp. 307–21.

Campbell, B. *et al.* (2013), 'International Society of Sports Nutrition position stand: energy drinks', *Journal of the International Society of Sports Nutrition*, 10(1), p. 1. doi: 10.1186/1550-2783-10-1.

Campbell, W. W. *et al.* (1995), 'Effects of resistance training and dietary protein intake in protein metabolism in older adults', *Am. J. Physiol.*, Vol 268, pp. 1143–53.

Candow, D. G. *et al.* (2001), 'Effect of glutamine supplementation combined with resistance training in young adults', *Eur. J. Appl. Physiol.*, vol. 86(2), pp. 142–9.

Candow, D. G. *et al.* (2006), 'Effect of whey and soya protein supplementation combined with resistance training in young adults', *Int. J. Sports Nutr. Exerc. Metab.*, vol. 16, pp. 233–44.

Candow, D. G., Chilibeck, P. D. and Forbes, S. C. (2014), 'Creatine supplementation and aging musculoskeletal health', *Endocrine*, 45(3), pp. 354–coyle361. doi: 10.1007/s12020-013-0070-4.

Cann, C. E. *et al.* (1984), 'Decreased spinal mineral content in amenhorreic women', *JAMA,* vol. 251, pp. 626–9.

Cannell, J. *et al.* (2009), 'Athletic performance and vitamin D', *Med. Sci. Sports Exerc.*, vol. 41, pp. 1102–10.

Carbon, R. (2002), 'The female athlete triad does not exist', *Sports Care News,* 26, pp. 3–5.

Carr, A. J. (2011), 'Effects of acute alkalosis and acidosis on performance: a meta-analysis', *Sports Med.*, vol. 41(10), pp. 801–14.

Carswell, A. T. *et al.* (2018), 'Influence of Vitamin D Supplementation by Sunlight or Oral D3 on Exercise Performance', *Medicine and Science in Sports and Exercise*, 50(12), pp. 2555–2564. doi: 10.1249/MSS.0000000000001721.

Carter, J. M. *et al.* (2004), 'The effect of carbohydrate mouth rinse on 1-h cycle time-trial performance', *Med. Sci. Sports Exerc.*, vol. 36, pp. 2107–11.

Castell, L. M. and Newsholme, E. A. (1997), 'The effects of oral glutamine supplementation on athletes after prolonged exhaustive exercise', *Nutrition*, vol. 13, pp. 738–42.

Castell, L. M., Poortmans, J. R. and Newsholme, E. A. (1996), 'Does glutamine have a role in reducing infections in athletes?', *European Journal of Applied Physiology and Occupational Physiology*, 73(5), pp. 488–490. doi: 10.1007/BF00334429.

Cermak N. M. *et al.* (2012), 'Nitrate supplementation's improvement of 10 km time-trial performance in trained cyclists'. *Int. J. Sport Nutr. Exerc. Metab.*, vol. 1, pp. 64–71.

Chaix, A. *et al.* (2014), 'Time-restricted feeding is a prevencole tative and therapeutic intervention against diverse nutritional challenges', *Cell Metabolism*, 20(6), pp. 991–1005. doi: 10.1016/j.cmet.2014.11.001.

Chen, Z. *et al.* (2005), 'Postmenopausal hormone therapy and body composition--a substudy of the estrogen plus progestin trial of the Women's Health Initiative', *The American Journal of Clinical Nutrition*, 82(3), pp. 651–656. doi: 10.1093/ajcn.82.3.651.

Cheung, S. S. *et al.* (2015), 'Separate and combined effects of dehydration and thirst sensation on exercise performance in the heat'. *Scand. J. Med. Sci. Sports,* vol. 25, Suppl. 1, pp. 104–11.

Cheuvront, S. N., Carter, R., and and Sawka, M. N. (2003), 'Fluid balance and endurance exercise performance', *Current Sports Medicine Reports,* vol. 2 pp. 202–8.

Cheuvront, S. N., Montain, S. J. and Sawka, M. N. (2007), 'Fluid replacement and performance during the marathon', *Sports Medicine (Auckland, N.Z.),* 37(4–5), pp. 353–357. doi: 10.2165/00007256-200737040-00020.

Chowdhury, E. A. *et al.* (2015), 'Carbohydrate-rich breakfast attenuates glycaemic, insulinaemic and ghrelin response to *ad libitum* lunch relative to morning fasting in lean adults'. *Br. J. Nutr.,* vol. 114(1), pp. 98–107.

Chowdhury, R. *et al.* (2014), 'Association of dietary, circulating, and supplement fatty acids with coronary risk: A systematic review and meta-analysis', *Ann. Intern. Med.,* vol. 160(6), pp. 398–406.

Christensen, E. H. and Hansen, O. (1939), 'Arbeitsfähigheit und Ernährung', *Skand. Arch. Physiol.,* vol. 81, pp. 160–71.

Chryssanthopoulos, C. *et al.* (2002), 'The effect of a high carbohydrate meal on endurance running capacity', *Int. J. Sport Nutr.,* vol. 12, pp. 157–71.

Churchward-Venne, T. A. *et al.* (2012), 'Supplementation of a suboptimal protein dose with leucine or essential amino acids: effects on myofibrillar protein synthesis at rest and following resistance exercise in men', *The Journal of Physiology,* 590(11), pp. 2751–2765. doi: 10.1113/jphysiol.2012.228833.

Churchward-Venne, T. A. *et al.* (2020), 'Dose-response effects of dietary protein on muscle protein synthesis during recovery from endurance exercise in young men: a double-blind randomized trial', *The American Journal of Clinical Nutrition,* 112(2), pp. 303–317. doi: 10.1093/ajcn/nqaa073.

Churuangsuk, C. *et al.* (2018), 'Low-carbohydrate diets for overweight and obesity: a systematic review of the systematic reviews', *Obesity Reviews: An Official Journal of the International Association for the Study of Obesity,* 19(12), pp. 1700–1718. doi: 10.1111/obr.12744.

Ciuris, C. *et al.* (2019), 'A Comparison of Dietary Protein Digestibility, Based on DIAAS Scoring, in Vegetarian and Non-Vegetarian Athletes', *Nutrients,* 11(12). doi: 10.3390/nu11123016.

Clark, J. F. (1997), 'Creatine and phosphocreatine: a review'. , *J. Athletic Training,* vol. 32(1), pp. 45–50.

Clark, N. (1995), 'Nutrition quackery: when claims are too good to be true'. , *Phys. Sports Med.,* vol. 23, pp. 7–8.

Clayton D. J. *et al.* (2015), 'Effect of breakfast omission on energy intake and evening exercise performance', *Med. Sci. Sports Exerc.,* vol. 47(12), pp. 2645–52.

Clayton, D. J. and James, L. (2015), 'The effect of breakfast on appetite regulation, energy balance and exercise performance', *Proc. Nutr. Soc.,* vol. 14, pp. 1–9 (Epub ahead of print).

Close, G. L., Cobley, R. J., Owens, D. J. *et al.* (2013a8), 'Assessment of vitamin D concentration in non-supplemented professional athletes and healthy adults during the winter months in the UK: implications for skeletal muscle function', *J. Sports Sci.,* vol. 31(4), pp. 344–53.

Close, G. L., *et al.* (2013b), 'The effects of vitamin D3 supplementation on serum total 25(OH) D concentration and physical performance: a randomised dose-response study', *Br. J. Sports Med.,* vol. 47, pp. 692–6.

Close, G. L., Kasper, A. M. and Morton, J. P. (2019), 'From Paper to Podium: Quantifying the Translational Potential of Performance Nutrition Research', *Sports Medicine,* 49(1), pp. 25–37. doi: 10.1007/s40279-018-1005-2.

Cobb, K. L. *et al.* (2003), 'Disordered eating, menstrual irregularity and bone mineral density in female runners', *Med. Sci. Sports Exerc.,* vol. 35, pp. 711–19.

Cochran, A. J. R. *et al.* (2010), 'Carbohydrate feeding during recovery alters the skeletal muscle metabolic response to repeated sessions of high-intensity interval exercise in humans', *Journal of Applied Physiology (Bethesda, Md.: 1985),* 108(3), pp. 628–636. doi: 10.1152/japplphysiol.00659.2009.

Cockburn, E. *et al.* (2008), 'Acute milk-based protein-CHO supplementation attenuates exercise-induced muscle damage', *Appl. Physiol. Nutr. Metab.,* Aug; 33(4): 775–83.

Cockburn, E., Robson-Ansley, P., Hayes, P. R., Stevenson, E. (2012), 'Effect of volume of milk consumed on the attenuation of exercise-induced muscle damage', *Eur. J. Appl. Physiol.,* Jan 7. (Epub ahead of print.)

Coggan, A. R. and Coyle, E. F. (1987), 'Reversal of fatigue during prolonged exercise by carbohydrate infusion or ingestion'. *J. Appl. Physiol.,* vol. 63, pp. 2388–95.

Coggan, A. R. and Coyle, E. F. (1991), 'Carbohydrate ingestion during prolonged exercise: effects on metabolism and performance'. In J. Holloszy (ed.), *Exercise and Sports Science Reviews*, vol. 19 (Williams and Wilkins), pp. 1–40.

Cole, T. J., Bellizzi, M., Flegal, K. and Dietz, W. H. (2000), 'Establishing a standard definition for child overweight and obesity worldwide: international survey'. *British Medical Journal*, vol. 320, pp. 1240–3.

Collins, J. *et al.* (2021), 'UEFA expert group statement on nutrition in elite football. Current evidence to inform practical recommendations and guide future research', *British Journal of Sports Medicine*, 55(8), p. 416. doi: 10.1136/bjsports-2019-101961.

Cook, M. D. *et al.* (2015), 'New Zealand blackcurrant extract improves cycling performance and fat oxidation in cyclists'. *Eur. J. Appl. Physiol.,* vol. 115(11), pp. 2357–65.

Cooper, R. *et al.* (2012), 'Creatine supplementation with specific view to exercise/sports performance: an update'. *J. Int. Soc. Sports Nutr.,* vol. 9, p. 33.

Corder, K. E. *et al.* (2016), 'Effects of short-term docosahexaenoic acid supplementation on markers of inflammation after eccentric strength exercise in women'. *J. Sports Sci. Med.,* vol 15, pp. 176–83.

Costa, R. J. S. *et al.* (2017) (a) 'Systematic review: exercise-induced gastrointestinal syndrome-implications for health and intestinal disease', *Alimentary Pharmacology & Therapeutics*, 46(3), pp. 246–265. doi: 10.1111/apt.14157.

Costa, Ricardo J. S. *et al.* (2017) (b), 'Gut-training: the impact of two weeks repetitive gut-challenge during exercise on gastrointestinal status, glucose availability, fuel kinetics, and running performance', *Applied Physiology, Nutrition, and Metabolism = Physiologie Appliquee, Nutrition Et Metabolisme*, 42(5), pp. 547–557. doi: 10.1139/apnm-2016-0453.

Costill, D. L. (1985), 'Carbohydrate nutrition before, during and after exercise'. *Fed. Proc.,* vol. 44, pp. 364–368.

Costill, D. L. (1986), *Inside Running: Basics of Sports Physiology* (Benchmark Press), p. 189.

Costill, D. L. (1988), 'Carbohydrates for exercise: dietary demands for optimal performance'. *Int. J. Sports Med.,* vol. 9, pp. 1–18.

Costill, D. L. and Hargreaves, M. (1992), 'Carbohydrate nutrition and fatigue'. *Sports Med.,* vol. 13, pp. 86–92.

Costill, D. L. *et al.* (1971), 'Muscle glycogen utilisation during prolonged exercise on successive days'. *J. Appl. Physiol.,* vol. 31, pp. 834–8.

Cox, A. J., Pyne, D. B., Saunders, P. U., and and Fricker, P. A. (2008), 'Oral administration of the probiotic Lactobacillus fermentum VRI-003 and mucosal immunity in endurance athletes'. Br. *J. Sports Med.* (Epub Feb. 13).

Cox, G. *et al.* (2002), 'Acute creatine supplementation and performance during a field test simulating match play in elite female soccer players'. *Int. J. Sport Nutr.,* vol. 12, pp. 33–46.

Cox, G. R. *et al.* (2010), 'Daily training with high carbohydrate availability increases exogenous carbohydrate oxidation during endurance cycling', *Journal of Applied Physiology*, 109(1), pp. 126–134. doi: 10.1152/japplphysiol.00950.2009.

Cox, P. J. *et al.* (2016), 'Nutritional Ketosis Alters Fuel Preference and Thereby Endurance Performance in Athletes', *Cell Metabolism*, 24(2), pp. 256–268. doi: 10.1016/j.cmet.2016.07.010.

Coyle, E. (2004), 'Fluid and fuel intake during exercise'. *J. Sports Sci.,* vol. 22, pp. 39–55.

Coyle, E. F. (1988), 'Carbohydrates and athletic performance'. *Sports Sci. Exch. Sports Nutr.,* Gatorade Sports Science Institute, vol. 1.

Coyle, E. F. (1991), 'Timing and method of increased carbohydrate intake to cope with heavy training, competition and recovery'. *J. Sports Sci.,* vol. 9 (suppl.), pp. 29–52.

Coyle, E. F. (1995), 'Substrate utilization during exercise in active people'. *Am. J. Clin. Nutr.,* vol. 61 (suppl), pp. 968–79.

Coyle, E. F. and Coggan, A. R. (1984), 'Effectiveness of carbohydrate feeding in delaying fatigue during prolonged exercise', *Sports Medicine (Auckland, N.Z.)*, 1(6), pp. 446–458. doi: 10.2165/00007256-198401060-00004.

Coyle, E. F. *et al.* (1986), 'Muscle glycogen utilization during prolonged strenuous exercise when fed carbohydrate', *Journal of Applied Physiology (Bethesda, Md.: 1985)*, 61(1), pp. 165–172. doi: 10.1152/jappl.1986.61.1.165.

Craddock, J. *et al.* (2015), 'Vegetarian and omnivorous nutrition – comparing physical performance'. *Int. J. Sport Nutr. Exerc. Metab.,* Nov 16 (Epub ahead of print).

Craig, W. J., Mangels, A. R.; American Dietetic Association (2009), Position of the American Dietetic Association: vegetarian diets'. *J. Am. Diet. Assoc.,* vol. 109(7), pp. 1266–82.

Craven, J. *et al.* (2021), 'The Effect of Consuming Carbohydrate With and Without Protein on the Rate of Muscle Glycogen Re-synthesis During Short-Term Post-exercise Recovery: a Systematic Review and

Meta-analysis', *Sports Medicine – Open*, 7(1), p. 9. doi: 10.1186/s40798-020-00297-0.

Cribb P. J. *et al.* (2006), 'The effect of whey isolate and resistance training on strength, body composition and plasma glutamine'. *Int. J. Sports Nutr. Exerc. Metab.*, vol. 16, pp. 494–509.

Cronise, R. J., Sinclair, D. A. and Bremer, A. A. (2017), 'Oxidative Priority, Meal Frequency, and the Energy Economy of Food and Activity: Implications for Longevity, Obesity, and Cardiometabolic Disease', *Metabolic Syndrome and Related Disorders*, 15(1), pp. 6–17. doi: 10.1089/met.2016.0108.

Crooks, C. V. *et al.* (2006), 'The effect of bovine colostrum supplementation on salivary IgA in distance runners'. *Int. J. Sport Nutr. Exerc. Metab.*, vol. 16, pp. 47–64.

Crowe, F. L. *et al.* (2013), 'Risk of hospitalization or death from ischemic heart disease among British vegetarians and nonvegetarians: results from the EPIC-Oxford cohort study', *The American Journal of Clinical Nutrition*, 97(3), pp. 597–603. doi: 10.3945/ajcn.112.044073.

Crowe, M. J., Weatherson, J. N., Bowden, B. F. (2006), 'Effects of dietary leucine supplementation on exercise performance'. *Eur. J. Appl. Physiol.*, vol. 97(6), p. 664.

Cupisti, A. *et al.* (2002), 'Nutrition knowledge and dietary composition in Italian female athletes and non-athletes'. *Int. J. Sport Nutr.*, vol. 12, pp. 207–19.

Currell, K. and Jeukendrup, A. E. (2008), 'Superior endurance performance with ingestion of multiple transportable carbohydrates'. *Med. Sci. Sports Exerc.*, vol. 40(2), pp. 275–81.

Dangin, M. *et al.* (2001), 'The digestion rate of protein is an independent regulating factor of postprandial protein retention'. *Am. Physiol. Soc. Abstracts*, vol. 7: 022E.

Danz, M. *et al.* (2016), 'Hyponatremia among triathletes in the Ironman European Championship'. *N. Engl. J. Med.*, vol. 374, pp. 997–9.

Daries, H. N., Noakes, T. D. and Dennis, S. C. (2000), 'Effect of fluid intake volume on 2-h running performances in a 25 degrees C environment', *Medicine and Science in Sports and Exercise*, 32(10), pp. 1783–1789. doi: 10.1097/00005768-200010000-00019.

Darling, A. L. *et al.* (2019), 'Dietary protein and bone health across the life-course: an updated systematic review and meta-analysis over 40 years', *Osteoporosis international: a journal established as result of cooperation between the European Foundation for Osteoporosis and the National Osteoporosis Foundation of the USA*, 30(4), pp. 741–761. doi: 10.1007/s00198-019-04933-8.

Davey, G. K. *et al.* (2003), 'EPIC-Oxford: Lifestyle characteristics and nutrient intakes in a cohort of 33,883 meat-eaters and 31,546 non-meat-eaters in the UK'. *Public Health Nutrition*, vol. 6(3), pp. 259–68.

David, L. A. *et al.* (2014), 'Diet rapidly and reproducibly alters the human gut microbiome', *Nature*, 505(7484), pp. 559–563. doi: 10.1038/nature12820.

Davis, C. (1993), 'Body image, dieting behaviours and personality factors: a study of high-performance female athletes'. *Int. J. Sport Psych.*, vol. 23, pp. 179–92.

Davis, J. M. *et al.* (1988), 'Carbohydrate-electrolyte drinks: effects on endurance cycling in the heat'. *Am. J. Clin. Nutr.*, vol. 48, pp. 1023–30.

Davis, S. R. *et al.* (2012), 'Understanding weight gain at menopause', *Climacteric*, 15(5), pp. 419–429. doi: 10.3109/13697137.2012.707385.

Davison, G. (2012), 'Bovine colostrum and immune function after exercise'. *Med. Sport Sci.* vol. 59, pp. 62–9.

de Ataide e Silva, T. *et al.* (2013), 'Can carbohydrate mouth rinse improve performance during exercise? A systematic review'. *Nutrients*, Dec 19, 6(1), pp. 1–10. doi: 10.3390/nu6010001.

de Oliveira Otto, M. C., Mozaffarian, D., Kromhout, D. *et al.* (2012), 'Dietary intake of saturated fat by food source and incident cardio vascular disease: the multi-ethnic study of atherosclerosis'. *Am. J. of Clin. Nutr.*, vol. 96(2), pp. 397–404.

de Oliveira, E. P. and Burini, R. C. (2014), 'Carbohydrate-dependent, exercise-induced gastrointestinal distress', *Nutrients*, 6(10), pp. 4191–4199. doi: 10.3390/nu6104191.

de Oliveira, E. P., Burini, R. C. and Jeukendrup, A. (2014), 'Gastrointestinal Complaints During Exercise: Prevalence, Etiology, and Nutritional Recommendations', *Sports Medicine (Auckland, N.z.)*, 44(Suppl 1), pp. 79–85. doi: 10.1007/s40279-014-0153-2.

De Souza, M. J. *et al.* (2007), 'Drive for thinness score is a proxy indicator of energy deficiency in exercising women', *Appetite*, 48(3), pp. 359–367. doi: 10.1016/j.appet.2006.10.009.

De Souza, R. J. *et al.* (2015), 'Intake of saturated and trans unsaturated fatty acids and risk of all cause mortality, cardiovascular disease, and type 2 diabetes: systematic review and meta-analysis of observational studies'. *BMJ*, vol. 351, h3978.

De Souza, R. J. *et al.* (2015), 'Intake of saturated and trans unsaturated fatty acids and risk of all cause mortality, cardiovascular disease, and type 2 diabetes: systematic review and meta-analysis of observational studies'. *BMJ*, vol. 351, h3978.

DellaValle, D. M. (2013), 'Iron supplementation for female athletes: effects on iron status and performance outcomes', *Current Sports Medicine Reports*, 12(4), pp. 234–239. doi: 10.1249/JSR.0b013e31829a6f6b.

DeMarco, H. M. *et al.* (1999), *Med. Sci. Sports Ex.*, vol. 31(1), pp. 164–70.

Department of Health & Social Care (2016), 'UK Chief Medical Officers' Low Risk Drinking Guidelines'.

Department of Health & Social Care (2019), 'UK Chief Medical Officers' Physical Activity Guidelines'.

Department of Health (1991), 'Dietary Reference Values for Food Energy and Nutrients for the United Kingdom'. London: HMSO.

Department of Health (2004), 'At least five a week: Evidence on the impact of physical activity and its relationship to health. A report from the Chief Medical Officer'.

Derave, W. *et al.* (2007), 'Beta-alanine supplementation augments muscle carnosine content and attenuates fatigue during repeated isokinetic contraction bouts in trained sprinters'. *J. Appl. Physiol.*, vol. 103, pp. 1736–43.

Desbrow, B. *et al.* (2004), 'Carbohydrate-electrolyte feedings and 1 h time-trial cycling performance'. *Int. J. Sport Nutr. Exerc. Metab.*, vol. 14, pp. 541–9.

Desbrow, B. *et al.* (2012), 'The effects of different doses of caffeine on endurance cycling time trial performance', *Journal of Sports Sciences*, 30(2), pp. 115–120. doi: 10.1080/02640414.2011.632431.

Desbrow, B. *et al.* (2014a), 'Comparing the rehydration potential of different milk-based drinks to a carbohydrate-electrolyte beverage'. *Appl. Physiol. Nutr. Metab.*, vol. 39(12), pp. 1366–72.

Desbrow, B. *et al.* (2014b), 'Sports Dietitians Australia position statement: sports nutrition for the adolescent athlete', *International Journal of Sport Nutrition and Exercise Metabolism*, 24(5), pp. 570–584. doi: 10.1123/ijsnem.2014-0031.

Deutz, N. E. P. *et al.* (2014), 'Protein intake and exercise for optimal muscle function with aging: Recommendations from the ESPEN Expert Group'. *Clin. Nutr.*, vol. 33(6), pp. 929–36.

Devries, M. C. and Phillips, S. M. (2014), 'Creatine supplementation during resistance training in older adults-a meta-analysis', *Medicine and Science in Sports and Exercise*, 46(6), pp. 1194–1203. doi: 10.1249/MSS.0000000000000220.

Devries, M. C. *et al.* (2018), 'Changes in Kidney Function Do Not Differ between Healthy Adults Consuming Higher- Compared with Lower- or Normal-Protein Diets: A Systematic Review and Meta-Analysis', *The Journal of Nutrition*, 148(11), pp. 1760–1775. doi: 10.1093/jn/nxy197.

Dodd, H. *et al.* (2011), 'Calculating meal glycaemic index by using measured and published food values compared with directly measured meal glycaemic index'. *Am. J. Clin. Nutr.*, vol. 95, pp. 992–6.

Dodd, S. L. *et al.* (1993), 'Caffeine and exercise performance'. *Sports Med.*, vol. 15, pp. 14–23.

Donnelly, J. E. *et al.* (2009), 'American College of Sports Medicine Position Stand. Appropriate physical activity intervention strategies for weight loss and prevention of weight regain for adults', *Medicine and Science in Sports and Exercise*, 41(2), pp. 459–471. doi: 10.1249/MSS.0b013e3181949333.

Downes, J. W. (2002), 'The master's athlete: Defying aging'. *Topics in Clinical Chiropractic*, vol. 9(2), pp. 53–9.

Drew, M. *et al.* (2018), 'Prevalence of illness, poor mental health and sleep quality and low energy availability prior to the 2016 Summer Olympic Games', *British Journal of Sports Medicine*, 52(1), pp. 47–53. doi: 10.1136/bjsports-2017-098208.

Drew, M. *et al.* (2018), 'Prevalence of illness, poor mental health and sleep quality and low energy availability prior to the 2016 Summer Olympic Games', *British Journal of Sports Medicine*, 52(1), pp. 47–53. doi: 10.1136/bjsports-2017-098208.

Drew, M. K. *et al.* (2017), 'A multifactorial evaluation of illness risk factors in athletes preparing for the Summer Olympic Games', *Journal of Science and Medicine in Sport*, 20(8), pp. 745–750. doi: 10.1016/j.jsams.2017.02.010.

Drinkwater, B. L. (1986), 'Bone mineral content after resumption of menses in amenorrheic athletes'. *JAMA*, vol. 256, pp. 380–2.

Drinkwater, B. L. *et al.* (1984), 'Bone mineral content of amenorrheic and eumenorrheic athletes'. *New England. J. Med.*, vol. 311, pp. 277–81.

Drouin-Chartier, J.-P. *et al.* (2016), 'Comprehensive Review of the Impact of Dairy Foods and Dairy Fat on Cardiometabolic Risk', *Advances in Nutrition*, 7(6), pp. 1041–1051. doi: 10.3945/an.115.011619.

Drummond, M. J. and Rasmussen, B. B. (2008), 'Leucine-enriched nutrients and the regulation of mammalian target of rapamycin signalling and human skeletal muscle protein synthesis. *Curr. Opin. Clin. Nutr. Metab. Care,* vol. 11, pp. 222–6.

Ducker, K. J., Dawson, B., Wallman, K. E. (2013), 'Effect of beta-alanine supplementation on 800-m running performance'. *Int. J. Sport Nutr. Exerc. Metab.*, vol. 23(6), pp. 554–61.

Dueck, C. A. *et al.* (1996), 'Role of energy balance in athletic menstrual dysfunction'. *Int. J. Sport Nutr.*, vol. 6, pp. 165–90.

Duiven, E. *et al.* (2021), 'Undeclared Doping Substances are Highly Prevalent in Commercial Sports Nutrition Supplements', *Journal of Sports Science and Medicine*, pp. 328–338. doi: 10.52082/jssm.2021.328.

Dulloo, A. G. and Jacquet, J. (1998), 'Adaptive reduction in basal metabolic rate in response to food deprivation in humans: a role for feedback signals from fat stores', *The American Journal of Clinical Nutrition*, 68(3), pp. 599–606. doi: 10.1093/ajcn/68.3.599.

Dulloo, A. G. *et al.* (1999), 'Efficacy of a green tea extract rich in catechin polyphenols and caffeine in increasing 24 hour energy expenditure and fat oxidation in humans'. *Am. J. Clin. Nutr.*, vol. 70, pp. 1040–5.

Durnin, J. V. G. A. and Womersley, J. (1974), 'Body fat assessed from total body density and its estimation from skinfold thickness: measurements on 481 men and women ages from 16 to 72 Years'. *Brit. J. Nutr.*, vol. 32, p. 77.

Easton, C. *et al.* (2007), 'Creatine and glycerol hyperhydration in trained subjects before exercise in the heat'. *Int. J. Sports Nutr. Exerc. Metab.*, vol. 17, pp. 70–91.

Eckerson, J. M., Bull, A. J., Baechle, T. R., Fischer, C. A., O'Brien, D. C., Moore, G. A., Yee, J. C., Pulverenti, T. S. (2013), 'Acute ingestion of sugar-free Red Bull energy drink has no effect on upper body strength and muscular endurance in resistance trained men'. *J. Strength Cond. Res.*, vol. 27(8), pp. 2248–54.

Edwards, J. R. *et al.* (1993), 'Energy balance in highly trained female endurance runners'. *Med. Sci. Sports Ex.,* vol. 25(12), pp. 1398–404.

EFSA (2015), 'Scientific and technical assistance on food intended for sportspeople'. http://www.efsa.europa.eu/sites/default/files/scientific_output/files/main_documents/871e.pdf accessed March 2016.

EFSA Panel on Dietetic Products, Nutrition, and Allergies (2010), 'Scientific opinion on Dietary Reference Values for water'. *EFSA Journal,* vol. 8(3), p. 1459.

Egli, L. *et al.* (2013), 'Exercise prevents fructose-induced hypertriglyceridemia in healthy young subjects'. *Diabetes,* vol. 62(7), pp. 2259–65.

Eisinger, M. (1994), 'Nutrient intake of endurance runners with lacto-ovo vegetarian diet and regular Western diet'. *Z. Ernahrungswiss,* vol. 33, pp. 217–29.

Elliot, T. A. *et al.* (2006), 'Milk ingestion stimulates net muscle protein synthesis following resistance exercise,', ' *Med. Sci. Sports Exer.,* vol. 384, pp. 667–74.

English, K. L. *et al.* (2016), 'Leucine partially protects muscle mass and function during bed rest in middle-aged adults', *The American Journal of Clinical Nutrition*, 103(2), pp. 465–473. doi: 10.3945/ajcn.115.112359.

Erlenbusch, M. *et al.* (2005), 'Effect of high fat or high carbohydrate diets on endurance exercise: a meta-analysis'. *Int. J. Sport Nutr. Exerc. Metab.*, vol. 14, pp. 1–14.

Estaki, M. *et al.* (2016), 'Cardiorespiratory fitness as a predictor of intestinal microbial diversity and distinct metagenomic functions', *Microbiome*, 4. doi: 10.1186/s40168-016-0189-7.

Estruch, R. *et al.* (2013), 'Primary prevention of cardiovascular disease with a Mediterranean diet'. *N. Engl. J. Med.,* vol. 368, pp. 1279–90.

European Food Safety Authority EFSA (2009),. 'Scientific Opinion: Labelling reference intake values for n-3 and n-6 polyunsaturated fatty acids', *The EFSA Journal,*. 2009; 1176, 1–11.

Evans, G. H. *et al.* (2017), 'Optimizing the restoration and maintenance of fluid balance after exercise-induced dehydration', *Journal of Applied Physiology (Bethesda, Md.: 1985)*, 122(4), pp. 945–951. doi: 10.1152/japplphysiol.00745.2016.

Evans, M. *et al.* (2019), 'No Benefit of Ingestion of a Ketone Monoester Supplement on 10-km Running Performance', *Medicine and Science in Sports and Exercise*, 51(12), pp. 2506–2515. doi: 10.1249/MSS.0000000000002065.

Fagerberg, P. (2018), 'Negative Consequences of Low Energy Availability in Natural Male Bodybuilding: A Review', *International Journal of Sport Nutrition and Exercise Metabolism*, 28(4), pp. 385–402. doi: 10.1123/ijsnem.2016-0332.

Fairchild, T. J. *et al.* (2002), 'Rapid carbohydrate loading after a short bout of near maximal-intensity exercise'. *Med. Sci. Sports Exer.*, pp. 980–6.

Farajian, P. *et al.* (2004), 'Dietary intake and nutritional practices of elite Greek aquatic athletes'. *Int. J. Sport Nutr. Exerc. Metab.*, vol 14, pp. 574–85.

Febbraio, M. A. and Stewart, K. L. (1996), 'CHO feeding before prolonged exercise: effect of glycaemic index on muscle glycogenolysis and exercise performance'. *J. Appl. Phsyiol.*, vol. 81, pp. 1115–20.

Febbraio, M. A. *et al.* (2000), 'Effects of carbohydrate ingestion before and during exercise on glucose kinetics and performance'. *J. Appl. Physiol.*, vol. 89, pp. 2220–6.

Feinman, R. D. *et al.* (2015), 'Dietary carbohydrate restriction as the first approach in diabetes management: critical review and evidence base', *Nutrition (Burbank, Los Angeles County, Calif.)*, 31(1), pp. 1–13. doi: 10.1016/j.nut.2014.06.011.

Ference, B. A. *et al.* (2017), 'Low-density lipoproteins cause atherosclerotic cardiovascular disease. 1. Evidence from genetic, epidemiologic, and clinical studies. A consensus statement from the European Atherosclerosis Society Consensus Panel', *European Heart Journal*, 38(32), pp. 2459–2472. doi: 10.1093/eurheartj/ehx144.

Ferguson-Stegall, L. *et al.* (2011), 'Aerobic exercise training adaptations are increased by post-exercise carbohydrate-protein supplementation'. *J. Nutr. Metab.*, Epub Jun 9.

Fiala, K. A. *et al.* (2004), 'Rehydration with a caffeinated beverage during the non-exercise periods of 3 consecutive days of 2-a-day practices'. *Int. J. Sport Nutr. Exerc. Metab.*, vol 14. pp. 419–29.

Fleck, S. J. and Reimers, K. J. (1994), 'The practice of making weight: does it affect performance?' *Strength and Cond.*, vol. 1, pp. 66–7.

Flood, T. R. *et al.* (2020), 'Addition of pectin-alginate to a carbohydrate beverage does not maintain gastrointestinal barrier function during exercise in hot-humid conditions better than carbohydrate ingestion alone', *Applied Physiology, Nutrition, and Metabolism = Physiologie Appliquee, Nutrition Et Metabolisme*, 45(10), pp. 1145–1155. doi: 10.1139/apnm-2020-0118.

Fogelholm, M. (1994), 'Effects of bodyweight reduction on sports performance'. *Sports Med.*, vol. 18(14), pp. 249–67.

Fogelholm, M. (1995), 'Indicators of vitamin and mineral status in athletes' blood: a review'. *Int. J. Sports Nutr.*, vol. 5, pp. 267–84.

Food Standards Agency (2003), *Safe upper levels for vitamins and minerals* (HMSO).

Forbes, G. B. (2000), 'Body fat content influences the body composition response to nutrition and exercise', *Annals of the New York Academy of Sciences*, 904, pp. 359–365. doi: 10.1111/j.1749-6632.2000.tb06482.x.

Forbes, S. C., Candow, D. G., Little, J. P., *et al.* (2007), 'Effect of Red Bull energy drink on repeated Wingate cycle performance and bench-press muscle endurance'. *Int. J. Sport Nutr. Exerc. Metab.*, vol. 17(5), pp. 433–44.

Foster-Powell, K., Holt, S. and Brand-Miller, J. C. (2002), 'International table of glycaemic index and glycaemic load values: 2002'. *Am. J. Clin. Nutr.,* vol. 76, pp. 5–56.

Frankenfield D. C. *et al.* (2005), 'Comparison of predictive equations for Resting Metabolic Rate in healthy nonobese and obese adults: a systematic review'. *J. Am. Diet. Assoc.*, vol. 105, pp. 775–89.

Frentsos, J. A. and Baer, J. T. (1997), 'Increased energy and nutrient intake during training and competition improves elite triathletes' endurance performance'. *Int. J. Sport Nutr.*, vol. 7, pp. 61–71.

Funnell, M. P. *et al.* (2019), 'Blinded and unblinded hypohydration similarly impair cycling time trial performance in the heat in trained cyclists', *Journal of Applied Physiology (Bethesda, Md.: 1985)*, 126(4), pp. 870–879. doi: 10.1152/japplphysiol.01026.2018.

Gabel, K. *et al.* (2018), 'Effects of 8-hour time restricted feeding on body weight and metabolic disease risk factors in obese adults: A pilot study', *Nutrition and Healthy Aging*, 4(4), pp. 345–353. doi: 10.3233/NHA-170036.

Gaeini, A. A., Rahnama, N., Hamedinia, M. R. (2006), 'Effects of vitamin E supplementation on oxidative stress at rest and after exercise to exhaustion in athletic students'. *J. Sports Med. Phys. Fitness*, vol. 46(3), pp. 458–61.

Gallagher, D. et al. (2000) 'Healthy percentage body fat ranges: an approach for developing guidelines based on body mass index', *The American Journal of Clinical Nutrition*, 72(3), pp. 694–701. doi:10.1093/ajcn/72.3.694.

Gallagher, J. *et al.* (2018), 'Oral health and performance impacts in elite and professional athletes', *Community Dentistry and Oral Epidemiology*, 46(6), pp. 563–568. doi: https://doi.org/10.1111/cdoe.12392.

Galloway, S. D. R. and Maughan, R. (2000), 'The effects of substrate and fluid provision on thermoregulatory and metabolic responses to prolonged exercise in a hot environment'. *J. Sports Sci.*, vol. 18(5), pp. 339–51.

Ganio, M. S. *et al.* (2009), 'Effect of caffeine on sport-specific endurance performance: a systematic review', *Journal of Strength and Conditioning Research*, 23(1), pp. 315–324. doi: 10.1519/JSC.0b013e31818b979a.

Gant, N., Ali, A. and Foskett, A. (2010), 'The influence of caffeine and carbohydrate coingestion on simulated soccer performance'. *Int. J. Sport Nutr. Exerc. Metab.*, vol. 20, pp. 191–7.

Gardner, C. D. *et al.* (2018), 'Effect of Low-Fat vs Low-Carbohydrate Diet on 12-Month Weight Loss in Overweight Adults and the Association With Genotype Pattern or Insulin Secretion: The DIETFITS Randomized Clinical Trial', *JAMA*, 319(7), pp. 667–679. doi: 10.1001/jama.2018.0245.

Gardner, C. D. *et al.* (2019), 'Maximizing the intersection of human health and the health of the environment with regard to the amount and type of protein produced and consumed in the United States', *Nutrition Reviews*, 77(4), pp. 197–215. doi: 10.1093/nutrit/nuy073.

Garfinkel, P. E. and Garner, D. M. (1982), *Anorexia nervosa: a multidimensional perspective.* (Brunner/Mazel).

Garthe, I. and Maughan, R. J. (2018), 'Athletes and Supplements: Prevalence and Perspectives', *International Journal of Sport Nutrition and Exercise Metabolism*, 28(2), pp. 126–138. doi: 10.1123/ijsnem.2017-0429.

Garthe, I. *et al.* (2011), 'Effect of two different weight-loss rates on body composition and strength and power-related performance in elite athletes', *International Journal of Sport Nutrition and Exercise Metabolism*, 21(2), pp. 97–104. doi: 10.1123/ijsnem.21.2.97.

Garvican-Lewis, L. A. *et al.* (2018), 'Intravenous Iron Does Not Augment the Hemoglobin Mass Response to Simulated Hypoxia', *Medicine and Science in Sports and Exercise*, 50(8), pp. 1669–1678. doi: 10.1249/MSS.0000000000001608.

Gaskell, S. K. *et al.* (2020), 'Impact of 24-h high and low fermentable oligo-, di-, monosaccharide, and polyol diets on markers of exercise-induced gastrointestinal syndrome in response to exertional heat stress', *Applied Physiology, Nutrition, and Metabolism = Physiologie Appliquee, Nutrition Et Metabolisme*, 45(6), pp. 569–580. doi: 10.1139/apnm-2019-0187.

GBD 2016 Alcohol Collaborators (20182016), 'Alcohol use and burden for 195 countries and territories, 1990-2016: a systematic analysis for the Global Burden of Disease Study 2016', *Lancet (London, England)*, 392(10152), pp. 1015–1035. doi: 10.1016/S0140-6736(18)31310-2.

Gejl, K. D. and Nybo, L. (2021), 'Performance effects of periodized carbohydrate restriction in endurance trained athletes – a systematic review and meta-analysis', *Journal of the International Society of Sports Nutrition*, 18(1), p. 37. doi: 10.1186/s12970-021-00435-3.

German, J. B. *et al.* (2009), 'A reappraisal of the impact of dairy foods and milk fat on cardiovascular disease risk'. *European Journal of Nutrition*, vol. 48(4), pp. 191–203.

Geyer, H., Parr. M. K., Mareck, U., *et al.* (2004), 'Analysis of non-hormonal nutritional supplements for anabolic-androgenic steroids – results of an international study'. *Int. J. Sports Med.*, vol. 25(2), pp. 124–9.

Gibala, M. J. (2000), 'Nutritional supplementation and resistance exercise: what is the evidence for enhanced skeletal muscle hypertrophy?' *Can. J. Appl. Physiol.*, vol. 25(6), pp. 524–35.

Gilchrist, M., Winyard, P. G., and and Benjamin, N. (2010), 'Dietary nitrate – good or bad?' *Nitric Oxide*, vol. 22, pp. 104–9.

Gill, S. and Panda, S. (2015), 'A smartphone app reveals erratic diurnal eating patterns in humans that can be modulated for health benefits', *Cell metabolism*, 22(5), pp. 789–798. doi: 10.1016/j.cmet.2015.09.005.

Gilson, S. F. *et al.* (2009), 'Effects of chocolate milk consumption on markers of muscle recovery during intensified soccer training'. *Medicine and Science in Sports and Exercise*, vol. 41, p. S577.

Gisolphi, C. V. *et al.* (1992), 'Intestinal water absorption from select carbohydrate solutions in humans'. *J. Appl. Physiol.*, vol. 73, pp. 2142–50.

Gisolphi, C. V. *et al.* (1995), 'Effect of sodium concentration in a carbohydrate-electrolyte solution on intestinal absorption', *Med. Sci. Sports Ex.*, vol. 27(10), pp. 1414–20.

Gleeson, M. (2011), 'Nutrition and immunity', In *Diet, Immunity and Inflammation*, Calder, P. C. and Yaqoob, P (eds)) ,(Woodhead Publishing).

Gleeson, M. (2016), 'Immunological aspects of sport nutrition', *Immunology & Cell Biology*, 94(2), pp. 117–123. doi: https://doi.org/10.1038/icb.2015.109.

Gleeson, M. *et al.* (2008), 'Exercise and immune function: is there any evidence for probiotic benefit for sportspeople?' *Complete Nutrition*, vol. 8, pp. 35–7.

Gleeson, M., Nieman, D. C. and Pedersen, B. K. (2004), 'Exercise, nutrition and immune function', *Journal of Sports Sciences*, 22(1), pp. 115–125. doi: 10.1080/0264041031000140590.

Goldstone, A. P. *et al.* (2009), 'Fasting biases brain reward systems towards high-calorie foods', *Eur. J. Neurosci.*, vol 30(8), pp. 1625–35.

Gombart, A. F., Pierre, A. and Maggini, S. (2020), 'A Review of Micronutrients and the Immune System-Working in Harmony to Reduce the Risk of Infection', *Nutrients*, 12(1). doi: 10.3390/nu12010236.

Gomez-Cabrera *et al.* (2008), 'Oral administration of vitamin C decreases muscle mitochondrial biogenesis and hampers training-induced adaptations in endurance performance', *Am. J. Clin. Nutr.* 87(1), pp. 142–9.

Gontzea, I. *et al.* (1975), 'The influence of adaptation to physical effort on nitrogen balance in man', *Nutr. Rep. Int.*, vol. 22, pp. 213–16.

Gonzalez, J. T. *et al.* (2017), 'Glucose Plus Fructose Ingestion for Post-Exercise Recovery—Greater than the Sum of Its Parts?', *Nutrients*, 9(4), p. 344. doi: 10.3390/nu9040344.

Gonzalez-Alonzo, J. *et al.* (1992), 'Rehydration after exercise with common beverages and water', *Int. J. Sports Med.*, vol. 13, pp. 399–406.

Gordon, C. M. *et al.* (2017), 'Functional Hypothalamic Amenorrhea: An Endocrine Society Clinical Practice Guideline', *The Journal of Clinical Endocrinology and Metabolism*, 102(5), pp. 1413–1439. doi: 10.1210/jc.2017-00131.

Goulet, E. D. B. (2011), 'Effects of exercise-induced dehydration on time-trial exercise performance: a metaanalysis', *Brit. J. Sports Med.*, vol. 45, pp. 1149–56.

Goulet, E. D. B. (2013), 'Effect of exercise-induced dehydration on endurance performance: evaluating the impact of exercise protocols on outcomes using a meta-analytic procedure'. *Br. J. Sports Med.*, vol. 47(11), pp. 679–86.

Graham, T. E. and Spriet, L. L. (1991), 'Performance and metabolic responses to a high caffeine dose during prolonged exercise', *J. Appl. Physiol.*, vol. 71(6), pp. 2292–8.

Grandjean, A. (2000), 'The effect of caffeinated, non-caffeinated, caloric and non-caloric beverages on hydration', *J. Am. Coll. Nutr.*, vol. 19, pp. 591–600.

Gray-Donald, K. *et al.* (2014), 'Protein intake protects against weight loss in healthy community-dwelling older adults', *J. Nutr.* vol. 144, pp. 321–6.

Green, A. L. *et al.* (1996), 'Carbohydrate augments creatine accumulation during creatine supplementation in humans', *Am. J. Physiol.*, vol. 271, E821–6.

Greenhaff, P. L. (1997), 'Creatine supplementation and implications for exercise performance and guidelines for creatine supplementation', In A. Jeukendrup *et al.* (eds), *Advances in Training and Nutrition for Endurance Sports* (Maastricht: Novertis Nutrition Research Unit), pp. 8–11.

Greenwood, M. *et al.* (2003), 'Creatine supplementation during college football training does not increase the incidence of cramping or injury', *Molecular and Cellular Biochemistry*, 244(1–2), pp. 83–88.

Grgic, J. and Pickering, C. (2019), 'The effects of caffeine ingestion on isokinetic muscular strength: A meta-analysis', *Journal of Science and Medicine in Sport*, 22(3), pp. 353–360. doi: 10.1016/j.jsams.2018.08.016.

Grgic, J. *et al.* (2018), 'Effects of caffeine intake on muscle strength and power: a systematic review and meta-analysis', *Journal of the International Society of Sports Nutrition*, 15, p. 11. doi: 10.1186/s12970-018-0216-0.

Groen, B. *et al.* (2012), 'Intragastric protein administration stimulates overnight muscle protein synthesis in elderly men', *Am. J. Physiol. Endocrinol. Metab.*, vol. 302, pp. 52–60.

GSSI (1995), 'Roundtable on methods of weight gain in athletes'. *Sports Science Exchange*, vol. 6(3), pp. 1–4.

Gualano, B., *et al.* (2012), 'In sickness and in health: The widespread application of creatine supplementation', *Amino Acids*, vol. 43, pp. 519–29.

Guest, N. *et al.* (2018), 'Caffeine, CYP1A2 Genotype, and Endurance Performance in Athletes', *Medicine and Science in Sports and Exercise*, 50(8), pp. 1570–1578. doi: 10.1249/MSS.0000000000001596.

Guest, N. S. and Barr, S. (2005), 'Cognitive dietary restraint is associated with stress fractures in women runners', *Int. J. Sports Nutr. Exerc. Metab.*, vol. 15, pp. 147–59.

Guest, N. S. *et al.* (2021), 'International society of sports nutrition position stand: caffeine and exercise performance', *Journal of the International Society of Sports Nutrition*, 18(1), p. 1. doi: 10.1186/s12970-020-00383-4.

Hackney, A. C., Sinning, W. E. and Bruot, B. C. (1988), 'Reproductive hormonal profiles of endurance-trained and untrained males', *Medicine and Science in Sports and Exercise*, 20(1), pp. 60–65. doi: 10.1249/00005768-198802000-00009.

Haghighatdoost, F. *et al.* (2017), 'Association of vegetarian diet with inflammatory biomarkers: a systematic review and meta-analysis of observational studies',

Public Health Nutrition, 20(15), pp. 2713–2721. doi: 10.1017/S1368980017001768.

Hall, K. D. and Guo, J. (2017), 'Obesity Energetics: Body Weight Regulation and the Effects of Diet Composition', *Gastroenterology*, 152(7), pp. 1718-1727.e3. doi: 10.1053/j.gastro.2017.01.052.

Hall, Kevin D. *et al.* (2015), 'Calorie for calorie, dietary fat restriction results in more body fat loss than carbohydrate restriction in people with obesity', *Cell Metabolism*, vol. 22(3), pp. 427–36.

Halliday, T. *et al.* (2011), 'Vitamin D status relative to diet, lifestyle, injury and illness in college athletes', *Med. Sci. Sports Exerc.*, vol. 43, pp. 335–43.

Halliwell, B. and Gutteridge, J. M. C. (1985), *Free Radicals in Biology and Medicine* (Clarendon Press), pp. 162–4.

Hamilton, B. (2011), 'Vitamin D and athletic performance: the potential role of muscle', *Asian J. Sports Med.*, vol. 2(4), pp. 211–19.

Hammond, K. M. *et al.* (2019), 'Post-exercise carbohydrate and energy availability induce independent effects on skeletal muscle cell signalling and bone turnover: implications for training adaptation', *The Journal of Physiology*, 597(18), pp. 4779–4796. doi: https://doi.org/10.1113/JP278209.

Hanne, N., Dlin, R. and Rotstein, A. (1986), 'Physical fitness, anthropometric and metabolic parameters in vegetarian athletes'. *J. Sports Med. Phys. Fitness.*, vol. 26, pp. 180–5.

Hansen, A. K. *et al.* (2005), 'Skeletal muscle adaptation: training twice every second day vs. training once daily', *J. Appl. Physiol.*, vol 98(1), pp. 93–9.

Hao, Q. *et al.* (2011), 'Probiotics for preventing acute upper respiratory tract infections', *The Cochrane Database of Systematic Reviews*, (9), p. CD006895. doi: 10.1002/14651858.CD006895.pub2.

Hao, Q. *et al.* (2011), 'Probiotics for preventing acute upper respiratory tract infections', *The Cochrane Database of Systematic Reviews*, (9), p. CD006895. doi: 10.1002/14651858.CD006895.pub2.

Hao, Q., Dong, B. R. and Wu, T. (2015), 'Probiotics for preventing acute upper respiratory tract infections', *The Cochrane Database of Systematic Reviews*, (2), p. CD006895. doi: 10.1002/14651858.CD006895.pub3.

Hargreaves, M. and Snow, R. (2001), 'Amino acids and endurance exercise', *Int. J. Sport Nutr.*, vol. 11, pp. 133–145.

Hargreaves, M. *et al.* (2004), 'Pre-exercise carbohydrate and fat ingestion: effects on metabolism and performance', *J. Sports Sci.*, vol. 22(1), pp. 31–38.

Harris, R. C. (1998), 'Ergogenics 1', *Peak Performance*, vol. 112, pp. 2–6.

Harris, R. C. *et al.* (2006), 'The absorption of orally supplied beta-alanine and its effect on muscle carnosine synthesis in human vastus lateralis', *Amino Acids*, vol. 30(3), pp. 279–89.

Harrison, S. E. *et al.* (2021), 'Influence of Vitamin D Supplementation by Simulated Sunlight or Oral D3 on Respiratory Infection during Military Training', *Medicine and Science in Sports and Exercise*. doi: 10.1249/MSS.0000000000002604.

Hartman, J. W. *et al.* (2007), 'Consumption of fat-free fluid milk after resistance exercise promotes greater lean mass accretion than does consumption of soysoya or carbohydrate in young, novice, male weightlifters', *Am. J. Clin. Nutr.*, vol. 86(2), pp. 373–81.

Harvey, K. L., Holcomb, L. E. and Kolwicz, S. C. (2019), 'Ketogenic Diets and Exercise Performance', *Nutrients*, 11(10), p. 2296. doi: 10.3390/nu11102296.

Hatori, M. *et al.* (2012), 'Time-Restricted Feeding without Reducing Caloric Intake Prevents Metabolic Diseases in Mice Fed a High-Fat Diet', *Cell Metabolism*, 15(6), pp. 848–860. doi: 10.1016/j.cmet.2012.04.019.

Haub, M. D. (1998), 'Acute l-glutamine ingestion does not improve maximal effort exercise', *J. Sport Med. Phys. Fitness*, vol. 38, pp. 240–4.

Haub, M. D. *et al.* (2002), 'Effect of protein source on resistive-training-induced changes in body composition and muscle size in older men', *Am. J. Clin. Nutr.*, vol. 76, pp. 511–17.

Haussinger, D. *et al.* (1996), 'The role of cellular hydration in the regulation of cell functioning', *Biochem. J.*, vol. 31, pp. 697–710.

Havemann, L. *et al.* (2006), 'Fat adaptation followed by carbohydrate loading compromises high-intensity sprint performance', *J. Appl. Physiol.*, vol. 100(1), pp. 194–202.

Hawley, J. A. and Burke, L. M. (2010), 'Carbohydrate availability and training adaptation: effects on cell metabolism', *Exerc. Sports Sci. Rev.*, vol. 38, pp. 152–160.

Hawley, J. A. and Leckey, J. (2015), 'Carbohydrate dependence during prolonged, intense endurance exercise', *Sports Med.*, vol 45 (Suppl 1), pp. S5–S12.

Hawley, J. A. and Lessard, S. J. (2008), 'Exercise training-induced improvements in insulin action', *Acta Physiol* (Oxf), vol 192(1), pp. 127–35.

Hawley, J. *et al.* (1997), 'Carbohydrate loading and exercise performance', *Sports Med.*, vol. 24(1), pp. 1–10.

Hawley, J. *et al.* (2011), 'Nutritional modulation of training-induced skeletal muscle adaptations', *J. Appl. Physiol.*, vol. 100, pp. 834–45.

He, C.-S. *et al.* (2013), 'Influence of vitamin D status on respiratory infection incidence and immune function during 4 months of winter training in endurance sport athletes', *Exercise Immunology Review*, 19, pp. 86–101.

Heaney, R. P. (2011), 'Assessing vitamin D status', *Curr. Opin. Clin. Nutr. Metab. Care*, vol. 14, pp. 440–4.

Heaney, R. P. (2013), 'Health is better at serum 25(OH) D above 30ng/mL', *J. Steroid Biochem. Mol. Biol.*, vol. 136, pp. 224–8.

Hector, A. J. and Phillips, S. M. (2018), 'Protein Recommendations for Weight Loss in Elite Athletes: A Focus on Body Composition and Performance', *International Journal of Sport Nutrition and Exercise Metabolism*, 28(2), pp. 170–177. doi: 10.1123/ijsnem.2017-0273.

Heikura, I. A., Burke, L. M., *et al.* (2018) (a), 'Impact of Energy Availability, Health, and Sex on Hemoglobin-Mass Responses Following Live-High-Train-High Altitude Training in Elite Female and Male Distance Athletes', *International Journal of Sports Physiology and Performance*, 13(8), pp. 1090–1096. doi: 10.1123/ijspp.2017-0547.

Heikura, I. A., Uusitalo, A. L. T., *et al.* (2018) (b), 'Low Energy Availability Is Difficult to Assess but Outcomes Have Large Impact on Bone Injury Rates in Elite Distance Athletes', *International Journal of Sport Nutrition and Exercise Metabolism*, 28(4), pp. 403–411. doi: 10.1123/ijsnem.2017-0313.

Helge, J. W. *et al.* (2001), 'Fat utilisation during exercise: adaptation to a fat rich diet increases utilisation of plasma fatty acids and very low density lipoprotein-triacylglycerol in humans', *J. Physiol.*, vol. 537; 3, pp. 1009–20.

Helms, E. R. *et al.* (2014) (a), 'A systematic review of dietary protein during caloric restriction in resistance trained lean athletes: a case for higher intakes', *International Journal of Sport Nutrition and Exercise Metabolism*, 24(2), pp. 127–138. doi: 10.1123/ijsnem.2013-0054.

Helms, E. R. *et al.* (2014), 'A systematic review of dietary protein during caloric restriction in resistance trained lean athletes: a case for higher intakes'. *Int. J. Sport Nutr. Exerc. Metab.*, vol. 24(2), pp. 127–38.

Helms, E. R., Aragon, A. A. and Fitschen, P. J. (2014) (b), 'Evidence-based recommendations for natural bodybuilding contest preparation: nutrition and supplementation', *Journal of the International Society of Sports Nutrition*, 11(1), p. 20. doi: 10.1186/1550-2783-11-20.

Hemilä, H. (2011), Zinc lozenges may shorten the duration of colds: a systematic review. The open respiratory medicine journal, 5(1).

Hemilä, H. (2017), 'Zinc lozenges and the common cold: a meta-analysis comparing zinc acetate and zinc gluconate, and the role of zinc dosage', *JRSM open*, 8(5), p. 2054270417694291. doi: 10.1177/2054270417694291.

Hemilä, H. and Chalker, E. (2013), 'Vitamin C for preventing and treating the common cold', *The Cochrane Database of Systematic Reviews*, (1), p. CD000980. doi: 10.1002/14651858.CD000980.pub4.

Herman, P. and Polivy, J. (1991), 'Fat is a psychological issue', *New Scientist*, 16 Nov., pp. 41–5.

Hespel, P. *et al.* (2001), 'Oral creatine supplementation facilitates the rehabilitation of disuse atrophy and alters the expression of muscle myogenic factors in humans', *The Journal of Physiology*, 536(Pt 2), pp. 625–633. doi: 10.1111/j.1469-7793.2001.0625c.xd.

Hevia-Larraín, V. *et al.* (2021), 'High-Protein Plant-Based Diet Versus a Protein-Matched Omnivorous Diet to Support Resistance Training Adaptations: A Comparison Between Habitual Vegans and Omnivores', *Sports Medicine*. doi: 10.1007/s40279-021-01434-9.

Hew-Butler, T. *et al.* (2015), 'Statement of the Third International Exercise-Associated Hyponatremia Consensus Development Conference, Carlsbad, California, 2015', *Clinical Journal of Sport Medicine*, 25(4), pp. 303–320. doi: 10.1097/JSM.0000000000000221.

Hickey, H. S. *et al.* (1994), 'Drinking behaviour and exercise-thermal stress: role of drink carbonation', *Int. J. Sport Nutr.*, vol. 4, pp. 8–12.

Higgins, S. *et al.* (2015), 'The effects of pre-exercise caffeinated-coffee ingestion on endurance performance: an evidence-based review', *Int. J. Sport Nutr. Exerc. Metab.*, Nov 16 (Epub ahead of print).

Hill, A. M. *et al.* (2007), 'Combining fish-oil supplements with regular aerobic exercise improves body composition and cardiovascular disease risk factors'. *Am. J. Clin. Nutr.*, vol. 85(5), pp. 1267–74..

Hingley, L. *et al.* (2017), 'DHA-rich Fish Oil Increases the Omega-3 Index and Lowers the Oxygen Cost of Physiologically Stressful Cycling in Trained Individuals.

International journal of sport nutrition and exercise metabolism. doi: 10.1123/ijsnem.2016-0150.

Hitchins, S. *et al.* (1999), 'Glycerol hyperhydration improves cycle time-trial performance in hot humid conditions', *Eur. J. Appl. Physiol. Occup. Physiol.*, vol. 80(5), pp. 494–501.

Hobson, R. M. *et al.* (2012), 'Effects of -alanine supplementation on exercise performance: a meta-analysis', *Amino Acids*, vol. 43(1), pp. 25–37.

Hodgson, A. B., Randell, R. K. and Jeukendrup, A. E. (2013) (a), 'The metabolic and performance effects of caffeine compared to coffee during endurance exercise', *PloS One*, 8(4), p. e59561. doi: 10.1371/journal.pone.0059561.

Hodgson, A. B., Randell, R. K. and Jeukendrup, A. E. (2013) (b), 'The Effect of Green Tea Extract on Fat Oxidation at Rest and during Exercise: Evidence of Efficacy and Proposed Mechanisms', *Advances in Nutrition*, 4(2), pp. 129–140. doi: 10.3945/an.112.003269.

Hoffman, J. R. *et al.* (2008), 'Short-duration beta-alanine supplementation increases training volume and reduces subjective feelings of fatigue in college football players', *Nutr. Res.*, vol. 28, pp. 31–5.

Hoffman, M. D. *et al.* (2016), 'VIEW: Is Drinking to Thirst Adequate to Appropriately Maintain Hydration Status During Prolonged Endurance Exercise? Yes', *Wilderness & Environmental Medicine*, 27(2), pp. 192–195. doi: 10.1016/j.wem.2016.03.003.

Holt, S. J. (1992), 'Relationship of satiety to postprandial glycaemic, insulin and cholecystokinin responses'. *Appetite*, vol. 18, pp. 129–41.

Hoon, M. W. *et al.* (2014), 'Nitrate supplementation and high-intensity performance in competitive cyclists', *Applied Physiology, Nutrition, and Metabolism*, 0, 0, 10.1139/apnm-2013-0574.

Hoon, MW1, Johnson NA, Chapman PG, Burke LM (2013), The effect of nitrate supplementation on exercise performance in healthy individuals: a systematic review and meta-analysis. Int J Sport Nutr Exerc Metab. 2013 Oct; 23(5):522–32. Epub 2013 Apr 9.

Hooper, L. *et al.* (2012), 'Reduced or modified dietary fat for preventing cardiovascular disease', *Cochrane Database Syst. Rev.*, May 16;5.

Hooper, L. *et al.* (2015) (a), 'Effects of total fat intake on body weight', *The Cochrane Database of Systematic Reviews*, (8), p. CD011834. doi: 10.1002/14651858. CD011834.

Hooper, L. *et al.* (2015) (b), 'Reduction in saturated fat intake for cardiovascular disease', *The Cochrane Database of Systematic Reviews*, (6), p. CD011737. doi: 10.1002/14651858.CD011737.

Hooper, L. *et al.* (2020), 'Reduction in saturated fat intake for cardiovascular disease', *Cochrane Database of Systematic Reviews*, (5). doi: 10.1002/14651858. CD011737.pub2.

Hord N. G., Tang, Y. and Bryan, N. S. (2009), 'Food sources of nitrates and nitrites: the physiologic context for potential health benefits', *Am. J. Clin. Nutr.*, vol. 90(1), pp. 1–10.

Houtkooper, L. B. (2000), 'Body composition', in Manore, M. M. and Thompson, J. L., *Sport Nutrition for Health and Performance*, Human Kinetics, pp. 199–219.

Howarth, K. R. *et al.* (2009), 'Coingestion of protein with carbohydrate during recovery from endurance exercise stimulates skeletal muscle protein synthesis in humans', *J. Appl. Physiol.*, vol. 106, pp. 1394–1402.

Howatson, G., McHugh, M. P., Hill, J. A., *et al.* (2010), 'Influence of tart cherry juice on indices of recovery following marathon running', *Scand. J. Med. Sci. Sports*, vol. 20(6), pp. 843–52.

Howe, S. T. *et al.* (2013), 'The effect of beta-alanine supplementation on isokinetic force and cycling performance in highly trained cyclists', *Int. J. Sport Nutr. Exerc. Metab.* Dec, vol. 23(6), pp. 562–70 (Epub 2013 Apr 18).

Hu, T. *et al.* (2012), 'Effects of low-carbohydrate diets versus low-fat diets on metabolic risk factors: a meta-analysis of randomized controlled clinical trials', Am. J. Epidemiol., vol 176 Suppl 7, pp. S44–54.

Hudson, J. L. *et al.* (2020), 'Protein Intake Greater than the RDA Differentially Influences Whole-Body Lean Mass Responses to Purposeful Catabolic and Anabolic Stressors: A Systematic Review and Meta-analysis', *Advances in Nutrition (Bethesda, Md.)*, 11(3), pp. 548–558. doi: 10.1093/advances/nmz106.

Hughes, R. L. (2019), 'A Review of the Role of the Gut Microbiome in Personalized Sports Nutrition', *Frontiers in Nutrition*, 6, p. 191. doi: 10.3389/fnut.2019.00191.

Hulston C. J. *et al.* (2010), 'Training with low muscle glycogen enhances fat metabolism in well-trained cyclists', *Med. Sci. Sports Exerc.*, vol. 42, pp. 2046–55.

Hultman, E. *et al.* (1996), 'Muscle creatine loading in man', *J. Appl. Physiol.*, vol. 81, pp. 232–9.

Igwe, E. O. *et al.* (2019), 'A systematic literature review of the effect of anthocyanins on gut microbiota populations', *Journal of Human Nutrition and Dietetics:*

The Official Journal of the British Dietetic Association, 32(1), pp. 53–62. doi: 10.1111/jhn.12582.

Ihalainen, J. K. *et al.* (2021), 'Body Composition, Energy Availability, Training, and Menstrual Status in Female Runners', *International Journal of Sports Physiology and Performance*, pp. 1–6. doi: 10.1123/ijspp.2020-0276.

Impey, S. G. *et al.* (2016), 'Fuel for the work required: a practical approach to amalgamating train-low paradigms for endurance athletes', *Physiological Reports*, 4(10). doi: 10.14814/phy2.12803.

Impey, S. G. *et al.* (2018), 'Fuel for the Work Required: A Theoretical Framework for Carbohydrate Periodization and the Glycogen Threshold Hypothesis', *Sports Medicine (Auckland, N.Z.)*, 48(5), pp. 1031–1048. doi: 10.1007/s40279-018-0867-7.

International Olympic Committee (IOC) (2005), 'IOC Position Stand on the female athlete triad' http://www.olympic.org/assets/importednews/documents/en_report_917.pdf (Accessed March 2016).

International Olympic Committee (IOC) (2011), Consensus Statement on Sports Nutrition 2010, Sports Sci 4,29 Suppl 1: S3–4. http://www.olympic.org/Documents/Reports/EN/CONSENSUSFINAL-v8-en.pdf.

Ivy, J. L. *et al.* (1988), 'Muscle glycogen synthesis after exercise: effect of time of carbohydrate ingestion', *J. Appl. Physiol.*, vol. 64, pp. 1480–5.

Ivy, J. L. *et al.* (2002), 'Early post-exercise muscle glycogen recovery is enhanced with carbohydrate-protein supplement', *J. Appl. Physiol.*, vol. 93, pp. 1337–44.

Ivy, J. L. *et al.* (2003), 'Effect of a carbohydrate-protein supplement on endurance performance during exercise of varying intensity'. *Int. J. Sport Nutr. Exerc. Metab.*, vol. 13, pp. 388–401.

Ivy, J. L. *et al.* (2009), 'Improved cycling time-trial performance after ingestion of a caffeine energy drink', *Int. J. Sport Nutr. Exerc. Metab.*, vol. 19(1), pp. 61–78.

Jäger, R. *et al.* (2011), 'Analysis of the efficacy, safety, and regulatory status of novel forms of creatine', *Amino Acids*, vol. 40(5), pp. 1369–83.

Jäger, R. *et al.* (2017), 'International Society of Sports Nutrition Position Stand: protein and exercise', *Journal of the International Society of Sports Nutrition*, 14(1), p. 20. doi: 10.1186/s12970-017-0177-8.

Jäger, R. *et al.* (2019), 'International Society of Sports Nutrition Position Stand: Probiotics', *Journal of the International Society of Sports Nutrition*, 16(1), p. 62. doi: 10.1186/s12970-019-0329-0.

Jakobsen, M. U. *et al.* (2009), 'Major types of dietary fat and risk of coronary heart disease: a pooled analysis of 11 cohort studies', *Am. J. Clin. Nutr.*, vol. 89, pp. 1425–32.

Jakubowski, J. S. *et al.* (2020), ' ki, J. S. –32. Supplementation with the Leucine Metabolite β-hydroxy-β-methylbutyrate (HMB) does not Improve Resistance Exercise-Induced Changes in Body Composition or Strength in Young Subjects: A Systematic Review and Meta-Analysis', on with the Leucine Metabolite ry fat and risk of coronary heart disease: a pooled analysis of 11 cohort studies'. y'. –4. http://, abolic Stressors: A Systematic Review and Meta-analysis', S44–54.nalysis th*Nutrients*, 12(5), p. 1523. doi: 10.3390/nu12051523.

James, L. J. *et al.* (2017), 'Hypohydration impairs endurance performance: a blinded study', *Physiological Reports*, 5(12). doi: 10.14814/phy2.13315.

James, L. J. *et al.* (2019) (a), 'Cow's milk as a post-exercise recovery drink: implications for performance and health', *European Journal of Sport Science*, 19(1), pp. 40–48. doi: 10.1080/17461391.2018.1534989.

James, L. J. *et al.* (2019) (b), 'Does Hypohydration Really Impair Endurance Performance? Methodological Considerations for Interpreting Hydration Research', *Sports Medicine (Auckland, N.Z.)*, 49(Suppl 2), pp. 103–114. doi: 10.1007/s40279-019-01188-5.

Jamurtas, A. Z. *et al.* (2011), 'The effects of low and high glycemic index foods on exercise performance and beta-endorphin responses', *J. Int. Soc. Sports Nutr.*, vol. 8, p. 15.

Janelle, K. C. and Barr, S. I. (1995), 'Nutrient intakes and eating behavior scores of vegetarian and non-vegetarian women', *J. Am. Diet. Assoc.*, vol. 95, pp. 180–6, 189.

Jang, L.-G. *et al.* (2019), 'The combination of sport and sport-specific diet is associated with characteristics of gut microbiota: an observational study', *Journal of the International Society of Sports Nutrition*, 16(1), p. 21. doi: 10.1186/s12970-019-0290-y.

Janssen, I. *et al.* (2000), 'Skeletal muscle mass and distribution in 468 men and women aged 18–88 yr', *J. Appl. Physiol.*, vol. 89(1), pp. 81–8.

Jentjens, R. L. *et al.* (2001), 'Addition of protein and amino acids to carbohydrates does not enhance postexercise muscle glycogen synthesis', *Journal of Applied Physiology (Bethesda, Md.: 1985)*, 91(2), pp. 839–846. doi: 10.1152/jappl.2001.91.2.839.

Jentjens, R. L. P. G. *et al.* (2004), 'Oxidation of combined ingestion of glucose and fructose during exercise', *Journal of Applied Physiology*, 96(4), pp. 1277–1284. doi: 10.1152/japplphysiol.00974.2003.

Jéquier, E. (2002), 'Pathways to obesity', *International Journal of Obesity and Related Metabolic Disorders: Journal of the International Association for the Study of Obesity*, 26 Suppl 2, pp. S12-17. doi: 10.1038/sj.ijo.0802123.

Jeukendrup, A. E. (2004), 'Carbohydrate intake during exercise and performance', *Nutrition*, 20(7–8), pp. 669–677. doi: 10.1016/j.nut.2004.04.017.

Jeukendrup, A. E. (2004), 'Carbohydrate intake during exercise and performance', *Nutrition*, vol. 20, pp. 669–77.

Jeukendrup, A. E. (2008), 'Carbohydrate feeding during exercise', *Eur. J. Sports Sci.*, vol. 8(2), pp. 77–86.

Jeukendrup, A. E. (2017), 'Training the Gut for Athletes', *Sports Medicine (Auckland, N.Z.)*, 47(Suppl 1), pp. 101–110. doi: 10.1007/s40279-017-0690-6.

Jeukendrup, A. E. A. (2014), 'A step towards personalized sports nutrition: carbohydrate intake during exercise', *Sports Med.*, vol. 44 (Suppl 1), pp. 25–33.

Jeukendrup, A. E. A. et al. (1997), 'Carbohydrate-electrolyte feedings improve 1-hour time trial cycling performance', *Int. J. Sports Med.*, vol. 18, pp. 125–9.

Jeukendrup, A. E. A., et al. (2000), 'Relationship between gastro-intestinal complaints and endotoxaemia, cytokine release and the acute-phase reaction during and after a long-distance triathlon in highly trained men', *Clin. Sci.* (Lond.), vol. 98(1), pp. 47–55.

Jeukendrup, A. E.A. (2010), 'Carbohydrate and exercise performance: the role of multiple transportable carbohydrates', *Curr. Opin. Clin. Nutr. Metab. Care*, vol. 13(4), pp. 452–57.

Jeukendrup, A. E.A. (2014), 'A step towards personalized sports nutrition: carbohydrate intake during exercise', *Sports Medicine (Auckland, N.Z.)*, 44 Suppl 1, pp. S25-33. doi: 10.1007/s40279-014-0148-z.

Johnston, B. C. et al. (2014), 'Comparison of weight loss among named diet programs in overweight and obese adults: a meta-analysis', *JAMA*, 312(9), pp. 923–933. doi: 10.1001/jama.2014.10397.

Johnston, C. S. et al. (2006), 'Ketogenic low-carbohydrate diets have no metabolic advantage over nonketogenic low-carbohydrate diets', *Am. J. Clin. Nutr.*, vol 83(5), pp. 1055–61.

Jonnalagadda, S. S. et al. (2004), 'Food preferences, dieting behaviours, and body image perceptions of elite figure skaters', *Int. J. Sports Nutr. Exerc. Metab.*, vol. 14, pp. 594–606.

Josse, A. R. et al. (2010), 'Body composition and strength changes in women with milk and resistance exercise', *Med. Sci. Sports Exerc.*, vol. 42(6), pp. 1122–30.

Jouris K. et al. (2011), 'The effect of omega-3 fatty acid supplementation on the inflammatory response to eccentric strength exercise'. *J. Sports Sci. Med.*, vol. 10, pp. 432–38.

Jowko, E. et al. (2001), 'Creatine and HMB additively increase lean body mass and muscle strength during a weight training programme'. *Nutrition,* vol. 17(7), pp. 558–66.

Joyce, S., et al. (2012), 'Acute and chronic loading of sodium bicarbonate in highly trained swimmers', *Eur. J. Appl. Physiol.*, vol. 112(2), pp. 461–9.

Judkins, C. (2008), 'Investigation into supplementation contamination levels in the UK market', *HFL Sport Science.* www.informed-sport.com

Kamber, M. et al. (2001), 'Nutritional supplements as a source for positive doping cases?' *Int. J. Sports Nutr.*, vol. 11, pp. 258–63.

Kammer L. et al. (2009), 'Cereal and non-fat milk support muscle recovery following exercise', *J. Int. Soc. Sports Nutr.*, vol. 6, p. 11.

Kannel, W. B. et al. (1986), 'Overall and coronary heart disease mortality rates in relation to major risk factors in 325,348 men screened for the MRFIT. Multiple Risk Factor Intervention Trial', *American Heart Journal*, 112(4), pp. 825–836. doi: 10.1016/0002-8703(86)90481-3.

Karlsson, J. and Saltin, B. (1971), 'Diet, muscle glycogen and endurance performance', *J. Appl. Physiol.*, vol. 31, pp. 201–6.

Karp, J. R. et al. (2006), 'Chocolate milk as a post-exercise recovery aid', *Int. J. Sport Nutr. Exerc. Metab.*, vol. 16, pp. 78–91.

Karsch--Völk, M., Barrett, B., Kiefer, D., Bauer, R., Ardjomand--Woelkart, K., & Linde, K. (2014), *Echinacea for preventing and treating the common cold.* , The Cochrane Library.

Kasper, A. M. et al. (2015), 'Carbohydrate mouth rinse and caffeine improves high-intensity interval running capacity when carbohydrate restricted', *Eur. J. Sport Sci.*, vol. 2, pp. 1–9 (Epub ahead of print).

Kasper, A. M. et al. (2019), 'Case Study: Extreme Weight Making Causes Relative Energy Deficiency, Dehydration, and Acute Kidney Injury in a Male Mixed Martial Arts Athlete', *International Journal of Sport Nutrition and Exercise Metabolism*, 29(3), pp. 331–338. doi: 10.1123/ijsnem.2018-0029.

Kasper, A. M. *et al.* (2020), 'High Prevalence of Cannabidiol Use Within Male Professional Rugby Union and League Players: A Quest for Pain Relief and Enhanced Recovery', *International Journal of Sport Nutrition and Exercise Metabolism*, 30(5), pp. 315–322. doi: 10.1123/ijsnem.2020-0151.

Katsanos, C. S. *et al.* (2006), 'A high proportion of leucine is required for optimal stimulation of the rate of muscle protein synthesis by essential amino acids in the elderly', *Am. J. Physiol. Endocrinol. Metab.*, vol. 291, pp. E381–E387.

Kawabata, F. *et al.* (2014), 'Supplementation with eicosapentaenoic acid-rich fish oil improves exercise economy and reduces perceived exertion during submaximal steady-state exercise in normal healthy untrained men', *Bioscience, Biotechnology, and Biochemistry*, 78(12), pp. 2081–2088. doi: 10.1080/09168451.2014.946392.

Kay, C. D. *et al.* (2012), 'Relative impact of flavonoid composition, dose and structure on vascular function: a systematic review of randomised controlled trials of flavonoid-rich food products', *Molecular Nutrition & Food Research*, 56(11), pp. 1605–1616. doi: 10.1002/mnfr.201200363.

Keane, K. M. *et al.* (2018), 'Effects of montmorency tart cherry (L. Prunus Cerasus) consumption on nitric oxide biomarkers and exercise performance', *Scandinavian Journal of Medicine & Science in Sports*, 28(7), pp. 1746–1756. doi: 10.1111/sms.13088.

Keay, N. *et al.* (2019), 'Clinical evaluation of education relating to nutrition and skeletal loading in competitive male road cyclists at risk of relative energy deficiency in sports (RED-S): 6-month randomised controlled trial', *BMJ Open Sport — Exercise Medicine*, 5(1). doi: 10.1136/bmjsem-2019-000523.

Keay, N., Fogelman, I. and Blake, G. (1997), 'Bone mineral density in professional female dancers.', *British Journal of Sports Medicine*, 31(2), pp. 143–147. doi: 10.1136/bjsm.31.2.143.

Keay, N., Francis, G. and Hind, K. (2018), 'Low energy availability assessed by a sport-specific questionnaire and clinical interview indicative of bone health, endocrine profile and cycling performance in competitive male cyclists', *BMJ Open Sport & Exercise Medicine*, 4(1), p. e000424. doi: 10.1136/bmjsem-2018-000424.

Keay, N., Overseas, A. and Francis, G. (2020), 'Indicators and correlates of low energy availability in male and female dancers', *BMJ Open Sport & Exercise Medicine*, 6(1), p. e000906. doi: 10.1136/bmjsem-2020-000906.

Keizer, H. A. *et al.* (1986), 'Influence of liquid or solid meals on muscle glycogen resynthesis, plasma fuel hormone response and maximal physical working capacity', *Int. J. Sports Med.*, vol. 8, pp. 99–104.

Kenefick, R. W. and Cheuvront, S. N. (2012), 'Hydration for recreational sport and physical activity', *Nutrition Reviews*, 70(s2), pp. S137–S142. doi: https://doi.org/10.1111/j.1753-4887.2012.00523.x.

Kennerly, K. *et al.* (2011), Influence of banana versus sports beverage ingestion on 75 km cycling performance and exercise-induced inflammation', *Med. Sci. Sports Exerc.*, vol. 43(5), pp. 340–341.

Kenney, W. L. and Chiu, P. (2001), 'Influence of age on thirst and fluid intake', *Med. Sci. Sports Exerc.*, vol. 33(9), pp. 1524–32.

Keohane, D. M. *et al.* (2019), 'Four men in a boat: Ultra-endurance exercise alters the gut microbiome', *Journal of Science and Medicine in Sport*, 22(9), pp. 1059–1064. doi: 10.1016/j.jsams.2019.04.004.

Kerksick, C. M. *et al.* (2018), 'ISSN exercise & sports nutrition review update: research & recommendations', *Journal of the International Society of Sports Nutrition*, 15(1), p. 38. doi: 10.1186/s12970-018-0242-y.

Key, T. J. A. *et al.* (1996), 'Dietary habits and mortality in a cohort of 11,000 vegetarians and health conscious people: results of a 17-year follow-up', *Br. Med. J.*, vol. 313, pp. 775–9.

Keys, A.B. (1980), Seven Countries: A Multivariate Analysis of Death and Coronary Heart Desease (Harvard University Press, 1980).

Kiens, B. *et al.* (1990), 'Benefit of simple carbohydrates on the early post-exercise muscle glycogen repletion in male athletes', *Med. Sci. Sports Ex.* (suppl.), S88.

Killer, S.C. *et al.* (2014), 'No Evidence of Dehydration with Moderate Daily Coffee Intake: A Counterbalanced Cross-Over Study in a Free-Living Population', *PLoS ONE*, vol. 9 (1): e84154.

Kim, H., Caulfield, L. E. and Rebholz, C. M. (2018), 'Healthy Plant-Based Diets Are Associated with Lower Risk of All-Cause Mortality in US Adults', *The Journal of Nutrition*, 148(4), pp. 624–631. doi: 10.1093/jn/nxy019.

King, D. S. *et al.* (1999), 'Effects of oral androstenedione on serum testosterone and adaptations to resistance training in young men', *J. Am. Med. Assoc.*, vol. 281 (21), pp. 2020–8.

King, S. *et al.* (2014), 'Effectiveness of probiotics on the duration of illness in healthy children and adults who develop common acute respiratory infectious conditions: a systematic review and meta-analysis', *The

British Journal of Nutrition, 112(1), pp. 41–54. doi: 10.1017/S0007114514000075.

Kirkpatrick, C. F. *et al.* (2019), 'Review of current evidence and clinical recommendations on the effects of low-carbohydrate and very-low-carbohydrate (including ketogenic) diets for the management of body weight and other cardiometabolic risk factors: A scientific statement from the National Lipid Association Nutrition and Lifestyle Task Force', *Journal of Clinical Lipidology*, 13(5), pp. 689-711. e1. doi: 10.1016/j.jacl.2019.08.003.

Knez, W. L. and Peake, J. M. (2010), 'The prevalence of vitamin supplementation in ultra-endurance triathletes', *Int. J. Sport Nutr. Exerc. Metab.*, vol. 20(6), pp. 507–14.

Koopman, R. (2011), 'Dietary protein and exercise training in ageing', *Proc. Nutr. Soc.*, vol. 70, pp. 104–13.

Koopman, R. *et al.* (2005), 'Combined ingestion of protein and free leucine with carbohydrate increases post-exercise muscle protein synthesis in vivo in male subjects', *Am. J. Physiol. Endocrinol. Metab.*, vol. 288(4), pp. E645–653.

Kreider, R. (2003) (a), 'Effects of whey protein supplementation with casein or BCAA and glutamine on training adaptations: body composition', *Med. Sci. Sport Exerc.*, vol. 35(5), suppl. 1, p. S395.

Kreider, R. B. (2003) (b), 'Effects of creatine supplementation on performance and training adaptations', *Mol. Cell Biochem.*, vol. 244(1–2), pp. 89–94.

Kreider, R. B. *et al.* (1996), 'Effects of ingesting supplements designed to promote lean tissue accretion on body composition during resistance training', *Int. J. Sport Nutr.*, vol. 63, pp. 234–46.

Kreider, R. B. *et al.* (2000), 'Effects of calcium-HMB supplementation during training on markers of catabolism, body composition, strength and sprint. performance', *J. Exerc. Physiol.*, vol. 3 (4), pp. 48–59.

Kreider, R. B. *et al.* (2002), 'Effects of conjugated linoleic acid supplementation during resistance training on body composition, bone density, strength, and selected hematological markers', *J. Strength Cond. Res.*, vol. 16(3), pp. 325–34.

Kreider, R. B. *et al.* (2017), 'International Society of Sports Nutrition position stand: safety and efficacy of creatine supplementation in exercise, sport, and medicine', *Journal of the International Society of Sports Nutrition*, 14(1), p. 18. doi: 10.1186/s12970-017-0173-z.

Kristensen, K. *et al.* (1999), 'Hormone replacement therapy affects body composition and leptin differently in obese and non-obese postmenopausal women', *The Journal of Endocrinology*, 163(1), pp. 55–62. doi: 10.1677/joe.0.1630055.

Kristiansen, M. *et al.* (2005), 'Dietary supplement use by varsity athletes at a Canadian University', *Int. J. Sport Nutr. Exerc. Metab.*, vol. 15, pp. 195–210.

Lambert, E. V. *et al.* (1994), 'Enhanced endurance in trained cyclists during moderate intensity exercise following 2 weeks adaptation to a high fat diet', *Eur. J. Appl. Physiol.*, vol. 69, pp. 287–293.

Lane, S. C. *et al.* (2013) (a), 'Effect of a carbohydrate mouth rinse on simulated cycling time-trial performance commenced in a fed or fasted state', *Applied Physiology, Nutrition, and Metabolism = Physiologie Appliquee, Nutrition Et Metabolisme*, 38(2), pp. 134–139. doi: 10.1139/apnm-2012-0300.

Lane, S. C. *et al.* (2013) (b), 'Caffeine ingestion and cycling power output in a low or normal muscle glycogen state', *Med. Sci. Sports Exerc.*, Aug. 45(8), pp. 1577–84.

Lane, S. C. *et al.* (2013) (c), 'Single and combined effects of beetroot juice and caffeine supplementation on cycling time-trial performance', *Appl. Physiol. Nutr. Metab.*, 10.1139/apnm-2013-0336

Lane, S. C. *et al.* (2015), 'Effects of sleeping with reduced carbohydrate availability on acute training responses', *J. Appl. Physiol.*, vol. 119(6), pp. 643–55.

Langan-Evans, C., Close, G. L. and Morton, J. P. (2011), 'Making Weight in Combat Sports', *Strength & Conditioning Journal*, 33(6), pp. 25–39. doi: 10.1519/SSC.0b013e318231bb64.

Lansley, K. I. *et al.* (2011) (a), 'Dietary nitrate supplementation reduces the O2 cost of walking and running: a placebo-controlled study', *J. Appl. Physiol.*, vol. 110, pp. 591–600.

Lansley, K. I., *et al.* (2011) (b), 'Acute dietary nitrate supplementation improves cycling time-trial performance', *Med. Sci. Sports Exerc.*, vol. 43, pp. 1125–31.

Lantzouni, E. *et al.* (2002), 'Reversibility of growth stunting in early onset anorexia nervosa: a prospective study', *The Journal of Adolescent Health: Official Publication of the Society for Adolescent Medicine*, 31(2), pp. 162–165. doi: 10.1016/s1054-139x(02)00342-7.

Lanza, I. R. *et al.* (2008), 'Endurance exercise as a countermeasure for aging', *Diabetes,* vol. 57(11), pp. 2933–42.

Larson-Meyer, D. E. and Willis, K. S. (2010), 'Vitamin D and athletes', *Curr. Sports Med. Rep.*, vol. 9(4), pp. 220–6.

Lassale Camille, et al.*et al.* (2015), '"Abstract 16: A Pro-Vegetarian Food Pattern and Cardiovascular Mortality in the Epic Study."' Circulation, vol. 131, no. suppl_1, Mar. 2015, pp. A16–A16. ahajournals. org (Atypon), doi:10.1161/circ.131.suppl_1.16.

Laursen, P. B. *et al.* (2006), 'Core temperature and hydration status during an Ironman triathlon', *Br. J. Sports Med.* 2006 Apr; 40(4), pp. 320–5; discussion 325.

Layman, D. K. *et al.* (2005), 'Dietary protein and exercise have additive effects on body composition during weight loss in adult women', *J. Nutr.* vol. 35(8), pp. 1903–10.

Le, L. T. and Sabaté, J. (2014), 'Beyond meatless, the health effects of vegan diets: findings from the Adventist cohorts', *Nutrients*, 6(6), pp. 2131–2147. doi: 10.3390/nu6062131.

Lean, M. E. J. *et al.* (1995), 'Waist circumference as a measure for indicating need for weight management', *BMJ*, vol. 311, pp. 158–61.

Leckey, J. J. *et al.* (2016), 'Altering fatty acid availability does not impair prolonged, continuous running to fatigue: Evidence for carbohydrate dependence'. *J. Appl. Physiol.*, vol. 120(2), pp. 107–13.

Leckey, J. J. *et al.* (2017), 'Ketone Diester Ingestion Impairs Time-Trial Performance in Professional Cyclists', *Frontiers in Physiology*, 8, p. 806. doi: 10.3389/fphys.2017.00806.

Leddy, J. *et al.* (1997), 'Effect of a high or a low fat diet on cardiovascular risk factors in male and female runners', *Medicine & Science in Sports & Exercise*, 29(1), pp. 17–25.

Leeds, A., Brand Miller, J., Foster-Powell, K. and Colagiuri, S. (2000), *The Glucose Revolution* (London: Hodder and Stoughton), p. 29.

Leenders, M. *et al.* (2013), 'Elderly men and women benefit equally from prolonged resistance-type exercise training', *J. Gerontol. A. Biol. Sci. Med. Sci.*, vol. 68(7), pp. 769–79.

Lehnen, T. E. *et al.* (2015), 'A review on effects of conjugated linoleic fatty acid (CLA) upon body composition and energetic metabolism', *J. Int. Soc. Sports Nutr.*, vol. 12, p. 36.

Lemon, P. W. R. (1992), 'Protein requirements and muscle mass/strength changes during intensive training in novice bodybuilders, *J. Appl. Physiol.*, vol. 73, pp. 767–75.

Lemon, P. W. R. (1995), 'Do athletes need more dietary protein and amino acids?', *Int. J. Sport Nutr.*, vol. 5 pp. s39–61.

Lemon, P. W. R. (1998), 'Effects of exercise on dietary protein requirements', *Int. J. Sport Nutr.*, vol. 8, pp. 426–47.

Lenn, J. *et al.* (2002), 'The effects of fish oil and isoflavones on delayed onset muscle soreness'. *Med. Sci. Sports Exerc.*, vol. 34(10), pp. 1605–13.

Levine, S. A., Gordon, B. and Derick, C. L. (1924), 'Some changes in the chemical constituents of the blood following a marathon race: with special reference to the development of hypoglycemia', *Journal of the American Medical Association*, 82(22), pp. 1778–1779. doi: 10.1001/jama.1924.02650480034015.

Levitsky, D. A. and Pacanowski, C. R. (2013), 'Effect of skipping breakfast on subsequent energy intake', *Physiol Behav.* vol. 119, pp. 9–16.

Lewis, N. A. *et al.* (2020), 'Are There Benefits from the Use of Fish Oil Supplements in Athletes? A Systematic Review', *Advances in Nutrition (Bethesda, Md.)*, 11(5), pp. 1300–1314. doi: 10.1093/advances/nmaa050.

LGC (2015), Clean Sport http://www.informed-sport.com/sites/default/files/LGC_Clean_Sport_trifold_0315_EN_4336_digital2_0.pdf. Accessed March 2016.

Li, Y., Hruby, A., Bernstein, A. M., *et al.* (2015), 'Saturated fats compared with unsaturated fats and sources of carbohydrates in relation to risk of coronary heart disease: a prospective cohort study', *J. Am. Coll. Cardiol.*, vol. 66(14), pp. 1538–48.

Lis, D. *et al.* (2016), 'Food avoidance in athletes: FODMAP foods on the list', *Applied Physiology, Nutrition, and Metabolism = Physiologie Appliquee, Nutrition Et Metabolisme*, 41(9), pp. 1002–1004. doi: 10.1139/apnm-2015-0428.

Lis, D. M. and Baar, K. (2019), 'Effects of Different Vitamin C-Enriched Collagen Derivatives on Collagen Synthesis', *International Journal of Sport Nutrition and Exercise Metabolism*, 29(5), pp. 526–531. doi: 10.1123/ijsnem.2018-0385.

Lis, D. M. *et al.* (2018), 'Low FODMAP: A Preliminary Strategy to Reduce Gastrointestinal Distress in Athletes', *Medicine & Science in Sports & Exercise*, 50(1), pp. 116–123. doi: 10.1249/MSS.0000000000001419.

Lissner, L. *et al.* (1987), 'Dietary fat and the regulation of energy intake in human subjects', *The American Journal of Clinical Nutrition*, 46(6), pp. 886–892. doi: 10.1093/ajcn/46.6.886.

Liu, T.-H. *et al.* (2009), 'No effect of short-term arginine supplementation on nitric oxide production, metabolism and performance in intermittent exercise in athletes', *The Journal of Nutritional Biochemistry*, 20(6), pp. 462–468. doi: 10.1016/j.jnutbio.2008.05.005.

Lloyd, T. *et al.* (1986), 'Women athletes with menstrual irregularity have increased musculoskeletal injuries', *Med. Sci. Sports Ex.*, vol. 18, pp. 3427–9.

Logan-Sprenger, H. M. *et al.* (2015), 'The effect of dehydration on muscle metabolism and time trial performance during prolonged cycling in males', *Physiological Reports*, 3(8). doi: 10.14814/phy2.12483.

Logue, D. *et al.* (2018), 'Low Energy Availability in Athletes: A Review of Prevalence, Dietary Patterns, Physiological Health, and Sports Performance', *Sports Medicine (Auckland, N.Z.)*, 48(1), pp. 73–96. doi: 10.1007/s40279-017-0790-3.

Logue, D. M. *et al.* (2020), 'Low Energy Availability in Athletes 2020: An Updated Narrative Review of Prevalence, Risk, Within-Day Energy Balance, Knowledge, and Impact on Sports Performance', *Nutrients*, 12(3), p. 835. doi: 10.3390/nu12030835.

Lohman, T. G. (1992), 'Basic concepts in body composition assessment', In *Advances in Body Composition Assessment*, Human Kinetics, pp. 109–118.

Longland, T. M. *et al.* (2016), 'Higher compared with lower dietary protein during an energy deficit combined with intense exercise promotes greater lean mass gain and fat mass loss: a randomized trial', *Am. J. Clin. Nutr.* Jan 27 (Epub ahead of print).

Loucks, A. B. (2003), 'Energy availability, not body fatness, regulates reproductive function in women', *Exerc. Sport Sci. Rev.*, vol. 31, pp. 144–148.

Loucks, A. B. and Thuma, J. R. (2003), 'Luteinizing hormone pulsatility is disrupted at a threshold of energy availability in regularly menstruating women', *The Journal of Clinical Endocrinology and Metabolism*, 88(1), pp. 297–311. doi: 10.1210/jc.2002-020369.

Loucks, A. B. *et al.* (1989), 'Alterations in the hypothalamic-pituitary-ovarian and the hypothalamic-pituitary axes in athletic women', *J. Clinical Endocrinol. Metab.*, vol. 68, pp. 402–22.

Loucks, A. B., Kiens, B. and Wright, H. H. (2011), 'Energy availability in athletes', *Journal of Sports Sciences*, 29 Suppl 1, pp. S7-15. doi: 10.1080/02640414.2011.588958.

Lovell, G. (2008), 'Vitamin D status of females in an elite gymnastic programme', *Clin. J. Sports Med.*, vol. 18, pp. 159–61.

Luden, N. D. *et al.* (2007), 'Post-exercise carbohydrate-protein-antioxidant ingestion increase CK and muscle soreness in cross-country runners', *Int. J. Sports Exerc. Metab.*, vol. 17, pp. 109–122.

Lukaski, H.C. (2004), 'Vitamin and mineral status: effects on physical performance'. *Nutrition*, vol. 20, 632–44.

Lun, V. *et al.* (2012), 'Dietary supplementation practices in Canadian high-performance athletes', *Int. J. Sport Nutr. Exerc. Metab.*, vol. 22(1), pp. 31–7.

Lynch, Heidi M., et al.*et al.* (2016), '"Cardiorespiratory Fitness and Peak Torque Differences between Vegetarian and Omnivore Endurance Athletes: A Cross-Sectional Study."', *Nutrients*, vol. 8, no. 11, Nov. 2016, p. 726. www.mdpi.com, doi:10.3390/nu8110726.

MacConnie, S. E. *et al.* (1986), 'Decreased hypothalamic gonadotropin-releasing hormone secretion in male marathon runners', *The New England Journal of Medicine*, 315(7), pp. 411–417. doi: 10.1056/NEJM198608143150702.

Mach, N. and Fuster-Botella, D. (2017), 'Endurance exercise and gut microbiota: A review', *Journal of Sport and Health Science*, 6(2), pp. 179–197. doi: 10.1016/j.jshs.2016.05.001.

Macintosh, B. R. *et al.* (1995), 'Caffeine ingestion and performance of a 1500-metre swim'. *Can. J. Appl. Physiol.*, vol. 20 (2): pp. 168–77.

Mackie, G. M., Samocha-Bonet, D. and Tam, C. S. (2017), 'Does weight cycling promote obesity and metabolic risk factors?', *Obesity Research & Clinical Practice*, 11(2), pp. 131–139. doi: 10.1016/j.orcp.2016.10.284.

Macnaughton, L. S. *et al.* (2016), 'The response of muscle protein synthesis following whole-body resistance exercise is greater following 40 g than 20 g of ingested whey protein', *Physiol. Rep.* vol. 4 (15). pii: e12893.

Mäestu, J. *et al.* (2010), 'Anabolic and catabolic hormones and energy balance of the male bodybuilders during the preparation for the competition', *Journal of Strength and Conditioning Research*, 24(4), pp. 1074–1081. doi: 10.1519/JSC.0b013e3181cb6fd3.

Mäestu, J. *et al.* (2010), 'Anabolic and catabolic hormones and energy balance of the male bodybuilders during the preparation for the competition', *Journal of Strength and Conditioning Research*, 24(4), pp. 1074–1081. doi: 10.1519/JSC.0b013e3181cb6fd3.

Maffucci, D. M. and McMurray, R. G. (2000), 'Towards optimising the timing of the pre-exercise meal', *Int. J. Sport Nutr.*, vol. 10, pp. 103–13.

Maggini, S., Pierre, A. and Calder, P. C. (2018), 'Immune Function and Micronutrient Requirements Change over the Life Course', *Nutrients*, 10(10). doi: 10.3390/nu10101531.

Mamerow, M. M. *et al.* (2014), 'Dietary Protein Distribution Positively Influences 24-h Muscle Protein Synthesis in Healthy Adults', *J. Nutrition,* vol. 144, pp. 876–80.

Margolis, L. M. *et al.* (2021), 'Congestion of Carbohydrate and Protein on Muscle Glycogen Synthesis after Exercise: A Meta-analysis', *Medicine and Science in Sports and Exercise*, 53(2), pp. 384–393. doi: 10.1249/MSS.0000000000002476.

Mariotti, FrançoisF., and Christopher D. Gardner (2019), '"Dietary Protein and Amino Acids in Vegetarian Diets—A Review."', *Nutrients*, vol. 11, no. 11, Nov. 2019, p. 2661. www.mdpi.com, doi:10.3390/nu11112661.

Marquet, L. A. *et al.* (2016) (a), 'Enhanced endurance performance by periodization of cho intake: 'sleep low' strategy', Med. Sci. Sports Exerc., vol. 48(4), pp. 663–72.

Marquet, L.-A. *et al.* (2016) (b), 'Periodization of Carbohydrate Intake: Short-Term Effect on Performance', *Nutrients*, 8(12), p. 755. doi: 10.3390/nu8120755.

Martin, W. F., Armstrong, L. E. and Rodriguez, N. R. (2005), 'Dietary protein intake and renal function', *Nutrition & Metabolism*, 2(1), p. 25. doi: 10.1186/1743-7075-2-25.

Martinez, L. R. and Haymes, E. M. (1992), 'Substrate utilisation during treadmill running in prepubescent girls and women', *Med. Sci. Sports Exerc.*, vol. 24, pp. 975–83.

Martinsen, M. *et al.* (2010), 'Dieting to win or to be thin? A study of dieting and disordered eating among adolescent elite athletes and non-athlete controls', *British Journal of Sports Medicine*, 44(1), pp. 70–76. doi: 10.1136/bjsm.2009.068668.

Mason, W. L. *et al.* (1993), 'Carbohydrate ingestion during exercise: liquid vs solid feedings', *Med. Sci. Sports Ex.*, vol. 25, pp. 966–9.

Maughan, R. J. (1995), 'Creatine supplementation and exercise performance', *Int. J. Sport Nutr.*, vol. 5, pp. 94–101.

Maughan, R. J. and Shirreffs, S. M. (2012), 'Nutrition for sports performance: issues and opportunities', *Proc. Nutr. Soc.;* vol. 71 (1), pp. 112–19.

Maughan, R. J. *et al.* (1996), 'Rehydration and recovery after exercise', *Sports Sci. Ex.*, vol. 9(62), pp. 1–5.

Maughan, R. J. *et al.* (2016), 'A randomized trial to assess the potential of different beverages to affect hydration status: development of a beverage hydration index', *Am J. Clin. Nutr.*, vol. 103, pp. 717–23.

Maughan, R. J. *et al.* (2018), 'IOC consensus statement: dietary supplements and the high-performance athlete', *British Journal of Sports Medicine*, 52(7), pp. 439–455. doi: 10.1136/bjsports-2018-099027.

Mayhew, D. L. *et al.* (2002), 'Effects of long term creatine supplementation on liver and kidney function in American Football players', *Int. J. Sport Nutr.*, vol. 12, pp. 453–60.

McConnell, G. K. *et al.* (1997), 'Influence of ingested fluid volume on physiological responses during prolonged exercise', *Acta. Phys. Scand.*, vol. 160, pp. 149–56.

McCubbin, A. J. *et al.* (2020), 'Hydrogel Carbohydrate-Electrolyte Beverage Does Not Improve Glucose Availability, Substrate Oxidation, Gastrointestinal Symptoms or Exercise Performance, Compared With a Concentration and Nutrient-Matched Placebo', *International Journal of Sport Nutrition and Exercise Metabolism*, 30(1), pp. 25–33. doi: 10.1123/ijsnem.2019-0090.

McDonald, D. *et al.* (2018), 'American Gut: an Open Platform for Citizen Science Microbiome Research', *mSystems*, 3(3). doi: 10.1128/mSystems.00031-18.

McGlory, C. *et al.* (2016), 'Fish oil supplementation suppresses resistance exercise and feeding-induced increases in anabolic signaling without affecting myofibrillar protein synthesis in young men', *Physiological Reports*, 4(6). doi: 10.14814/phy2.12715.

McLeay, Y. *et al.* (2012), 'Effect of New Zealand blueberry consumption on recovery from eccentric exercise-induced muscle damage', *Journal of the International Society of Sports Nutrition*, 9(1), p. 19. doi: 10.1186/1550-2783-9-19.

Mears, S. A. *et al.* (2020), 'Addition of sodium alginate and pectin to a carbohydrate-electrolyte solution does not influence substrate oxidation, gastrointestinal comfort, or cycling performance', *Applied Physiology, Nutrition, and Metabolism = Physiologie Appliquee, Nutrition Et Metabolisme*, 45(6), pp. 675–678. doi: 10.1139/apnm-2019-0802.

Meier, C. *et al.* (2004), 'Supplementation with oral vitamin D and calcium during winter prevents seasonal bone loss: a randomnised controlled open-label prospective trial', *J. Bone Mineral Res.*, vol. 19, pp. 1221–30.

Melby, C. *et al.* (1993), 'Effect of acute resistance exercise on resting metabolic rate', *J. Appl. Physiol.*, vol. 75, pp. 1847–53.

Melin, A. *et al.* (2015), 'Energy availability and the female athlete triad in elite endurance athletes', *Scandinavian Journal of Medicine & Science in Sports*, 25(5), pp. 610–622. doi: https://doi.org/10.1111/sms.12261.

Melina, V., Craig, W. and Levin, S. (2016), 'Position of the Academy of Nutrition and Dietetics: Vegetarian Diets', *Journal of the Academy of Nutrition and Dietetics*, 116(12), pp. 1970–1980. doi: 10.1016/j.jand.2016.09.025.

Mensink, R.P *et al.* (2003), 'Effects of dietary fatty acids and carbohydrate on the ratio of serum total to HDL cholesterol and on serum lipids and apolipo proteins: a meta-analysis of 60 controlled trials', American Journal of Clinical Nutrition, 77 (5), pp. 1146–1155.

Menzies, C. *et al.* (2020), 'Frequent Carbohydrate Ingestion Reduces Muscle Glycogen Depletion and Postpones Fatigue Relative to a Single Bolus', *International Journal of Sport Nutrition and Exercise Metabolism*, pp. 1–7. doi: 10.1123/ijsnem.2019-0291.

Mercuro, G. *et al.* (2006), 'Impairment of physical exercise capacity in healthy postmenopausal women', *American Heart Journal*, 151(4), pp. 923–927. doi: 10.1016/j.ahj.2005.06.027.

Mero, A. A. *et al.* (2010), 'Moderate energy restriction with high protein diet results in healthier outcome in women', *Journal of the International Society of Sports Nutrition*, 7(1), p. 4. doi: 10.1186/1550-2783-7-4.

Messina, Mark, et al.*et al.* (2018), '"No Difference Between the Effects of Supplementing With Soya Protein Versus Animal Protein on Gains in Muscle Mass and Strength in Response to Resistance Exercise."', *International Journal of Sport Nutrition and Exercise Metabolism*, vol. 28, no. 6, Nov. 2018, pp. 674–85. journals.humankinetics.com, doi:10.1123/ijsnem.2018-0071.

MHRA (2012), http://www.mhra.gov.uk/home/groups/comms-po/documents/news/con174847.pdf

Middleton, N., Jelen, P. and Bell, G. (2004), 'Whole blood and mononuclear cell glutathione response to dietary whey protein supplementation in sedentary and trained male human subjects', *International journal of food sciences and nutrition*. doi: 10.1080/09637480410001666504.

Miescher, E. and Fortney, S. M. (1989), 'Responses to dehydration and rehydration during heat exposure in young and older men', *Am. J. Physiol.*, vol. 257, pp. R1050–R1056.

Mifflin, M. D. *et al.* (1990), 'A new predictive equation for resting energy expenditure in healthy individuals', *J. Am. Diet. Assoc.*, vol. 51, pp. 241–7.

Mihic, S. *et al.* (2000), 'Acute creatine loading increases fat free mass but does not affect blood pressure, plasma creatinine or CK activity in men and women', *Med. Sci. Sport. Exerc.*, vol. 32, pp. 291–6.

Miller, S. L. *et al.* (2002), 'Metabolic responses to provision of mixed protein-carbohydrate supplementation during endurance exercise attenuate the increases in cortisol', *Int. J. Sport Nutr.*, vol. 12, pp. 384–97.

Minehan, M. R. *et al.* (2002), 'Effect of flavour and awareness of kilojoule content of drinks on preference and fluid balance in teAm. sports', *Int. J. Sport Nutr.*, vol. 12, pp. 81–92.

Minetto, M. A. *et al.* (2013), 'Origin and development of muscle cramps', *Exercise and Sport Sciences Reviews*, 41(1), pp. 3–10. doi: 10.1097/JES.0b013e3182724817.

Misra, M. *et al.* (2004), 'Effects of anorexia nervosa on clinical, hematologic, biochemical, and bone density parameters in community-dwelling adolescent girls', *Pediatrics*, 114(6), pp. 1574–1583. doi: 10.1542/peds.2004-0540.

Mitchell, C. M. *et al.* (2019), 'Does Exercise Alter Gut Microbial Composition? A Systematic Review', *Medicine and Science in Sports and Exercise*, 51(1), pp. 160–167. doi: 10.1249/MSS.0000000000001760.

Mitchell, W. K. *et al.* (2012), 'Sarcopenia, dynapenia, and the impact of advancing age on human skeletal muscle size and strength; a quantitative review', *Front Physiol.* vol. 3, p. 260.

Mizumura, K. and Taguchi, T. (2016) (b), 'Delayed onset muscle soreness: Involvement of neurotrophic factors', *The journal of physiological sciences: JPS*, 66(1), pp. 43–52. doi: 10.1007/s12576-015-0397-0.

Mohr, A. E. *et al.* (2020), 'The athletic gut microbiota', *Journal of the International Society of Sports Nutrition*, 17(1), p. 24. doi: 10.1186/s12970-020-00353-w.

Montain, S. J. and Coyle, E. F. (1992), 'The influence of graded dehydration on hyperthermia and cardiovascular drift during exercise', *J. Appl. Physiol.*, vol. 73, pp. 1340–50.

Moore, D. R. (2019), 'Maximizing Post-exercise Anabolism: The Case for Relative Protein Intakes', *Frontiers in Nutrition*, 6. doi: 10.3389/fnut.2019.00147.

Moore, D. R. *et al.* (2009), 'Ingested protein dose response of muscle and albumin protein synthesis after existence exercise in young men', *Am. J. Clin. Nutr.,* vol. 89, pp. 161–8.

Moore, D. R. *et al.* (2014), 'Beyond muscle hypertrophy: why dietary protein is important for endurance athletes', *Appl. Physiol. Nutr. Metab.,* vol 39(9), pp. 987–97

Moore, D. R. *et al.* (2015), 'Protein ingestion to stimulate myofibrillar protein synthesis requires greater relative protein intakes in healthy older versus younger men', *J. Gerontol. A. Biol. Sci. Med. Sci.* vol. 70(1), pp. 57–62.

Morehen, J. C. *et al.* (2020), 'Montmorency tart cherry juice does not reduce markers of muscle soreness, function and inflammation following professional male rugby League match-play', *European Journal of Sport Science*, pp. 1–10. doi: 10.1080/17461391.2020.1797181.

Morrison, L. J. *et al.* (2004), 'Prevalent use of dietary supplements among people who exercise at a commercial gym'. *Int. J. Sport Nutr. Exerc. Metab.,* vol. 14, pp. 481–92.

Morton, J. P. *et al.* (2009), 'Reduced carbohydrate availability does not modulate training-induced heat shock protein adaptations but does upregulate oxidative enzyme activity in human skeletal muscle', *Journal of Applied Physiology (Bethesda, Md.: 1985)*, 106(5), pp. 1513–1521. doi: 10.1152/japplphysiol.00003.2009.

Morton, R. W. *et al.* (2018), 'A systematic review, meta-analysis and meta-regression of the effect of protein supplementation on resistance training-induced gains in muscle mass and strength in healthy adults', *British Journal of Sports Medicine*, 52(6), pp. 376–384. doi: 10.1136/bjsports-2017-097608.

Mountjoy, M. *et al.* (2014), 'The IOC consensus statement: beyond the Female Athlete Triad--Relative Energy Deficiency in Sport (RED-S)', *British Journal of Sports Medicine*, 48(7), pp. 491–497. doi: 10.1136/bjsports-2014-093502.

Mountjoy, M. *et al.* (2015), 'Authors' 2015 additions to the IOC consensus statement: Relative Energy Deficiency in Sport (RED-S)', *British Journal of Sports Medicine*, 49(7), pp. 417–420. doi: 10.1136/bjsports-2014-094371.

Mountjoy, M. *et al.* (2018), 'IOC consensus statement on relative energy deficiency in sport (RED-S): 2018 update', *British Journal of Sports Medicine*, 52(11), pp. 687–697. doi: 10.1136/bjsports-2018-099193.

Mozaffarian, D. *et al.* (2006), 'Trans fatty acids and cardiovascular disease', *New Eng. J. Med.,* vol. 354, pp. 1601–13.

Mozaffarian, D. *et al.* (2011), muls 'Components of a cardioprotective diet: new insights', *Circulation*, vol. 123, pp. 2870–91.

Mullins, V. A. *et al.* (2001), 'Nutritional status of US elite female heptathletes during training', *Int. J. Sport Nutr.,* vol. 11, pp. 299–314.

Muls, E. *et al.* (1995), 'Is weight cycling detrimental to health? A review of the literature in humans', *International Journal of Obesity and Related Metabolic Disorders: Journal of the International Association for the Study of Obesity*, 19 Suppl 3, pp. S46-50.

Muoio, D. M. *et al.* (1994), 'Effect of dietary fat on metabolic adjustments to maximal VO_2 and endurance in runners', *Med. Sci. Sports Exerc.,* vol. 26(1), pp. 81–8.

Murphy, C. H. *et al.* (2015), 'Considerations for protein intake in managing weight loss in athletes', *Eur. J. Sport Sci.,* vol 15(1), pp. 21–8.

Murphy, M. *et al.* (2012), 'Whole beetroot consumption acutely improves running performance', *J. Acad. Nutr. Diet.,* vol. 112, pp. 548–52.

Murray, R. *et al.* (1999), 'A comparison of the gastric emptying characteristics of selected sports drinks', *Int. J. Sports Nutr.,* vol. 9, pp. 263–74.

Nattiv, A. *et al.* (2007), 'American College of Sports Medicine position stand. The female athlete triad', *Med. Sci. Sports Exerc.,* vol. 39, pp. 1867–82.

Nebl, Josefine, *et al.* (a2019), 'Exercise Capacity of Vegan, Lacto-Ovo-Vegetarian and Omnivorous Recreational Runners.', *Journal of the International Society of Sports Nutrition*, vol. 16, no. 1, May 2019, p. 23. BioMed Central, doi:10.1186/s12970-019-0289-4.

Needleman I *et al.* (2014), 'Oral health and impact on performance of athletes participating in the London 2012 Olympic Games: a cross-sectional study', *Br J Sports Med.,* vol. 47(16), pp. 1054–8.

Needleman, I. *et al.* (2015), 'Oral health and elite sport performance', *Br. J. Sports Med.,* vol. 49, pp. 3–6.

Nelson, A. *et al.* (1997), 'Creatine supplementation raises anaerobic threshold', FASEB J., vol. 11, A586 (abstract).

Nelson, M. E. *et al.* (1986), 'Diet and bone status in amenorrheic runners', *Am. J. Clin. Nutr.,* vol. 43, pp. 910–16.

Neufer, P. D. *et al.* (1987), 'Improvements in exercise performance: effects of carbohydrate feedings and diet', *J. Appl. Physiol.,* vol. 62, pp. 983–8.

Neychev, V. K. and Mitev VI. (2005), 'The aphrodisiac herb *Tribulus terrestris* does not influence the androgen production in young men', *J. Ethnopharmacol.*, vol. 101(1–3), pp. 319–20.

Nichols, J. F. *et al.* (2007), 'Disordered eating and menstrual irregularity in high school athletes in lean-build and non lean-build sports', *Int. J. Sport Nutr. Exerc. Metab.*, vol. 17, pp. 364–77.

Nielsen, F. H. and Lukaski, H. C. (2006), 'Update on the relationship between magnesium and exercise', *Magnesium Research*, 19(3), pp. 180–189.

Nieman, D. C. (1999), 'Physical fitness and vegetarian diets: is there a relation?', *The American Journal of Clinical Nutrition*, 70(3), pp. 570s–575s. doi: 10.1093/ajcn/70.3.570s.

Nieman, D. C. (1999), 'Physical fitness and vegetarian diets: is there a relation?' *Am. J. Clin. Nutr.*, (Sep) vol. 70 (3 suppl), pp. 570S–5S.

Nieman, D. C. *et al.* (1989), 'Hematological, anthropometric, and metabolic comparisons between vegetarian and nonvegetarian elderly women'. *Int. J. Sports Med.*, vol. 10, pp. 243–50.

Nieman, D. C. *et al.* (2007), 'Quercetin reduces illness but not immune perturbations after intense exercise', *Med. Sci. Sports Exerc.*, vol. 39, pp. 1561–69.

Nieman, D. C., Henson, D. A., McAnulty, S. R., *et al.* (2004), 'Vitamin E and immunity after the Kona Triathlon World Championship', *Med. Sci. Sports Exerc.*, Aug 36(8), pp. 1328–35.

Noakes, T. D. (1993), 'Fluid replacement during exercise', *Exerc. Sport Sci. Rev.*, vol. 21, pp. 297–330.

Noakes, T. D. (2000), 'Hyponatremia in distance athletes: pulling the IV on the dehydration myth', *Phys. Sportsmed.*, vol. 26 (Sept), pp. 71–6.

Noakes, T. D. (2007), 'Drinking guidelines for exercise: what evidence is there that athletes should drink as much as possible to replace the weight lost during exercise or ad libitum?', *J. Sports Sci.*, vol. 25 (7), pp. 781–96.

Noakes, T. D. (2010), 'Is drinking to thirst optimum?' *Ann. Nutr. Metab.*, vol, 57, Suppl 2, pp. S9–17.

Noakes, T. D. (2012), *Waterlogged: The Serious Problem of Overhydration in Endurance Sports*, (Champaign, IL:/Human Kinetics).

Noreen, E. E. *et al.* (2010), 'Effects of supplemental fish oil on resting metabolic rate, body composition, and salivary cortisol in healthy adults'. *J. Int. Soc. Sports Nutr.*, vol. 7, p. 31.

Norris, M. L. *et al.* (2016), 'Gastrointestinal complications associated with anorexia nervosa: A systematic review', *International Journal of Eating Disorders*, 49(3), pp. 216–237. doi: https://doi.org/10.1002/eat.22462.

Norton, L. E. and Layman, D. K. (2006), 'Leucine Regulates Translation Initiation of Protein Synthesis in Skeletal Muscle after Exercise', *The Journal of Nutrition*, 136(2), pp. 533S-537S. doi: 10.1093/jn/136.2.533S.

Nosaka, K. *et al.* (2006), 'Effects of amino acid supplementation on muscle soreness and damage'. *Int. J. Sports Nutr. Exerc. Metab.*, vol. 16, pp. 620–35.

Nyakayiru, J. *et al.* (2017), 'Beetroot Juice Supplementation Improves High-Intensity Intermittent Type Exercise Performance in Trained Soccer Players', *Nutrients*, 9(3). doi: 10.3390/nu9030314.

O'Donovan, C. M. *et al.* (2020), 'Distinct microbiome composition and metabolome exists across subgroups of elite Irish athletes', *Journal of Science and Medicine in Sport*, 23(1), pp. 63–68. doi: 10.1016/j.jsams.2019.08.290.

Oliver, J. M., Anzalone, A. J. and Turner, S. M. (2018), 'Protection Before Impact: the Potential Neuroprotective Role of Nutritional Supplementation in Sports-Related Head Trauma', *Sports Medicine (Auckland, N.Z.)*, 48(Suppl 1), pp. 39–52. doi: 10.1007/s40279-017-0847-3.

Onywera, V. O. *et al.* (2004), 'Food and macronutrient intake of elite kenyan distance runners'. *Int. J. Sport Nutr. Exerc. Metab.*, vol. 14(6), pp. 709–19.

Ostendorf, D. M. *et al.* (2018), 'No consistent evidence of a disproportionately low resting energy expenditure in long-term successful weight-loss maintainers', *The American Journal of Clinical Nutrition*, 108(4), pp. 658–666. doi: 10.1093/ajcn/nqy179.

Ostojic, S. (2004), 'Creatine supplementation in young soccer players'. *Int. J. Sport Nutr. Exerc. Metab.*, vol. 14, pp. 95–103.

Otis, C. L. *et al.* (1997), 'American College of *Sports Medicine* position stand. The Female Athlete Triad'. *Med. Sci. Sport Exerc.*, vol. 29, pp. i–ix.

Otte, J. A. *et al.* (2001), 'Exercise induces gastric ischemia in healthy volunteers: a tonometry study', *Journal of Applied Physiology (Bethesda, Md.: 1985)*, 91(2), pp. 866–871. doi: 10.1152/jappl.2001.91.2.866.

Owens, B. M. (2007), 'The potential effects of pH and buffering capacity on dental erosion'. *Gen. Dent.*, vol. 55(6), pp. 527–31.

Owens, D. J., Allison, R. and Close, G. L. (2018), 'Vitamin D and the Athlete: Current Perspectives and

New Challenges', *Sports Medicine*, 48(1), pp. 3–16. doi: 10.1007/s40279-017-0841-9.

Owens, D. J., Fraser, W. D. and Close, G. L. (2015), 'Vitamin D and the athlete: emerging insights', *European Journal of Sport Science*, 15(1), pp. 73–84. doi: 10.1080/17461391.2014.944223.

Paddon-Jones, D. *et al.* (2001), 'Short term HMB supplementation does not reduce symptoms of eccentric muscle damage'. *Int. J. Sport Nutr.*, vol. 11, pp. 442–50.

Pagoto, S. L. and Appelhans, B. M. (2013), 'A call for an end to the diet debates'. *JAMA*, vol 310(7), pp. 687–688.

Palmer-Green, D. *et al.* (2013), 'The Injury/Illness Performance Project (IIPP): A Novel Epidemiological Approach for Recording the Consequences of Sports Injuries and Illnesses', *Journal of Sports Medicine*, 2013, pp. 1–9. doi: 10.1155/2013/523974.

Pannemans, D. L. *et al.* (1997), 'Calcium excretion, apparent calcium absorption and calcium balance in young and elderly subjects: influence of protein intake'. *Brit. J. Nutr.*, vol. 77(5), pp. 721–9.

Papageorgiou, M. *et al.* (2018), 'Reduced energy availability: implications for bone health in physically active populations', *European Journal of Nutrition*, 57(3), pp. 847–859. doi: 10.1007/s00394-017-1498-8.

Parr, E. B. *et al.* (2014), 'Alcohol ingestion impairs maximal post-exercise rates of myofibrillar protein synthesis following a single bout of concurrent training', *PloS One*, 9(2), p. e88384. doi: 10.1371/journal.pone.0088384.

Parry-Billings, M. *et al.* (1992), 'Plasma amino acid concentrations in over-training syndrome: possible effects on the immune system'. *Med. Sci. Sport Ex.*, vol. 24, pp. 1353–8.

Pasiakos S. M. *et al.* (2013), 'Effects of high-protein diets on fat-free mass and muscle protein synthesis following weight loss: a randomized controlled trial'. *FASEB* J., vol 27(9), pp.3837–47.

Pasiakos, S. M, and and McClung, J. P. (2011), 'Supplemental dietary leucine and the skeletal muscle anabolic response to essential amino acids'. *Nutr. Rev.*, vol. 69(9), pp. 550–57.

Pasiakos, S. M. *et al.* (2010), 'Acute energy deprivation affects skeletal muscle protein synthesis and associated intracellular signaling proteins in physically active adults', *The Journal of Nutrition*, 140(4), pp. 745–751. doi: 10.3945/jn.109.118372.

Pasiakos, S. M., McClung, H. L., McClung, J. P. (2011), 'Leucine-enriched essential amino acid supplementa-

tion during moderate steady state exercise enhances post-exercise muscle protein synthesis'. *Am. J. Clin. Nutr.*, vol. 94(3), pp. 809–18.

Pasricha, S. R. *et al.* (2014), 'Iron Supplementation Benefits Physical Performance in Women of Reproductive Age: A Systematic Review and Meta-Analysis'. *J. Nutr. 2014* jn.113.189589; first published online April 9, 2014.

Passe, D. H. *et al.* (2004), 'Palatability and voluntary intake of sports beverages, diluted orange juice and water during exercise'. *Int. J. Sport Nutr. Exerc. Metab.*, vol. 14, pp. 272–84.

Patterson, S. D. and Gray, S. C. (2007), 'Carbohydrate-gel supplementation and endurance performance during intermittent high-intensity shuttle running'. *Int. J. Sports Nutr. Exerc. Metab.*, vol. 17, pp. 445–55.

Paulsen, G., Cumming, K. T. *et al.* (2013), 'Vitamin C and E supplementation hampers cellular adaptation to endurance training in humans: a double-blind randomized controlled trial'. *J. Physiol.* 2013.267419

Peeling, P. *et al.* (2008), 'Athletic induced iron deficiency: new insights into the role of inflammation, cytokines and hormones', *European Journal of Applied Physiology*, 103(4), pp. 381–391. doi: 10.1007/s00421-008-0726-6.

Pennings, B. *et al.* (2011), 'Exercising before protein intake allows for greater use of dietary protein-derived amino acids for de novo muscle protein synthesis in both young and elderly men'. *Am. J. Clin. Nutr.*, vol. 93, pp. 322–31.

Pennings, B. *et al.* (2012), 'Amino acid absorption and subsequent muscle protein accretion following graded intakes of whey protein in elderly men'. *Am. J. Physiol. Endocrinol. Metab.*, vol. 302, pp. E992–9.

Peternelj, T. T. and Coombes, J. S. (2011), 'Antioxidant supplementation during exercise training: beneficial or detrimental?' *Sports Med.*, vol. 41(12), pp. 1043–69.

Peters, E. M. *et al.* (1993), 'Vitamin C supplementation reduces the incidence of post-race symptoms of upper-respiratory-tract infection in ultra-marathon runners'. *Am. J. Clin. Nutr.*, vol. 57, pp. 170–4.

Peters, E. M. *et al.* (2001), 'Vitamin C supplementation attenuates the increases in circulating cortisol, adrenaline and anti-inflammatory polypeptides following ultra-marathon running'. *Int. J. Sports Med.*, vol. 22(7), pp. 537–43.

Petersen, L. M. *et al.* (2017), 'Community characteristics of the gut microbiomes of competitive cyclists', *Microbiome*, 5. doi: 10.1186/s40168-017-0320-4.

Petersen, L. M. *et al.* (2017), 'Community characteristics of the gut microbiomes of competitive cyclists', *Microbiome*, 5, p. 98. doi: 10.1186/s40168-017-0320-4.

Peterson, M. *et al.* (2011), 'Influence of resistance exercise on lean body mass in aging adults: a metaanalysis'. *Med. Sci. Sports Exerc.*, vol. 43, pp. 249–58.

Petkus, D. L., Murray-Kolb, L. E. and De Souza, M. J. (2017), 'The Unexplored Crossroads of the Female Athlete Triad and Iron Deficiency: A Narrative Review', *Sports Medicine*, 47(9), pp. 1721–1737. doi: 10.1007/s40279-017-0706-2.

Pfeiffer, B. *et al.* (2010a) (a), 'Oxidation of solid versus liquid CHO sources during exercise'. *Med. Sci. Sports Exerc.*, vol. 42(11), pp. 2030–7.

Pfeiffer, B. *et al.* (2010b) (b), 'CHO oxidation from a CHO gel compared with a drink during exercise'. *Med. Sci. Sports Exerc.*, vol. 42(11), pp. 2038–45.

Phillips, P. A. *et al.* (1984), 'Reduced thirst after water deprivation in healthy elderly men'. *N. Engl. J. Med.*, vol. 311, pp. 753–59.

Phillips, S. M. (2012), 'Dietary protein requirements and adaptive advantages in athletes'. *Br J. Nutr.*, vol. 108, Suppl. 2, pp. S158–67.

Phillips, S. M. and Van Loon, L. J. C. (2011) (a), 'Dietary protein for athletes: from requirements to optimum adaptation', *Journal of Sports Sciences*, 29 Suppl 1, pp. S29-38. doi: 10.1080/02640414.2011.619204.

Phillips, S. M. and Van Loon, L. J. C. (2011) (b), 'Dietary protein for athletes: from requirements to optimum adaptation', *Journal of Sports Sciences*, 29 Suppl 1, pp. S29-38. doi: 10.1080/02640414.2011.619204.

Phillips, S. M. *et al.* (1997), 'Mixed muscle protein synthesis and breakdown after resistance training in humans'. *Am. J. Physiol.*, vol. 273(1), pp. E99–E107.

Phillips, S. M. *et al.* (1999), 'Resistance training reduces acute exercise-induced increase in muscle protein turnover'. *Am. J. Physiol.*, vol. 276(1), pp. E118–24.

Phillips, S. M. *et al.* (2005), 'Dietary protein to support anabolism with resistance exercise in young men'. *J. Am. Coll. Nutr.*, vol. 24(2), pp. 134S–9S.

Phillips, S. M. *et al.* (2007), 'A critical examination of dietary protein requirements, benefits and excesses in athletes'. *Int. J. Sports Nutr. Exerc. Metab.*, vol. 17, pp. 58–78.

Phillips, S. M., Chevalier, S. and Leidy, H. J. (2016), 'Protein "requirements" beyond the RDA: implications for optimizing health', *Applied Physiology, Nutrition, and Metabolism = Physiologie Appliquee, Nutrition Et Metabolisme*, 41(5), pp. 565–572. doi: 10.1139/apnm-2015-0550.

Phillips, S. M., *et al.* (2011)(c), 'Nutrition for weight and resistance training'. In: Lanham-New, S. A. *et al.* (eds), *Sport and Exercise Nutrition* (Oxford: Wiley-Blackwell).

Phillips, T. *et al.* (2003), 'A dietary supplement attenuates IL-6 and CRP after eccentric exercise in untrained males'. *Med. Sci. Sports Exerc.*, vol. 35(12), pp. 2032–7.

Philpott, J. D., Witard, O. C. and Galloway, S. D. R. (2019), 'Applications of omega-3 polyunsaturated fatty acid supplementation for sport performance', *Research in Sports Medicine (Print)*, 27(2), pp. 219–237. doi: 10.1080/15438627.2018.1550401.

Phinney, S. D. *et al.* (1983), 'The human metabolic response to chronic ketosis without caloric restriction: preservation of submaximal exercise capability with reduced carbohydrate oxidation'. *Metabolism*, vol. 32(8), pp. 69–76.

Pilegaard, H. *et al.* (2005), 'Substrate availability and transcriptional regulation of metabolic genes in human skeletal muscle during recovery from exercise'. *Metabolism*, vol. 54(8), pp. 1048–55.

Pillay, S. *et al.* (2021), 'Longer race distance predicts gastrointestinal illness-related medical encounters in 153 208 endurance runner race starters – SAFER XVI', *The Journal of Sports Medicine and Physical Fitness*. doi: 10.23736/S0022-4707.21.12072-9.

Pinto, C. L. *et al.* (2016), 'Impact of creatine supplementation in combination with resistance training on lean mass in the elderly', *Journal of Cachexia, Sarcopenia and Muscle*, 7(4), pp. 413–421. doi: https://doi.org/10.1002/jcsm.12094.

Plotkin, D. L. *et al.* (2021), 'Isolated Leucine and Branched-Chain Amino Acid Supplementation for Enhancing Muscular Strength and Hypertrophy: A Narrative Review', *International Journal of Sport Nutrition and Exercise Metabolism*, pp. 1–10. doi: 10.1123/ijsnem.2020-0356.

Pöchmüller, M. *et al.* (2016), 'A systematic review and meta-analysis of carbohydrate benefits associated with randomized controlled competition-based performance trials'. *J. Int. Soc. Sports Nutr.* vVol. 13, pp 27.

Poffé, C. *et al.* (2020), 'Exogenous ketosis impacts neither performance nor muscle glycogen breakdown in prolonged endurance exercise', *Journal of Applied Physiology (Bethesda, Md.: 1985)*, 128(6), pp. 1643–1653. doi: 10.1152/japplphysiol.00092.2020.

Polidori, D. *et al.* (2016), 'How Strongly Does Appetite Counter Weight Loss? Quantification of the Feedback Control of Human Energy Intake', *Obesity (Silver*

Spring, Md.), 24(11), pp. 2289–2295. doi: 10.1002/oby.21653.

Pollock, M. L. and Jackson, A. S. (1984), 'Research progress invalidation of clinical methods of assessing body composition'. *Med. Sci. Sport Ex.*, vol. 16, pp. 606–13.

Poortmans, J. R. and Francaux, M. (1999), 'Longterm oral creatine supplementation does not impair renal function in healthy athletes'. *Med. Sci. Sports Ex.*, vol. 31(8), pp. 1103–10.

Pottier, A. *et al.* (2010), 'Mouth rinse but not ingestion of a carbohydrate solution improves 1-h cycle time trialtime-trial performance', *Scand. J. Med. Sci. Sports,* vol. 20(1), pp. 105–11.

Powers, M. E. (2002), 'The safety and efficacy of anabolic steroid precursors: what is the scientific evidence?'. *J. Athol. Training,* vol. 37(3), pp. 300–5.

Powers, S. *et al.* (2011), 'Antioxidant and vitamin D supplements for athletes: sense or nonsense?' *J. Sports Sci.*, vol. 29, Suppl. 1, S47–55.

Public Health England (2011), 'Government Dietary Recommendation's.

Public Health England (2016), 'The Eatwell Guide'.. Available at: https://www.gov.uk/government/publications/the-eatwell-guide(Accessed: 30 April 2021).

Pugh, J. N. *et al.* (2018), 'Prevalence, Severity and Potential Nutritional Causes of Gastrointestinal Symptoms during a Marathon in Recreational Runners', *Nutrients*, 10(7). doi: 10.3390/nu10070811.

Pugh, J. N. *et al.* (2019), 'Four weeks of probiotic supplementation reduces GI symptoms during a marathon race', *European Journal of Applied Physiology*, 119(7), pp. 1491–1501. doi: 10.1007/s00421-019-04136-3.

Pyne, D. B. *et al.* (2015), 'Probiotics supplementation for athletes – clinical and physiological effects', *European Journal of Sport Science*, 15(1), pp. 63–72. doi: 10.1080/17461391.2014.971879.

Quesnele, J. J. *et al.* (2014), 'The effects of Beta-alanine supplementation on performance: a systematic review of the literature'. *Int. J. Sport Nutr. Exerc. Metab.*, vol. 24(1), pp. 14–27.

Ravussin, E. *et al.* (2019), 'Early Time-Restricted Feeding Reduces Appetite and Increases Fat Oxidation But Does Not Affect Energy Expenditure in Humans', *Obesity (Silver Spring, Md.)*, 27(8), pp. 1244–1254. doi: 10.1002/oby.22518.

Rawson, E. S. and Volek, J. S. (2003), 'Effects of creatine supplementation and resistance training on muscle strength and weightlifting performance'. *J. Strength Cond. Res.*, vol. 17, pp. 822–31.

Ready, S. L. *et al.* (1999), 'The effect of two sports drink formulations on muscle stress and performance'. *Med. Sci. Sports Exerc.*, vol. 31(5), p. S119.

Reidy, P. T. *et al.* (2013), 'Protein blend ingestion following resistance exercise promotes human muscle protein synthesis'. *J. Nutr.*, vol. 143(4), pp. 410–16.

Rennie, M. J. (2009), 'Anabolic resistance: the effects of aging, sexual dimorphism, and immobilization on human muscle protein turnover'. *Appl. Physiol. Nutr. Metab.*, vol. 34, pp. 377–81.

Rennie, M. J. and Tipton, K. D. (2000), 'Protein and amino acid metabolism during and after exercise and the effects of nutrition', *Annual Review of Nutrition*, 20, pp. 457–483. doi: 10.1146/annurev.nutr.20.1.457.

Res, P. T. *et al.* (2012), 'Protein ingestion prior to sleep improves post-exercise overnight recovery'. *Med. Sci. Sports Exerc.*, Feb 9 (Epub ahead of print).

Reubinoff, B. E. *et al.* (1995), 'Effects of hormone replacement therapy on weight, body composition, fat distribution, and food intake in early post-menopausal women: a prospective study', *Fertility and Sterility*, 64(5), pp. 963–968. doi: 10.1016/s0015-0282(16)57910-2.

Ribeiro, A. S. *et al.* (2016), 'Effect of conjugated linoleic acid associated with aerobic exercise on body fat and lipid profile in obese women: a randomized, double-blinded, and placebo-controlled trial'. *Int. J. Sport Nutr. Exerc. Metab.*, vol. 26(2), pp. 135–44.

Richter, E. A. *et al.* (1991), 'Immune parameters in male athletes after a lacto-ovo-vegetarian diet and a mixed Western diet'. *Med. Sci. Sports Exerc.*, vol. 23, pp. 517–21.

Rickenlund, A. *et al.* (2005), 'Amenorrhea in Female Athletes Is Associated with Endothelial Dysfunction and Unfavorable Lipid Profile', *The Journal of Clinical Endocrinology & Metabolism*, 90(3), pp. 1354–1359. doi: 10.1210/jc.2004-1286.

Ritz, P and Rockwell, M (2021), Promoting Optimal Omega-3 Fatty Acid Status in Athletes Gatorade Sports Science Institute. Available at: http://www.gssi-web.org:80/en/sports-science-exchange/Article/promoting-optimal-omega-3-fatty-acid-status-in-athletes (Accessed: 13 July 2021).

Ritz, P. P. *et al.* (2020), 'Dietary and Biological Assessment of the Omega-3 Status of Collegiate Athletes: A Cross-Sectional Analysis', *PloS One*, 15(4), p. e0228834. doi: 10.1371/journal.pone.0228834.

Rivera-Brown, A. M. *et al.* (1999), 'Drink composition, voluntary drinking and fluid balance in exercising trained heat-acclimatized boys'. *J. Appl. Physiol.*, vol. 86, pp. 78–84.

Rizkalla, S. *et al.* (2004), 'Improved plasma glucose control, whole body glucose utilisation and lipid profile on a low glycaemic index diet in type 2 diabetic men: a randomised controlled trial'. *Diab. Care*, vol. 27, pp. 1866–72.

Roberts, J. D. *et al.* (2016), 'An Exploratory Investigation of Endotoxin Levels in Novice Long Distance Triathletes, and the Effects of a Multi-Strain Probiotic/Prebiotic, Antioxidant Intervention', *Nutrients*, 8(11). doi: 10.3390/nu8110733.

Robinson. T. M. *et al.* (2000), 'Dietary creatine supplementation does not affect some haematological indices, or indices of muscle damage and hepatic and renal function'. *Brit. J. Sports Med.*, vol. 34, pp. 284–8.

Rodriguez, N. R., Di Marco, N. M., Langley, S., *et al.* (2009), 'American College of Sports Medicine position stand: Nutrition and athletic performance', *Med. Sci. Sports Exerc.*, vol. 41(3), pp. 709–31.

Rogers, J. *et al.* (2005), 'Gastric emptying and intestinal absorption of a low carbohydrate sport drink during exercise'. *Int. J. Sport Nutr. Exerc. Metab.*, vol. 15, pp. 220–35.

Rogers, M. A. *et al.* (2021), 'Prevalence of impaired physiological function consistent with Relative Energy Deficiency in Sport (RED-S): an Australian elite and pre-elite cohort', *British Journal of Sports Medicine*, 55(1), pp. 38–45. doi: 10.1136/bjsports-2019-101517.

Rogerson, S. *et al.* (2007), 'The effect of five weeks of Tribulus terrestris supplementation on muscle strength and body composition during preseason training in elite rugby league players'. *J. Strength Cond. Res.*, vol. 21(2), pp. 348–53.

Rokitzki, L. *et al.* (1994), 'a-tocopherol supplementation in racing cyclists during extreme endurance training'. *Int. J. Sports Nutr.*, vol. 4, pp. 235–64.

Rollo, I. *et al.* (2008), 'The influence of carbohydrate mouth rinse on self-selected speeds during a 30-min treadmill run,', ' *Int. J. Sport Nutr. Exerc. Metab.*, vol 18(6), pp. 585–600.

Rolls, B. J. and Shide, D. J. (1992), 'The influence of fat on food intake and body weight'. *Nutr. Revs.*, vol. 50(10), pp. 283–90.

Romano-Ely, B. C. *et al.* (2006), 'Effects of an isocaloric carbohydrate-protein-antioxidant drink on cycling performance'. *Med. Sci. Sports Exerc.*, vol. 38, pp. 1608–16.

Rosen, L. W. *et al.* (1986), 'Pathogenic weightcontrol behavior in female athletes'. *Phys. Sports Med.*, vol. 14, pp. 79–86.

Rosenbaum, M. and Leibel, R. L. (2010), 'Adaptive thermogenesis in humans', *International Journal of Obesity (2005)*, 34 Suppl 1, pp. S47-55. doi: 10.1038/ijo.2010.184.

Rossow, L. M. *et al.* (2013), 'Natural bodybuilding competition preparation and recovery: a 12-month case study', *International Journal of Sports Physiology and Performance*, 8(5), pp. 582–592. doi: 10.1123/ijspp.8.5.582.

Rowbottom, D. G. *et al.* (1996), 'The energizing role of glutamine as an indicator of exercise stress and overtraining'. *Sports Med.*, vol. 21(2), pp. 80–97.

Ruddick-Collins, L. C., Morgan, P. J. and Johnstone, A. M. (2020), 'Mealtime: A circadian disruptor and determinant of energy balance?', *Journal of Neuroendocrinology*, 32(7), p. e12886. doi: https://doi.org/10.1111/jne.12886.

Rustad, P.I. *et al.* (2016), 'Intake of Protein Plus Carbohydrate during the First Two Hours after Exhaustive Cycling Improves Performance the following Day'. *PLoS One*, vol. 11(4) e0153229.

Rutherfurd, Shane M., et al.*et al.* (2015), "'Protein Digestibility-Corrected Amino Acid Scores and Digestible Indispensable Amino Acid Scores Differentially Describe Protein Quality in Growing Male Rats."', *The Journal of Nutrition*, vol. 145, no. 2, Feb. 2015, pp. 372–79. PubMed, doi:10.3945/jn.114.195438.

Rynders, C. A. *et al.* (2019), 'Effectiveness of Intermittent Fasting and Time-Restricted Feeding Compared to Continuous Energy Restriction for Weight Loss', *Nutrients*, 11(10), p. 2442. doi: 10.3390/nu11102442.

Sacks, F. M. *et al.* (2017), 'Dietary Fats and Cardiovascular Disease: A Presidential Advisory From the American Heart Association', *Circulation*, 136(3), pp. e1–e23. doi: 10.1161/CIR.0000000000000510.

SACN (2015), 'Carbohydrates and Health', https://assets.publishing.service.gov.uk/government/uploads/system/uploads/attachment_data/file/445503/SACN_Carbohydrates_and_Health.pdf Accessed May 2021.

SACN (2019) Saturated fats and health: SACN report (no date) *GOV.UK.* Available at: https://www.gov.

uk/government/publications/saturated-fats-and-health-sacn-report (Accessed: 30 April 2021).

Santos, V. C. *et al.* (2013), 'Effects of DHA-rich fish oil supplementation on lymphocyte function before and after a marathon race'. *Int. J. Sport Nutr. Exerc. Metab.*, vol. 23(2), pp. 161–9.

Santosa, S. and Jensen, M. D. (2013), 'Adipocyte fatty acid storage factors enhance subcutaneous fat storage in postmenopausal women', *Diabetes*, 62(3), pp. 775–782. doi: 10.2337/db12-0912.

Saunders, B. *et al.* (2017), 'β-alanine supplementation to improve exercise capacity and performance: a systematic review and meta-analysis', *British Journal of Sports Medicine*, 51(8), pp. 658–669. doi: 10.1136/bjsports-2016-096396.

Saunders, M. J. (2007), 'Coingestion of carbohydrate-protein during endurance exercise: influence on performance and recovery'. *Int. J. Sports Nutr. Exerc. Metab.*, vol. 17, S87–S103.

Saunders, M. J. *et al.* (2004), 'Effects of a carbohydrate-protein-beverage on cycling endurance and muscle damage'. *Med. Sci. Sports Exerc.*, vol. 36, pp. 1233–8.

Sawka, M. N. (1992), 'Physiological consequences of hypohydration: exercise performance and thermoregulation'. *Med. Sci. Sports Exerc.*, vol. 24, pp. 657–70.

Sawka, M. N. *et al.* (2007), 'American College of Sports Medicine Position stand. Exercise and fluid replacement'. *Med. Sci. Sports Exerc.*, vol. 39, pp. 377–90.

Sawka, M. N., Cheuvront, S. N. and Kenefick, R. W. (2015), 'Hypohydration and Human Performance: Impact of Environment and Physiological Mechanisms', *Sports Medicine (Auckland, N.z.)*, 45(Suppl 1), pp. 51–60. doi: 10.1007/s40279-015-0395-7.

Sawka, M. N., Coyle, E.F. (1999), 'Influence of body water and blood volume on thermoregulation and exercise performance in the heat', *Exerc. Sport. Sci. Rev.*, 1999;27:167-218. PMID: 10791017.

Schoenfeld, B. J. and Aragon, A. A. (2018), 'How much protein can the body use in a single meal for muscle-building? Implications for daily protein distribution', *Journal of the International Society of Sports Nutrition*, 15(1), p. 10. doi: 10.1186/s12970-018-0215-1.

Schoenfeld, B. J. *et al.* (2013), 'The effect of protein timing on muscle strength and hypertrophy: a meta-analysis'. *J. Int. Soc. Sports Nutr.*, vol. 10(1), p. 53.

Schoenfeld, B. J. *et al.* (2017) (a), 'Strength and Hypertrophy Adaptations Between Low- vs. High-Load Resistance Training: A Systematic Review and Meta-analysis', *Journal of Strength and Conditioning Research*, 31(12), pp. 3508–3523. doi: 10.1519/JSC.0000000000002200.

Schoenfeld, B. J. *et al.* (2017) (b), 'Pre- versus post-exercise protein intake has similar effects on muscular adaptations'. *PeerJ.*, vol. 5, e2825.

Schokman, C. P. *et al.* (1999), 'Pre- and post game macronutrient intake of a group of elite Australian Football Players'. *Int. J. Sport Nutr.*, vol. 9, pp. 60–9.

Seebohar, B. (2014), 'Metabolic efficiency training: teaching the body to burn more fat'. (2nd edn), www.enrgperformance.com.

Seiler, D. *et al.* (1989), 'Effects of long-distance running on iron metabolism and hematological parameters'. *Int. J. Sports Med.*, vol. 10, pp. 357–62.

Seip, R. L. and Semenkovich, C. F. (1998), 'Skeletal muscle lipoprotein lipase: molecular regulation and physiological effects in relation to exercise'. *Exerc. Sport Sci. Rev.*, vol. 26, pp. 191–218.

Sender, R., Fuchs, S. and Milo, R. (2016), 'Revised Estimates for the Number of Human and Bacteria Cells in the Body', *PLoS Biology*, 14(8). doi: 10.1371/journal.pbio.1002533.

Senefeld, J. W. *et al.* (2020), 'Ergogenic Effect of Nitrate Supplementation: A Systematic Review and Meta-analysis', *Medicine and Science in Sports and Exercise*, 52(10), pp. 2250–2261. doi: 10.1249/MSS.0000000000002363.

Shahidi, F. and Ambigaipalan, P. (2018), 'Omega-3 Polyunsaturated Fatty Acids and Their Health Benefits', *Annual Review of Food Science and Technology*, 9, pp. 345–381. doi: 10.1146/annurev-food-111317-095850.

Shaw, G. *et al.* (2017), 'Vitamin C–enriched gelatin supplementation before intermittent activity augments collagen synthesis12', *The American Journal of Clinical Nutrition*, 105(1), pp. 136–143. doi: 10.3945/ajcn.116.138594.

Sherman, W. M. *et al.* (1981), 'Effect of exercise-diet manipulation on muscle glycogen and its subsequent utilisation during performance'. *Int. J. Sports Med.*, vol. 2, pp. 114–18.

Sherman, W. M. *et al.* (1991), 'Carbohydrate feedings 1 hour before exercise improve cycling performance'. *Am. J. Clin. Nutr.*, vol. 54, pp. 866–70.

Sherman, W. M. *et al.* (1993), 'Dietary carbohydrate, muscle glycogen, and exercise performance during 7 d of training', *The American Journal of Clinical Nutrition*, 57(1), pp. 27–31. doi: 10.1093/ajcn/57.1.27.

Shi, X. *et al.* (2004), 'Gastrointestinal discomfort during intermittent high-intensity exercise: effect of carbohydrate-electrolyte beverage', *International Journal of Sport Nutrition and Exercise Metabolism*, 14(6), pp. 673–683. doi: 10.1123/ijsnem.14.6.673.

Shimizu, K. *et al.* (2011), 'Influences of weight loss on monocytes and T-cell subpopulations in male judo athletes', *Journal of Strength and Conditioning Research*, 25(7), pp. 1943–1950. doi: 10.1519/JSC.0b013e3181e4f9c6.

Shimomura, Y. *et al.* (2006), 'Nutraceutical effects of branched chain amino acids on skeletal muscle'. *J. Nutr.*, vol. 136, pp. 529–32.

Shing, C. M., Hunter, D. C. and, Stevenson, L. M. (2009), 'Bovine colostrum supplementation and exercise performance: potential mechanisms'. *Sports Med.*, vol. 39(12), pp. 1033–54.

Shing, C.M. *et al.* (2007), 'Effects of bovine colostrum supplementation on immune variables in highly trained cyclists'. *J. Appl. Physiol.*, vol. 102, pp. 1113–22.

Shirreffs S. M. *et al.* (2004), 'Fluid and electrolyte needs for preparation and recovery from training and competition'. *J. Sports Sci.*, vol. 22(1), pp. 57–63.

Shirreffs, S. M. and Sawka, M. N. (2011), 'Fluid and electrolyte needs for training, competition, and recovery'. *J. Sports Sci.*, vol. 29, suppl 1, pp. S39–46.

Shirreffs, S. M. *et al.* (2007), 'Milk as an effective post-exercise rehydration drink'. *Br J. Nutr.*, vol. 98, pp. 173–180.

Shirreffs, S. M., *et al.* (1996), 'Post-exercise rehydration in man: effects of volume consumed. and drink sodium content'. *Med. Sci. Sports Ex.*, vol. 28, pp. 1260–71.

Short, S. H. and Short, W. R. (1983), 'Four-year study of university athletes' dietary intake'. *J. Am. Diet. Assoc.*, vol. 82, p. 632.

Siervo, M. *et al.* (2013), 'Inorganic nitrate and beetroot juice supplementation reduces blood pressure in adults: a systematic review and meta-analysis', *The Journal of Nutrition*, 143(6), pp. 818–826. doi: 10.3945/jn.112.170233.

Silva, M. R. G. and Paiva, T. (2015), 'Low energy availability and low body fat of female gymnasts before an international competition', *European Journal of Sport Science*, 15(7), pp. 591–599. doi: 10.1080/17461391.2014.969323.

Silva-Cavalcante, M. D. *et al.* (2013), 'Caffeine increases anaerobic work and restores cycling performance following a protocol designed to lower endogenous carbohydrate availability'. PLoS One, vol. 8(8), e72025.

Sim, M. *et al.* (2019), 'Iron considerations for the athlete: a narrative review', *European Journal of Applied Physiology*, 119(7), pp. 1463–1478. doi: 10.1007/s00421-019-04157-y.

Simopoulos, A. P. and Robinson, J. (1998), *The Omega Plan* (New York, HarperCollins).

Simpson, R. J. *et al.* (2020), 'Can exercise affect immune function to increase susceptibility to infection?', *Exercise Immunology Review*, 26, pp. 8–22.

Singh, Pramil N., et al.*et al.* "(2003), 'Does Low Meat Consumption Increase Life Expectancy in Humans?"', *The American Journal of Clinical Nutrition*, vol. 78, no. 3, Sept. 2003, pp. 526S-532S. academic.oup.com, doi:10.1093/ajcn/78.3.526S.

Sinning, W. E. (1998), 'Body composition in athletes'. , In Roche, A. F. *et al.* (eds.) *Human Body Composition*, (Champaign, IL: Human Kinetics), pp. 257–73.

Skaug, A., Sveen, O., and Raastad, T. (2014), 'An antioxidant and multivitamin supplement reduced improvements in VO2maxVO2 max'. *J. Sports Med. Phys. Fitness.*, vol. 54(1), pp. 63–9.

Slater, G. *et al.* (2001), 'HMB supplementation does not affect changes in strength or body composition during resistance training in trained men'. *Int. J. Sport Nutr.*, vol. 11, pp. 383–96.

Sloth, B. *et al.* (2004), 'No difference in body weight decrease between a low GI and high GI diet but reduced LDL cholesterol after 10 wk ad libitum intake of the low GI diet'. *Am. J. Clin Nutr.*, vol. 80, pp. 337–47.

Smith, G. I. *et al.* (2011) (a), 'Dietary omega-3 fatty acid supplementation increases the rate of muscle protein synthesis in older adults: a randomized controlled trial', *The American Journal of Clinical Nutrition*, 93(2), pp. 402–412. doi: 10.3945/ajcn.110.005611.

Smith, G. I. *et al.* (2011) (b), 'Omega-3 polyunsaturated fatty acids augment the muscle protein anabolic response to hyperinsulinaemia-hyperaminoacidaemia in healthy young and middle-aged men and women', *Clinical Science (London, England: 1979)*, 121(6), pp. 267–278. doi: 10.1042/CS20100597.

Smith, J. W. *et al.* (2010), 'Fuel selection and cycling endurance performance with ingestion of [13C] glucose: evidence for a carbohydrate dose response', *Journal of Applied Physiology (Bethesda, Md.: 1985)*, 108(6), pp. 1520–1529. doi: 10.1152/japplphysiol.91394.2008.

Snijders, T. *et al.* (2015), 'Protein ingestion before sleep increases muscle mass and strength gains during prolonged resistance-type exercise training in healthy young men'. *J. Nutr.* In press, Apr 29, 2015.

Snyder, A. C. *et al.* (1989), 'Influence of dietary iron source on measures of iron status among female runners'. *Med. Sci. Sports Exerc.*; vol. 21, pp. 7–10.

Sobiecki, Jakub G., et al.*et al.* "(2016), 'High Compliance with Dietary Recommendations in a Cohort of Meat Eaters, Fish Eaters, Vegetarians, and Vegans: Results from the European Prospective Investigation into Cancer and Nutrition-Oxford Study.'", *Nutrition Research* (New York, N.Y.), vol. 36, no. 5, May 2016, pp. 464–77. PubMed, doi:10.1016/j.nutres.2015.12.016.

Soenen, S. *et al.* (2012), 'Relatively high-protein or "low-carb" energy-restricted diets for body weight loss and body weight maintenance?', *Physiology & Behavior*, 107(3), pp. 374–380. doi: 10.1016/j.physbeh.2012.08.004.

Somerville, V. S., Braakhuis, A. J. and Hopkins, W. G. (2016), 'Effect of Flavonoids on Upper Respiratory Tract Infections and Immune Function: A Systematic Review and Meta-Analysis12', *Advances in Nutrition*, 7(3), pp. 488–497. doi: 10.3945/an.115.010538.

Sorrenti, V. *et al.* (2020), 'Deciphering the Role of Polyphenols in Sports Performance: From Nutritional Genomics to the Gut Microbiota toward Phytonutritional Epigenomics', *Nutrients*, 12(5), p. 1265. doi: 10.3390/nu12051265.

Southward, K., Rutherfurd-Markwick, K. J. and Ali, A. (2018), 'The Effect of Acute Caffeine Ingestion on Endurance Performance: A Systematic Review and Meta-Analysis', *Sports Medicine (Auckland, N.Z.)*, 48(8), pp. 1913–1928. doi: 10.1007/s40279-018-0939-8.

Souza, D. B. *et al.* (2017), 'Acute effects of caffeine-containing energy drinks on physical performance: a systematic review and meta-analysis', *European Journal of Nutrition*, 56(1), pp. 13–27. doi: 10.1007/s00394-016-1331-9.

Spector, T. (2015), *The Diet Myth: The real science behind what we eat* (WBH).

Speedy, D. B. *et al.* (1999), 'Hyponatremia in ultra-distance triathletes'. *Med. Sci. Sports Exerc.*, vol. 31, pp. 809–15.

Spence, L. *et al.* (2007), 'Incidence, etiology, and symptomatology of upper respiratory illness in elite athletes', *Medicine and Science in Sports and Exercise*, 39(4), pp. 577–586. doi: 10.1249/mss.0b013e31802e851a.

Spencer, E. A. *et al.* (2003), 'Weight gain over 5 years in 21,966 meat-eating, fish-eating, vegetarian, and vegan men and women in EPIC-Oxford'. *Int. J. Obes. Relat. Metab. Disord.* Jun; 27(6), pp. 728–34.

Spriet, L. (1995), 'Caffeine and performance'. *Int. J. Sport Nutr.*, vol. 5, pp. S84–S99.

Spriet, L. L. (2014(a), 'Exercise and Sport Performance with Low Doses of Caffeine', *Sports Medicine*, 44(2), pp. 175–184. doi: 10.1007/s40279-014-0257-8.

Spriet, L. L. (2014(b)), 'New insights into the interaction of carbohydrate and fat metabolism during exercise', *Sports Medicine (Auckland, N.Z.)*, 44 Suppl 1, pp. S87-96. doi: 10.1007/s40279-014-0154-1.

Steen, S. N. and McKinney, S. (1986), 'Nutrition assessment of college wrestlers'. *Phys. Sports Med.*, vol. 14, pp. 100–6.

Steenge, G. R. *et al.* (1998), 'The stimulatory effect of insulin on creatine accummulation in human skeletal muscle'. *Am. J. Physiol.*, vol. 275, pp. E974–9.

Stegen, S. *et al.* (2014), 'The beta-alanine dose for maintaining moderately elevated muscle carnosine levels'. *Med. Sci. Sports Exerc.*, 1 (Epub ahead of print).

Stellingwerff, T. and Cox, G. R. (2014), 'Systematic review: Carbohydrate supplementation on exercise performance or capacity of varying durations', *Applied Physiology, Nutrition, and Metabolism = Physiologie Appliquee, Nutrition Et Metabolisme*, 39(9), pp. 998–1011. doi: 10.1139/apnm-2014-0027.

Stellingwerff, T. and Cox, G. R. (2014), 'Systematic review: Carbohydrate supplementation on exercise performance or capacity of varying durations', *Applied Physiology, Nutrition, and Metabolism = Physiologie Appliquee, Nutrition Et Metabolisme*, 39(9), pp. 998–1011. doi: 10.1139/apnm-2014-0027.

Stellingwerff, T. *et al.* (2006), 'Decreased PDH activation and glycogenolysis during exercise following fat adaptation with carbohydrate restoration'. *Am. J. Physiol. Endocrinol. Metab.*, vol. 290(2), pp. 380–8.

Stevenson, E. *et al.* (2005), 'Improved recovery from prolonged exercise following the consumption of low glycaemic index carbohydrate meals'. *Int. J. Sport Nutr. Exerc. Metab.*, vol. 15, pp. 333–49.

Stoffel, N. U. *et al.* (2020), 'Iron absorption from supplements is greater with alternate day than with consecutive day dosing in iron-deficient anemic women', *Haematologica*, 105(5), pp. 1232–1239. doi: 10.3324/haematol.2019.220830.

Strauss, R. H., Lanese, R. R. and Malarkey, W. B. (1985), 'Weight loss in amateur wrestlers and its effect on serum testosterone levels', *JAMA*, 254(23), pp. 3337–3338.

Stroehlein, J. K. *et al.* (2021), 'Vitamin D supplementation for the treatment of COVID-19: a living systematic review', *The Cochrane Database of Systematic Reviews*, 5, p. CD015043. doi: 10.1002/14651858. CD015043.

Sun, G. *et al.* (2005), 'Comparison of multifrequency bioelectrical impedance analysis with dual-energy X-ray absorptiometry for assessment of percentage body fat in a large, healthy population'. *Am. J. Clin Nutr.*, vol. 81, pp. 74–8.

Sundgot-Borgen, J. (1994a)(a), 'Eating disorders in female athletes'. *Sports Med.*, vol. 17(3), pp. 176–88.

Sundgot-Borgen, J. (1994b)(b), 'Risk and trigger factors for the development of eating disorders in female elite athletes'. *Med. Sci. Sports Ex.*, vol. 26, pp. 414–19.

Sundgot-Borgen, J. and Garthe, I. (2011), 'Elite athletes in aesthetic and Olympic weight-class sports and the challenge of body weight and body compositions', *Journal of Sports Sciences*, 29 Suppl 1, pp. S101-114. doi: 10.1080/02640414.2011.565783.

Sundgot-Borgen, J. and Larsen, S. (1993), 'Nutrient intake and eating behaviour in elite female athletes suffering from anorexia nervosa, anorexia athletica and bulimia nervosa'. *Int. J. Sport Nutr.*, vol. 3, pp. 431–42.

Sundgot-Borgen, J. and Torstveit M. K. (2004), 'Prevalence of eating disorders in elite athletes is higher than in the general population'. *Clin. J. Sport Nutr.*, vol. 14, pp. 25–32.

Sundgot-Borgen, J. and Torstveit, M. K. (2010), 'Aspects of disordered eating continuum in elite high-intensity sports', *Scandinavian Journal of Medicine & Science in Sports*, 20 Suppl 2, pp. 112–121. doi: 10.1111/j.1600-0838.2010.01190.x.

Sundgot-Borgen, J. and Torstveit, M. K. (2010), 'Aspects of disordered eating continuum in elite high-intensity sports'. *Scand. J. Med. Sci. Sports.*, vol. 20 (Suppl 2), pp. 112–21.

Sundgot-Borgen, J. *et al.* (2013), 'How to minimise the health risks to athletes who compete in weight-sensitive sports review and position statement on behalf of the Ad Hoc Research Working Group on Body Composition, Health and Performance, under the auspices of the IOC Medical Commission', *British Journal of Sports Medicine*, 47(16), pp. 1012–1022. doi: 10.1136/bjsports-2013-092966.

Sutehall, S. *et al.* (2020), 'Addition of an Alginate Hydrogel to a Carbohydrate Beverage Enhances Gastric Emptying', *Medicine and Science in Sports and Exercise*, 52(8), pp. 1785–1792. doi: 10.1249/MSS.0000000000002301.

Sutton, E. F. *et al.* (2018), 'Early Time-Restricted Feeding Improves Insulin Sensitivity, Blood Pressure, and Oxidative Stress Even without Weight Loss in Men with Prediabetes', *Cell Metabolism*, 27(6), pp. 1212-1221.e3. doi: 10.1016/j.cmet.2018.04.010.

Swaminathan, R. *et al.* (1985), 'Thermic effect of feeding carbohydrate, fat, protein and mixed meal in lean and obese subjects'. *Am. J. Clin. Nutr.*, vol. 42, pp. 177–81.

Talanian, J. L. and Spriet, L. L. (2016), 'Low and moderate doses of caffeine late in exercise improve performance in trained cyclists', *Applied Physiology, Nutrition, and Metabolism = Physiologie Appliquee, Nutrition Et Metabolisme*, 41(8), pp. 850–855. doi: 10.1139/apnm-2016-0053.

Tanaka, H. and Seals, D. R. (2008), 'Endurance exercise performance in Masters athletes: age-associated changes and underlying physiological mechanisms.' *J Physiol.*, Volvol. 586(1), p.55–63.

Tang, J. E. *et al.* (2009), 'Ingestion of whey hydrolysate, casein, or soya protein isolate: effects on mixed muscle protein synthesis at rest and following resistance exercise in young men'. *J. Appl. Physiol.*, vol. 107(3), pp. 987–92.

Tarnopolsky, M. and MacLennan, D. P. (1988), 'Influence of protein intake and training status in nitrogen balance and lean body mass'. *J. Appl. Physiol.*, vol. 64, pp. 187–93.

Tarnopolsky, M. and MacLennan, D. P. (1992), 'Evaluation of protein requirements for trained strength athletes'. *J. Appl. Physiol.*, vol. 73, pp. 1986–95.

Tarnopolsky, M. and MacLennan, D. P. (1997), 'Post exercise protein-carbohydrate and carbohydrate supplements increase muscle glycogen in males and females'. *J. Appl. Physiol.*, Abstracts, vol. 4, p. 332A.

Tarnopolsky, M. and MacLennan, D. P. (2000), 'Creatine monohydrate supplementation enhances high-intensity exercise performance in males and females'. *Int. J. Sport Nutr.*, vol. 10, pp. 452–63.

Terada, T. *et al.* (2019), 'Overnight fasting compromises exercise intensity and volume during sprint interval training but improves high-intensity aerobic endurance', *The Journal of Sports Medicine and Physical Fitness*, 59(3), pp. 357–365. doi: 10.23736/S0022-4707.18.08281-6.

Theodorou, A. A. *et al.* (2011), 'No effect of antioxidant supplementation on muscle performance and blood redox status adaptations to eccentric training'. *Am. J. Clin. Nutr.*, vol. 93(6), pp. 1373–83.

Thomas, D. E. *et al.* (1991), 'Carbohydrate feeding before exercise: effect of glycaemic index'. *Int. J. Sports Med.*, vol. 12, pp. 180–6.

Thomas, D. E. *et al.* (1994), 'Plasma glucose levels after prolonged strenuous exercise correlate inversely with glycaemic response to food consuMed. before exercise'. *Int. J. Sports Nutr.*, vol. 4, pp. 261–73.

Thomas, D. T., Erdman, K. A. and Burke, L. M. (2016), 'American College of Sports Medicine Joint Position Statement. Nutrition and Athletic Performance', *Medicine and Science in Sports and Exercise*, 48(3), pp. 543–568. doi: 10.1249/MSS.0000000000000852.

Thomas, M. H. and Burns, S. P. (2016), 'Increasing Lean Mass and Strength: A Comparison of High Frequency Strength Training to Lower Frequency Strength Training', *International Journal of Exercise Science*, 9(2), pp. 159–167.

Thompson, C. *et al.* (2016), 'Dietary nitrate supplementation improves sprint and high-intensity intermittent running performance'. *Nitric Oxide*, vol. 61, pp. 55–61.

Tipton K. D. *et al.* (2001), 'Timing of amino acid-carbohydrate ingestion alters anabolic response of muscle to resistance exercise'. *Am. J. Physiol.*, vol. 281(2), pp. E197–206.

Tipton, C. M. (1987), 'Commentary: physicians should advise wrestlers about weight loss'. *Phys. Sports Med.*, vol. 15, pp. 160–5.

Tipton, K. D. (2015), 'Nutritional Support for Exercise-Induced Injuries', *Sports Medicine (Auckland, N.Z.)*, 45 Suppl 1, pp. S93-104. doi: 10.1007/s40279-015-0398-4.

Tipton, K. D. and Witard, O. C. (2007), 'Protein requirements and recommendations for athletes: relevance of ivory tower arguments for practical recommendations'. *Clin. Sports Med.*, vol. 26(1), pp. 17–36.

Tipton, K. D. and Wolfe, R. (2007), 'Protein needs and amino acids for athletes'. *J. Sports Sci.*, vol 22(1), pp. 65–79.

Tipton, K. D. *et al.* (2004), 'Ingestion of casein and whey proteins result in muscle analbolism after resistance exercise'. *Med. Sci. Sports Exerc.*, vol. 36 (12), pp. 2073–81.

Tipton, K. D. *et al.* (2007), 'Stimulation of net protein synthesis by whey protein ingestion before and after exercise'. *Am. J. Physiol. Endocrinol. Metab.*, vol. 292(1), pp. E71–6.

Tobias, Deirdre K. *et al.* (2015), 'Effect of low-fat diet interventions versus other diet interventions on long-term weight change in adults: a systematic review and meta-analysis'. *The Lancet Diabetes & Endocrinology*, vol. 3(12), pp. 968–79.

Tornberg, Å. B. *et al.* (2017), 'Reduced Neuromuscular Performance in Amenorrheic Elite Endurance Athletes', *Medicine & Science in Sports & Exercise*, 49(12), pp. 2478–2485. doi: 10.1249/MSS.0000000000001383.

Torstveit, M. K. and J. Sundgot-Borgen (2005), 'Participation in leanness sports but not training volume is associated with menstrual dysfunction: a national survey of 1276 athletes and controls'. *Br. J. Sports Med.*, vol. 39, pp. 141–7.

Toth, M. J. *et al.* (2000), 'Menopause-related changes in body fat distribution', *Annals of the New York Academy of Sciences*, 904, pp. 502–506. doi: 10.1111/j.1749-6632.2000.tb06506.x.

Toth, P. P. (2005), 'The "good cholesterol": High-density lipoprotein', *Circulation*, vol. 111(5), pp. 89–91.

Trapp, D., Knez, W. and Sinclair, W. (2010), 'Could a vegetarian diet reduce exercise-induced oxidative stress? A review of the literature', *Journal of Sports Sciences*, 28(12), pp. 1261–1268. doi: 10.1080/02640414.2010.507676.

Trombold, J. R. *et al.* (2011), 'The Effect of Pomegranate Juice Supplementation on Strength and Soreness after Eccentric Exercise', *Journal of strength and conditioning research*. doi: 10.1519/JSC.0b013e318220d992.

Trommelen, J. *et al.* (2017), 'Fructose and Sucrose Intake Increase Exogenous Carbohydrate Oxidation during Exercise', *Nutrients*, 9(2). doi: 10.3390/nu9020167.

Truby, H. *et al.* (2008), 'Commercial weight loss diets meet nutrient requirements in free living adults over 8 weeks: a randomised controlled weight loss trial'. *Nutrition Journal* 2008, vol. 7, p. 25.

Tsintzas, O. K. *et al.* (1995), 'Influence of carbohydrate electrolyte drinks on marathon running performance'. *Eur. J. Appl. Physiol.*, vol. 70, pp. 154–60.

U.S. Department of Health and Human Services (2018). Physical Activity Guidelines for Americans, 2nd edition. Washington, DC.

Uauy, R. *et al.* (2009), 'WHO Scientific Update on trans fatty acids: summary and conclusions'. *Eur. J. Clin. Nutr.*, vol. 63, pp. S68–S75.

Unnithan, V. B. *et al.* (2001), 'Is there a physiologic basis for creatine use in children and adolescents?' *J. Strength Cond. Res.*, vol. 15(4), pp. 524–8.

Vahedi, K. (2000), 'Ischaemic stroke in a sportsman who consumed mahuang extract and creatine mono-hydrate for bodybuilding'. *J. Neur., Neurosurgery and Psych.*, vol. 68, pp. 112–13.

Valdes, A. M. *et al.* (2018), 'Role of the gut microbiota in nutrition and health', *BMJ*, 361, p. k2179. doi: 10.1136/bmj.k2179.

Van Elswyk, M. E., Weatherford, C. A. and McNeill, S. H. (2018), 'A Systematic Review of Renal Health in Healthy Individuals Associated with Protein Intake above the US Recommended Daily Allowance in Randomized Controlled Trials and Observational Studies', *Advances in Nutrition (Bethesda, Md.)*, 9(4), pp. 404–418. doi: 10.1093/advances/nmy026.

Van Essen M. and Gibala, M. J. (2006), 'Failure of protein to improve time-trial performance when added to a sports drink'. *Med. Sci. Sports Exerc.*, vol. 38(8), pp. 1476–83.

Van Loon, L. J. C. (2007), 'Application of protein or protein hydrolysates to improve postexercise recovery'. *Int. J. Sports Nutr. Exerc. Metab.*, vol. 17, S104–17.

Van Loon, L. J. C. (2014), 'Is there a need for protein ingestion during exercise?' *Sports Med.*, vol. 44 (Suppl. 1), pp. 105–11.

Van Proeyen, K. *et al.* (2011), 'Beneficial metabolic adaptations due to endurance exercise training in the fasted state'. *J. Appl. Physiol.*, vol. 110(1), pp. 236–45.

Van Someren, K. A. *et al.* (2005), 'Supplementation with HMB and KIC reduces signs and symptoms of exercise-induced muscle damage in man'. *Int. J. Sport Nutr. Exerc. Metab.*, vol. 15, pp. 413–24.

Van Thienen, R. *et al.* (2009), 'Beta-alanine improves sprint performance in endurance cycling'. *Med. Sci. Sports Exerc.*, vol. 41, pp. 898–903.

van Vliet, S. *et al.* (2017), 'Consumption of whole eggs promotes greater stimulation of postexercise muscle protein synthesis than consumption of isonitrogenous amounts of egg whites in young men', *The American Journal of Clinical Nutrition*, 106(6), pp. 1401–1412. doi: 10.3945/ajcn.117.159855.

van Vliet, S., Burd, N. A. and van Loon, L. J. C. (2015), 'The Skeletal Muscle Anabolic Response to Plant- versus Animal-Based Protein Consumption', *The Journal of Nutrition*, 145(9), pp. 1981–1991. doi: 10.3945/jn.114.204305.

Vandenbogaerde, T. J. and Hopkins, W. G. (2011), 'Effects of acute carbohydrate supplementation on endurance performance: a meta-analysis'. *Sports Med.*, vol. 41(9), pp. 773–92.

Venables, M. *et al.* (2005), 'Erosive effect of a new sports drink on dental enamel during exercise'. *Med. Sci. Sports Exerc.*, vol. 37(1), pp. 39–44.

Volek, J. S. (1997), 'Response of testosterone and cortisol concentrations to high-intensity resistance training following creatine supplementation'. *J. Strength Cond. Res.*, vol. 11, pp. 182–7.

Volek, J. S. *et al.* (1999), 'Performance and muscle fibre adaptations to creatine supplementation and heavy resistance training'. *Med. Sci. Sports Ex.*, vol. 31(8), pp. 1147–56.

Volek, J. S. *et al.* (2013), 'Whey protein supplementation during resistance training augments lean body mass'. *J. Am. Coll. Nutr.*, vol. 32(2), pp. 122–35.

Volpe, S. L. (2010), 'Alcohol and Athletic Performance', *ACSM's Health & Fitness Journal*, 14(3), pp. 28–30. doi: 10.1249/FIT.0b013e3181daa567.

Wackerhage, H. *et al.* (2019), 'Stimuli and sensors that initiate skeletal muscle hypertrophy following resistance exercise', *Journal of Applied Physiology (Bethesda, Md.: 1985)*, 126(1), pp. 30–43. doi: 10.1152/japplphysiol.00685.2018.

Waitrose Food and Drink Report 2018–2019 https://www.waitrose.com/content/dam/waitrose/Inspiration/Waitrose%20&%20Partners%20Food%20and%20Drink%20Report%202018.pdf

Wall, B. T. and van Loon, L. J. C. (2013) (a), 'Nutritional strategies to attenuate muscle disuse atrophy', *Nutrition Reviews*, 71(4), pp. 195–208. doi: 10.1111/nure.12019.

Wall, B. T. *et al.* (2013) (b), 'Disuse impairs the muscle protein synthetic response to protein ingestion in healthy men', *The Journal of Clinical Endocrinology and Metabolism*, 98(12), pp. 4872–4881. doi: 10.1210/jc.2013-2098.

Wall, B. T. *et al.* (2014), 'Substantial skeletal muscle loss occurs during only 5 days of disuse', *Acta Physiologica (Oxford, England)*, 210(3), pp. 600–611. doi: 10.1111/apha.12190.

Wallis, G. A. *et al.* (2005), 'Oxidation of combined ingestion of maltodextrins and fructose during exercise', *Medicine and Science in Sports and Exercise*, 37(3), pp. 426–432. doi: 10.1249/01.mss.0000155399.23358.82.

Walser, B., Giordano, R. M. and Stebbins, C. L. (2006), 'Supplementation with omega-3 polyunsaturated fatty acids augments brachial artery dilation and blood flow during forearm contraction'. *Eur. J. Appl. Physiol.* Jun; 97(3), pp. 347–54.

Walsh, N. P. (2018), 'Recommendations to maintain immune health in athletes', *European Journal of Sport Science,* 18(6), pp. 820–831. doi: 10.1080/17461391.2018.1449895.

Walsh, N. P. (2019), 'Nutrition and athlete immune health: a new perspective.' Available at: http://www.gssiweb.org:80/sports-science-exchange/article/nutrition-and-athlete-immune-health-a-new-perspective (Accessed: 6 May 2021).

Wang, Y. *et al.* (2005), 'Comparison of abdominal adiposity and overall obesity in predicting

Warburton, D. E., Nicol, C. W. and Bredin, S. S. (2006), 'Health benefits of physical activity: the evidence'. *CMAJ,* vol. 174(6), pp. 801–9.

Warren, J. *et al.* (2003), 'Low glycaemic index breakfasts and reduced food intake in preadolescent children'. *Paediatrics,* vol. 112, pp. 414–19.

Wasserfurth, P. *et al.* (2020), 'Reasons for and Consequences of Low Energy Availability in Female and Male Athletes: Social Environment, Adaptations, and Prevention', *Sports Medicine – Open.* doi: 10.1186/s40798-020-00275-6.

Watt, K. K. O. *et al.* (2004), 'Skeletal muscle total creatine content and creatine transporter gene expression in vegetarians prior to and following creatine supplementation', *Int. J. Sport Nutr. Exerc. Metab.,* vol. 14, pp. 517–31.

Watt, M. J. *et al.* (2002), 'Intramuscular triacylglycerol, glycogen and acetyl group metabolism during 4 h of moderate exercise in man', *The Journal of Physiology,* 541(Pt 3), pp. 969–978. doi: 10.1113/jphysiol.2002.018820.

WCRF/AICR (2007), 'Food, Nutrition, Physical Activity, and the Prevention of Cancer: a Global Perspective'.

Wee, S. L. *et al.* (1999), 'Influence of high and low glycemic index meals on endurance running capacity', *Medicine and Science in Sports and Exercise,* 31(3), pp. 393–399. doi: 10.1097/00005768-199903000-00007.

Weisgarber, K. D., Candow, D. G. and Vogt, E. S. M. (2012), 'Whey protein before and during resistance exercise has no effect on muscle mass and strength in untrained young adults'. *Int. J. Sport Nutr. Exerc. Metab.,* vol. 22(6), pp. 463–9.

Wellington, B. M., Leveritt, M. D. and Kelly, V. G. (2017), 'The Effect of Caffeine on Repeat-High-Intensity-Effort Performance in Rugby League Players', *International Journal of Sports Physiology and Performance,* 12(2), pp. 206–210. doi: 10.1123/ijspp.2015-0689.

Wells, K. R. *et al.* (2020), 'The Australian Institute of Sport (AIS) and National Eating Disorders Collaboration (NEDC) position statement on disordered eating in high performance sport', *British Journal of Sports Medicine,* 54(21), pp. 1247–1258. doi: 10.1136/bjsports-2019-101813.

Wemple, R. D. *et al.* (1997), 'Caffeine vs. caffeine-free sports drinks: effects on urine production at rest and during prolonged exercise'. *Int. J. Sports Med.,* vol. 18(1), pp. 40–6.

West, N. P. *et al.* (2011), 'Supplementation with Lactobacillus fermentum VRI (PCC) reduces lower respiratory illness in athletes and moderate exercise-induced immune perturbations'. *Nutrition Journal,* vol. 10, p. 30.

Westcott, W. L. (2012), 'Resistance training is medicine: effects of strength training on health', *Current Sports Medicine Reports,* 11(4), pp. 209–216. doi: 10.1249/JSR.0b013e31825dabb8.

Westerterp-Plantenga, M. S. *et al.* (2012), 'Dietary protein – its role in satiety, energetics, weight loss and health'. *Br. J. Nutr.,* vol. 108, Suppl 2, pp. S105–12.

Westman, E. C. *et al.* (2007), 'Low-carbohydrate nutrition and metabolism', *The American Journal of Clinical Nutrition,* 86(2), pp. 276–284. doi: 10.1093/ajcn/86.2.276.

Wilborn, C. D. *et al.* (2004), 'Effects of zinc magnesium aspartate (ZMA) supplementation on training adaptations and markers of anabolism and catabolism'. *J. Int. Soc. Sports Nutr.,* vol. 1(2), pp. 12–20.

Wilk, B. and Bar-Or, O. (1996), 'Effect of drink flavour and NaCl on voluntary drinking and rehydration in boys exercising in the heat'. *J. Appl. Physiol.,* vol. 80, pp. 1112–17.

Wilkinson, S. B. *et al.* (2007), 'Consumption of fluid skim milk promotes greater protein accretion after resistance exercise than does consumption of an isonitrogenous and isoenergetic soysoya-protein beverage'. *Am. J. Clin. Nutr.,* vol. 85(4), pp. 1031–40.

Wilkinson, S. B. *et al.* (2008), 'Differential effects of resistance and endurance exercise in the fed state on signalling molecule phosphorylation and protein synthesis in human muscle', *The Journal of Physiology,* 586(Pt 15), pp. 3701–3717. doi: 10.1113/jphysiol.2008.153916.

Williams, C. and Devlin, J. T. (eds) (1992), *Foods, Nutrition and Performance: An International Scientific Consensus* (London: Chapman and Hall).

Williams, M. (2005), 'Dietary supplements and sports performance: amino acids', *Journal of the International Society of Sports Nutrition,* 2, pp. 63–67. doi: 10.1186/1550-2783-2-2-63.

Williams, M. H. (1985), *Nutritional Aspects of Human Physical and Athletic Performance,* (Springfield, IL: Charles C Thomas Publisher).

Williams, M. H. (1992), *Nutrition for Fitness and Sport* (Dubuque, IO: WilliAm. C. Brown).

Williams, M. H. (1998), *The Ergogenics Edge* (Champaign, IL: Human Kinetics).

Williams, M. H. (1999), *Nutrition for Health, Fitness and Sport,* 5th ed. (New York: McGraw-Hill).

Williams, M. H. *et al.* (1999), *Creatine: The Power Supplement* (Champaign, IL: Human Kinetics).

Williams, T. D. *et al.* (2020), 'Effect of Acute Beetroot Juice Supplementation on Bench Press Power, Velocity, and Repetition Volume', *The Journal of Strength & Conditioning Research,* 34(4), pp. 924–928. doi: 10.1519/JSC.0000000000003509.

Williamson, D. A. *et al.* (1995), 'Structured equation modeling of risk factors for the development of eating disorder symptoms in female athletes'. *Int. J. Eating Disorders,* vol. 17(4), 387–93.

Willis, L. H. *et al.* (2012), 'Effects of aerobic and/ or resistance training on body mass and fat mass in overweight or obese adults'. *J. Appl. Physiol.* Dec, 113(12), pp. 1831–7. http://www.ncbi.nlm.nih.gov/pubmed/23019316

Willoughby, D. S. *et al.* (2011), 'Effects of 7 Days of Arginine-Alpha-Ketoglutarate Supplementation on Blood Flow, Plasma L-Arginine, Nitric Oxide Metabolites, and Asymmetric Dimethyl Arginine After Resistance Exercise', *International Journal of Sport Nutrition and Exercise Metabolism,* 21(4), pp. 291–299. doi: 10.1123/ijsnem.21.4.291.

Willoughby, D. S., Stout, J. R. and Wilborn, C. D. (2007), 'Effects of resistance training and protein plus amino acid supplementation on muscle anabolism, mass, and strength', *Amino Acids,* 32(4), pp. 467–477. doi: 10.1007/s00726-006-0398-7.

Wilmore, J. H. (1983), 'Body composition in sport and exercise'. *Med. Sci. Sports Ex.,* vol. 15, pp. 21–31.

Wilson, J. M. *et al.* (2013), 'International Society of Sports Nutrition Position Stand: beta-hydroxy-beta-methylbutyrate (HMB)', *Journal of the International Society of Sports Nutrition,* 10(1), p. 6. doi: 10.1186/1550-2783-10-6.

Wilson, P. B. (2017), 'Frequency of Chronic Gastrointestinal Distress in Runners: Validity and Reliability of a Retrospective Questionnaire', *International Journal of Sport Nutrition and Exercise Metabolism,* 27(4), pp. 370–376. doi: 10.1123/ijsnem.2016-0305.

Witard O. C,. *et al.* (2016), 'Protein Considerations for Optimising Skeletal Muscle Mass in Healthy Young and Older Adults.' Nutrients. Vol 8 (4), p. 181.

Witard, O. C. *et al.* (2011), 'Effect of increased dietary protein on tolerance to intensified training'. *Med. Sci. Sports Exerc.,* vol. 43(4), pp. 598–607.

Witard, O. C. *et al.* (2014) (a), 'High dietary protein restores overreaching induced impairments in leukocyte trafficking and reduces the incidence of upper respiratory tract infection in elite cyclists'. *Brain Behav. Immun.,* vol. 39, pp. 211–9.

Witard, O. C. *et al.* (2014) (b), 'Myofibrillar muscle protein synthesis rates subsequent to a meal in response to increasing doses of whey protein at rest and after resistance exercise'. *Am. J. Clin. Nutr.,* vol. 99(1), pp. 86–95.

Witard, O. C., Garthe, I. and Phillips, S. M. (2019), 'Dietary Protein for Training Adaptation and Body Composition Manipulation in Track and Field Athletes', *International Journal of Sport Nutrition and Exercise Metabolism,* 29(2), pp. 165–174. doi: 10.1123/ijsnem.2018-0267.

Wojtaszewski, J. F. P. *et al.* (2003), 'Regulation of 5'AMP-activated protein kinase activity and substrate utilization in exercising human skeletal muscle', *American Journal of Physiology. Endocrinology and Metabolism,* 284(4), pp. E813-822. doi: 10.1152/ajpendo.00436.2002.

Wolfe, R. R. (2017), 'Branched-chain amino acids and muscle protein synthesis in humans: myth or reality?', *Journal of the International Society of Sports Nutrition,* 14, p. 30. doi: 10.1186/s12970-017-0184-9.

Woods, A. L., Garvican-Lewis, L. A., Lundy, B., *et al.* (2017) (a), 'New approaches to determine fatigue in elite athletes during intensified training: Resting metabolic rate and pacing profile', *PloS One,* 12(3), p. e0173807. doi: 10.1371/journal.pone.0173807.

Woods, A. L., Garvican-Lewis, L. A., Rice, A., *et al.* (2017) (b), '12 days of altitude exposure at 1800 m does not increase resting metabolic rate in elite rowers', *Applied Physiology, Nutrition, and Metabolism = Physiologie Appliquee, Nutrition Et Metabolisme,* 42(6), pp. 672–676. doi: 10.1139/apnm-2016-0693.

World Cancer Research Fund (WCRF) (2018), 'Diet, Nutrition, Physical Activity and Cancer: A Global Perspective The Third Expert Report'.

World Health Organization (2003), 'Expert consultation on diet, nutrition and the prevention of chronic diseases'. WHO Technical Report Series No. 916, Geneva, Switzerland.

World Health Organization WHO (2016 no date), WHO *Effects of saturated fatty acids on serum lipids and lipoproteins: a systematic review and regression analysis* (no date) *WHO*. World Health Organization. Available at: http://www.who.int/nutrition/publications/nutrientrequirements/sfa_systematic_review/en/ (Accessed: 30 April 2021).

Wright, D. W. *et al.* (1991), 'Carbohydrate feedings before, during or in combination improve cycling endurance performance'. *J. Appl. Physiol.*, vol. 71, pp. 1082–88.

Wu, C. L. and Williams, C. (2006), 'A low glycaemic index meal before exercise improves endurance running capacity in men'. *Int. J. Sports Nutr. Exerc. Metab.*, vol 16, pp. 510–27.

Wu, C. L. *et al.* (2003), 'The influence of high carbohydrate meals with different glycaemic indices on substrate utilisation during subsequent exercise'. *Br. J. Nutr.*, vol. 90(6), pp. 1049–56.

Wu, G. D. *et al.* (2011), 'Linking long-term dietary patterns with gut microbial enterotypes', *Science (New York, N.Y.)*, 334(6052), pp. 105–108. doi: 10.1126/science.1208344.

Wylie, L. J. *et al.* (2013), 'Beetroot juice and exercise: pharmacodynamic and dose-response relationships'. *J. Appl. Physiol.*, vol 115(3), pp. 325–36.

Yang, Y. *et al.* (2012) (a), 'Myofibrillar protein synthesis following ingestion of soy protein isolate at rest and after resistance exercise in elderly men', *Nutrition & Metabolism*, 9(1), p. 57. doi: 10.1186/1743-7075-9-57.

Yang, Y. *et al.* (2012) (b), 'Resistance exercise enhances myofibrillar protein synthesis with graded intakes of whey protein in older men', *The British Journal of Nutrition*, 108(10), pp. 1780–1788. doi: 10.1017/S0007114511007422.

Yaspelkis, B. B., *et al.* (1993), 'Carbohydrate supplementation spares muscle glycogen during variable-intensity exercise'. *J. Appl. Physiol.* Oct, 75(4), pp. 1477–85.

Yeo, W. K. *et al.* (2008), 'Skeletal muscle adaptation and performance responses to once a day versus twice-every-second-day endurance training regimens'. *J. Appl. Physiol.*, vol. 105, pp. 1462–70.

Yeo, W. K. *et al.* (2010), 'Acute signalling responses to intense endurance training commenced with low or normal muscle glycogen', *Experimental Physiology*, 95(2), pp. 351–358. doi: 10.1113/expphysiol.2009.049353.

Yfanti, C. *et al.* (2010), 'Antioxidant supplementation does not alter endurance training adaptation'. *Med. Sci. Sports Exerc.*, vol. 42(7), pp. 1388–95.

Young, V. R., and and Pellett, P. L. (1994), Pellett. '"Plant Proteins in Relation to Human Protein and Amino Acid Nutrition."', *The American Journal of Clinical Nutrition*, vol. 59, no. 5, May 1994, pp. 1203S-1212S. academic.oup.com, doi:10.1093/ajcn/59.5.1203S.

Yüksel, H. *et al.* (2006) 'Effects of oral continuous 17β-estradiol plus norethisterone acetate replacement therapy on abdominal subcutaneous fat, serum leptin levels and body composition', *Gynecological endocrinology: the official journal of the International Society of Gynecological Endocrinology*, 22, pp. 381–7. doi: 10.1080/09513590600842281.

Zajac, A. *et al.* (2014), 'The effects of a ketogenic diet on exercise metabolism and physical performance in off-road cyclists'. *Nutrients,* vol. 6(7), pp. 2493–508.

Zawadzki, K. M. *et al.* (1992), 'Carbohydrate-protein complex increases the rate of muscle glycogen storage after exercise'. *J. Appl. Physiol.*, vol. 72, pp. 1854–9.

Ziberna, L. *et al.* (2013), 'The endothelial plasma membrane transporter bilitranslocase mediates rat aortic vasodilation induced by anthocyanins'. *Nutr. Metab. Cardiovasc. Dis.*, vol. 23(1), pp. 68–74.

Ziegenfuss, T. *et al.* (1997), 'Acute creatine ingestion: effects on muscle volume, anaerobic power, fluid volumes and protein turnover'. *Med. Sci. Sports Ex.*, vol. 29, supp. 127.

Ziegler, P. J. *et al.* (1999), 'Nutritional and physiological status of US National Figure Skaters'. *Int. J. Sport Nutr.*, vol. 9, pp. 345–60.

Zouhal, H. *et al.* (2011) 'Inverse relationship between percentage body weight change and finishing time in 643 forty-two-kilometre marathon runners', *British Journal of Sports Medicine*, 45(14), pp. 1101–1105. doi: 10.1136/bjsm.2010.074641.

Zouhal, H. *et al.* (2020), '<p>Exercise Training and Fasting: Current Insights</p>', *Open Access Journal of Sports Medicine*, 11, pp. 1–28. doi: 10.2147/OAJSM.S224919.

Zuhl, M. *et al.* (2014), 'Exercise regulation of intestinal tight junction proteins', *British Journal of Sports Medicine*, 48(12), pp. 980–986. doi: 10.1136/bjsports-2012-091585.

ONLINE RESOURCES

www.ausport.gov.au The website of AIS provides fact sheets on sports nutrition, recipes and comprehensive information on supplements ranked into four groups within the AIS Sports Supplement Framework.

www.sportsdietitians.com.au This website provides fact sheets on a wide range of sports nutrition topics.

www.mysportscience.com This website provides evidence-based articles and infographics on a wide range of sports nutrition topics.

www.eatright.org The website of the US Academy of Nutrition and Dietetics, provides articles on a variety of sport and exercise nutrition topics.

www.bda.uk.com The website of the British Dietetic Association includes fact sheets and information on a wide range of nutrition topics. It also provides details of Registered Dietitians working in private practice.

www.gssiweb.com This website includes Sports Science Exchange, a comprehensive library of sports nutrition articles written by world leading experts.

www.trainingpeaks.com This website provides articles on a variety of endurance training topics, including sports nutrition.

www.vegansociety.com The website of the UK Vegan Society provides comprehensive resources on the vegan lifestyle, nutrition, health and the environment, as well as tasty recipes.

www.vegsoc.org This website provides comprehensive information and fact sheets on vegetarian nutrition and health, as well as recipes.

www.healthstatus.com This US website provides useful health calculators for Body Mass Index, basal metabolic rate, and body fat percentage.

www.beateatingdisorders.org.uk The website of Beat, the UK's leading eating disorder charity, provides a national helpline, online support and a network of UK-wide self-help groups.

www.health4performance.co.uk This website provides evidence-based information on the symptoms and outcomes of RED-S with specific sections for athletes, coaches, parents and healthcare professionals.

TO FIND A SPORT AND EXERCISE NUTRITIONIST

www.associationfornutrition.org The UK voluntary register of nutritionists.

www.bda.uk.com/senr-sport-and-exercise-nutrition-register.html A voluntary competency-based register for sport and exercise nutritionists in the UK.

www.scandpg.org A register for dietitians specialising in sport nutrition in the US.

INDEX

adipose tissue 21, 28, 41, 171, 225

ADP (adenosine diphosphate) 16–17, 22

aerobic (glycolytic and lipolytic) energy systems 22, 24–5, 27–8, 30–1

alanine 66, 68

alcohol 17, 18, 19, 21, 164–6, 167

alpha-linolenic acid (ALA) 87, 88–9, 137, 272

amenorrhoea 177–8, 181, 214, 215, 224–6

amino acids 9, 18, 23, 26, 45, 66, 67, 68, 69, 72, 74, 88, 112, 114–15, 203, 205
  see also branched-chain amino acids

anabolism 18

anaerobic glycolytic/lactic system 22, 23–4, 25, 27, 28, 29, 31

anorexia nervosa 219, 221

antioxidant supplements 10–11, 98, 105, 110–12

antioxidants 13, 98, 104, 105, 122–3, 265

arginine 112, 115

'Athlete's Plate' 12–15

ATP (adenosine triphosphate) 7, 16–17, 21, 23, 24, 25, 30, 31, 33, 166, 280

ATP-PC (phosphagen) system 22–3, 24, 25, 27–8, 31, 268

banned substances 11, 108–9, 110, 121, 130–1, 143–4

basal metabolic rate (BMR) 6, 18, 182

beetroot juice 115–17

beta-alanine 11, 114–15

beta-carotene 13, 98, 187

bicarbonate 117–18

bioelectrical impedance analysis 174

blood fat levels 38, 84

blood glucose/sugar 7, 8, 11, 19–20, 24, 26, 30, 31, 32, 33, 36, 38–9, 40, 41, 42, 45, 64, 157, 158, 159, 167, 187, 195, 280

body composition 172
  body fat and performance 168–9, 179
  body fat distribution 170–1
  masters athletes 277–8
  measuring 171–5
  and microbiota 230
  minimum amount of fat 175–6, 177–9
  optimal body fat percentage in athletes 176–7, 179
  see also weight management

body mass index (BMI) 169–70, 229, 263

bone health/density 178, 208, 209, 214, 221–3, 225–6, 272, 278–9, 280, 288

branched-chain amino acids (BCAAs) 66, 68, 73, 112–14, 133, 136–7, 229

bulimia nervosa 219

butyrate 229

caffeine 11, 60–1, 118–21

calories 5–6, 18–19, 80, 183–4, 202

cannabidiol (CBD) 121–2

carbohydrate loading 11, 32, 58, 289–90, 302

carbohydrates 4, 6–7, 8, 9, 11, 13, 17, 18, 19–20, 21, 23, 24, 25–8, 29, 30, 31, 32–4, 36–7, 39, 42, 46, 49, 51, 56, 57, 58, 63, 64, 68, 83, 84, 86, 157, 158, 183, 185, 202, 203
  'Athlete's Plate' 13–14
  complex and simple 35–6, 40, 64
  fuelling for the work required 62, 63, 64
  intake during exercise 11–12, 31, 32, 37, 43–9, 64, 71, 157–8, 243
  mouth rinsing 8, 11, 43, 44, 62, 64, 157
  multiple transportable 8, 46, 158, 162–3, 167
  periodisation 8–9, 59, 60, 62–3, 64, 286
  post-exercise refuelling 7, 9, 49–54
  pre-exercise meals 7–8, 11, 39–43, 64, 71, 83
  recommended intake 34–5, 254–5, 284–5, 288
  see also glycogen stores; low-carbohydrate diets

cardiovascular health 84–6, 88, 89, 90, 91, 171, 209, 215, 278

carnosine 114

casein 72, 74, 76, 82, 141

catabolism 18

central nervous system 8, 11, 62, 130

cherry juice 122–3

chocolate milk 77–8

cholesterol 40, 84, 85–7, 88, 90–1, 104, 144, 171

Citrus aurantium 132

Coleus forskohlii 132

collagen 124–5, 248

colostrum 125

competition nutrition 11–12
  carbohydrate loading 289–90, 302
  endurance events >90 mins 289–95, 302
  endurance events < 90 mins/ multiple heats 300
  fluids/hydration 293, 294–5, 297, 298–9
  football and team sports 295–9, 302
  pre-competition and snacks 293
  short-duration events 299
  weight-class sports 299–302
conjugated linoleic acid (CLA) 123–4
cortisol 53, 54, 145, 179, 214, 216, 225, 226, 234, 242, 243
cramps 155, 235–6
creatine 11, 22, 126–9, 205, 247–8, 268, 276, 287, 288

de novo lipogenesis 20
dehydration see hypohydration
delayed onset muscle soreness (DOMS) 77, 122, 123
dietary reference values (DRVS) 93–4
digestible indispensable amino acid score (DIAAS) 67
disaccharides 35–6
disordered eating 178, 180, 181, 191, 208, 216, 218–20, 227
  commonality in athletes 220–1
  health and performance consequences 221–2
  people at risk 221
  warning signs and symptoms 221, 222, 224–5
docosahexaenoic acid (DHA) 87, 88, 89, 91, 137, 138, 272
doping risks 108–9, 110, 122
  see also banned substances
drinking to thirst 153, 156, 158, 166, 294
dual-energy X-ray absorptiometry (DEXA) 174

eating disorders 181, 211, 215, 216, 218–19, 223–4, 227
echinacea 245
eicosapentaenoic acid (EPA) 87, 88, 89, 91, 137, 138, 272
electrolytes 161, 162, 258, 295
endocrine system 176, 209, 214, 221
energy 5–6, 16
  ATP and ADP 16–17, 21
  food energy values 19
  measuring 18–19
  production systems 22–8, 31
  see also carbohydrates; fat; protein
energy availability (EA) 4, 5, 208, 209, 214–15, 217–18, 226–7
energy bars 129–30
ephedrine 130–1
ergogenic aids 11, 89, 107, 110, 116, 120, 121, 126, 139
essential amino acids (EAAs) 66, 67, 72, 73, 81, 82, 112, 136–7, 205, 207, 284
essential fat 175–6, 179
essential fatty acids 9, 87–8, 187
euhydration 148
excess post-exercise oxygen consumption (EPOC) 182, 198

fasted training 8, 39, 41, 56
fat 9–10, 11, 13, 17, 18, 19, 20, 21, 24, 25–8, 29, 30–1, 33, 41, 42–3, 45, 55, 56, 57, 58, 59, 64, 80, 83–4, 85–7, 91, 165, 183, 203
  see also under body composition; omega-3 fatty acids; omega-6 fatty acid
fat burners 130–2
fat mass (FM) 172, 173
fat-free mass (FFM) 5, 172, 173, 181, 209, 216
fatigue 5, 8, 11, 19, 24, 27, 29, 30–1, 32, 39, 44, 49, 58, 60–1, 63, 64, 152, 157, 185, 187, 213
fatty acids 18, 25, 27, 29, 68, 83, 84, 85, 135, 171
  see also individual fatty acids by name
Female Athlete Triad see RED-S

female athletes 5, 10, 94, 98, 100, 175, 177–8, 180, 181, 211
fermented foods 139, 140, 233
fertility 178, 179, 221
fibre 11, 13, 40, 42, 195–6, 232, 233, 265
FODMAP foods 237–8, 291, 297
folate 13, 106, 229
folic acid 98, 273
follicle-stimulating hormone (FSH) 178, 214, 225
food intake during exercise 43, 64
  exercise lasting 1–2½ hours 44–6
  exercise lasting 45–75 minutes 44
  exercise lasting longer than 2½ hours 46
  mouth rinsing 8, 11, 43, 44, 64
  what to eat/drink 47–9
  when to consume carbohydrates 47
  see also competition nutrition
free amino acid pool 68
free radicals 104–5, 111, 231
fructose 8, 12, 18, 35, 36, 38, 46, 47, 53, 64, 134, 158, 160
'fuelling for the work required' training model 62, 63, 64

galactose 18, 35, 36
gamma-linolenic acid (GLA) 87
gastrointestinal (GI) problems 46, 47, 53, 60, 101, 157, 159, 221, 238, 244
  alleviating 237
  causes 234–5
  commonality in athletes 234
  competition anxiety 291
  diarrhoea and defecation 236
  flatulence 236
  fullness and bloating 235
  leaky gut 230, 236
  nausea and vomiting 158, 235
  stomach cramps 235–6
genetics 21, 155, 182, 200, 225
glucagon 20
glucose 8, 12, 18, 19–20, 23–5, 29, 32–3, 35, 36, 39, 40, 46, 47, 48–9, 52, 53, 64, 68, 80, 158, 163, 203

glutamate 68
glutamine 66, 132–3, 245
glycaemic index (GI) 38–9
    high-GI foods 7, 8, 38–9, 42, 43, 47, 53–4, 64, 129, 255, 261
    low-GI foods 38–9, 42, 43, 47–8, 53–4, 64, 255
glycaemic load (GC) 39
glycerol and hyperhydration 151
glycogen stores 20, 22, 25, 29, 39, 43, 47, 56, 57, 60, 80, 83, 159, 165
    depletion 32, 34, 41, 44–5, 49–50, 51, 58, 60–1, 63, 64, 157, 185, 186, 187, 280
    liver 6–7, 11, 19, 24, 27, 28, 30, 31, 33, 40, 41, 45, 63, 64, 223, 284
    muscle 6–7, 8, 19, 23, 24, 26, 27, 28, 30, 31, 32, 33, 34, 35, 40, 44–5, 51, 58, 59, 63, 64, 66, 68, 157, 202, 206, 223, 284
    recovery 37, 49–54, 64, 77–8, 203
glycogen threshold hypothesis 58
glycogenesis 20, 68
glycogenolysis 20
glycolysis 24
gonadotrophin-releasing hormone (GnRH) 214, 225
green tea extract 132
growth hormone (GH) 77, 179, 203, 214, 215, 277
gut health 243–4, 265
    athletes' microbiota composition 229–30, 238
    diet and microbiome composition 231–2
    and exercise 230, 238
    impact on athletic performance 230–1
    improving 232–3, 238
    microbiota defined 228
    microbiota impact on health 229
    see also gastrointestinal (GI) problems

haematuria 100
haemoglobin 102, 105, 215, 269

haemoglobinuria 100
HDL cholesterol 84, 86, 87, 88, 90, 144
heart disease see cardiovascular risk
high-carbohydrate diets 32, 33–4, 36, 41, 51, 58, 59, 83, 195, 243
high-fibre diets 40
high-intensity interval training (HIIT) 199, 281
HMB (beta-hydroxy beta-methyl butyrate) 133–4
hormone replacement therapy (HRT) 280
hormones 5, 9, 21, 54, 83, 90, 98, 109, 110, 175–6, 177–9, 188, 200, 203, 208, 209, 225, 226, 227, 277–8, 279–80
horny goat weed 144–5
hydration plans 4, 153–4, 166
hydrogel energy drinks 134–5, 159
hydrogenated oils 90
hyperhydration 148, 151, 153, 295
hypertonic drinks 160, 163
hypoglycaemia 30, 41, 45
hypohydration 4, 10, 81, 120, 147, 148–51, 152, 153–4, 155, 157, 158, 166, 180, 181, 223, 257, 261, 287, 295
    see also water consumption
hyponatraemia 4, 10, 147, 152, 154–4, 167, 295
hypotonic drinks 160, 167

immune system/immunity 61, 87, 88, 94, 96, 97–8, 99, 121, 125, 132–3, 137, 165, 209, 215, 221, 227, 228, 229, 239–40, 265
    carbohydrate consumption 243
    importance of a balanced diet 241, 248
    influence of nutrition on 245–6
    matching energy intake to expenditure 242–3, 248
    polyphenol consumption 244–5, 248
    probiotics 243–4, 248
    recommendations for avoiding infection 245

reducing risk of infection 241
    risk factors for infection 240
    strenuous exercise and system suppression 240–1
    supplements 241–2, 243–4, 245, 248
    zinc lozenges 244
infections
    see immune system; injury and illness, nutrition and
inflammation 10, 13, 87, 88, 89, 91, 100, 111, 121, 122–3, 137, 139, 171, 229, 230, 231, 246, 248, 265
injury and illness, nutrition and 5, 58, 91, 97, 99, 125, 126, 137, 179, 213, 216, 223, 225, 226, 227, 239
    avoiding weight gain 246–7, 248
    minimising muscle loss 247, 248
    phases of recovery 246
    recovery promoting supplements 247–8
innate immunity 239–40
insulin 20, 37, 38, 39, 42, 185, 203, 280
insulin resistance 37, 171, 185
intramuscular fat 20, 28, 56
iodine 274
isoleucine 66, 68, 112
isotonic drinks 157, 159, 160, 167

ketogenic diets see low-carbohydrate diets; low-carbohydrate/high-fat diets
ketones/ketone esters 135–6, 185
ketosis 185
kilocalories and kilojoules 18–19

lactate 23, 24, 29, 30, 31
lactate threshold (LT) 281
lactic acid 24, 29, 30, 105
lactose 36
LDL cholesterol 40, 85–7, 88, 90, 91, 104
leaky gut 230, 236
leptin 183, 214, 225, 226
leucine 9, 66, 68, 72–3, 82, 112, 113, 133, 136–7, 207, 268, 284

libido 179, 213, 227
linoleic acid 87, 89, 187
lipase 27, 37–8, 123, 132
lipolysis 24
liver, the 20, 21, 23, 48, 68, 135, 166, 171
low energy availability (LEA) 6, 178, 180, 185, 187, 207, 208, 209–11, 214, 215, 216–17, 224–5, 242–3, 253, 269
low-carbohydrate diets 22, 27, 32, 185–6, 285–6
low-carbohydrate, high-fat diets 55–60, 64, 83, 84, 183
low-fat diets 87–8, 186
lower reference nutrient intake (LRNI) 93
luteinising hormone (LH) 178, 225

ma huang 130–1
magnetic resonance imaging (MRI) 175
maltodextrins 12, 36, 47, 49, 129, 134, 158, 160, 162, 167, 206
masters athletes 277
    ageing and performance 277, 288
    body composition 277–8
    carbohydrate requirements 284–5, 288
    endurance exercise 281
    energy requirements 282–3
    fluid intake 286–7, 288
    managing age related decline 280–1
    menopause/perimenopause 279–80, 288
    protein requirements 283–4, 288
    recovery 282, 288
    resistance and HIIT training 280–1, 282, 287, 288
    supplements 287–8
    weight management 285–6
maximal oxygen consumption (VO₂max) 223, 281
menopause/perimenopause 279
menstrual function and dysfunction 83, 100, 175, 177–8, 208, 209, 213, 214, 221, 227, 279
    commonality of dysfunction 224

consequences of dysfunction 225–6
dysfunction and performance 226
people at risk of dysfunction 224–5
treatment 226–7
mental wellbeing 58, 179, 221
metabolic flexibility 4, 60, 64
metabolic rate see basal metabolic rate (BMR); resting metabolic rate (RMR)
metabolism defined 18, 182
microbiota/microbiome 40, 228–9, 231–2, 238
    see also gut health
Mifflin-St Jeor equation 5, 282
milk recovery drinks 76–8, 156
minerals 92–3, 94, 101
    calcium 10, 94, 98–9, 272–3, 276
    chromium picolinate 102–3
    deficiencies 223, 241, 276
    exercise and increased requirement 94–5, 105
    high doses and imbalances 102–4, 105
    iodine 274
    iron and iron deficiency 10, 94, 99–101, 102, 103, 215, 269–71, 276
    magnesium 94, 145, 161, 227
    potassium 13, 161, 258
    supplements 10, 94, 101–4, 105, 110, 206, 227, 271, 274, 275, 276
    zinc 94, 144–5, 244, 248, 275
mitochondria 27, 56, 96
    biogenesis 56, 64
    enzyme activity 56, 64
monosaccharides 18, 35
monounsaturated fatty acids 86–7, 91
mouth rinsing, carbohydrate 8, 11, 43, 44, 62, 64, 157
muscle 10, 19, 20, 23, 41, 50, 60, 64, 66, 68, 72, 77, 82, 97, 110
    fast-twitch (FT) and slow-twitch (ST) fibres 23, 25, 200, 278

loss through dieting 182–3, 187, 193–4
muscle protein breakdown (MPB) 68, 82
sarcopenia 278, 279, 280
training to gain 198, 199–203
muscle protein synthesis (MPS) 9, 54, 58, 68, 69, 70–4, 82, 113, 142, 165, 198, 280, 283–4, 287
    and diet 74–8, 203–6, 207, 266, 268, 288

nandrolone 109
nausea during exercise 158
net protein balance (NPB) 68, 69
nitrates 11, 115–17
nitrogen 66, 68, 72, 80, 81, 202
non-essential amino acids 66, 68, 81, 112, 132–3, 144
nutrient reference values (NRVs) 104, 105, 274
nutrient timing 4, 203–5

oestrogen 98, 144, 171, 175, 208, 214, 216, 225, 226, 227, 277, 279, 280, 288
older athletes see masters athletes
omega-3 fatty acids 10, 84, 87, 88–9, 91
    and athletic performance 89–90
    supplementation 89, 91, 137–8, 248, 259, 272, 276, 287, 288
omega-6 fatty acids 87, 88, 89, 91
osmolality 159, 160
osteopenia 178, 221–2
osteoporosis 81, 178, 221–2, 226, 279
over-reaching 58
overhydration
    see hyponatraemia
oxidative stress 231, 264
oxygen 10, 18, 23, 24–5, 29, 59, 99, 115–16, 137, 138, 182, 215, 234, 278
    see also reactive oxygen species (ROS)

periodisation 4, 6, 282
  carbohydrate 8, 59, 60, 62–3, 64, 286
personal nutrition plans 4
  calculating carbohydrate requirement 304, 306
  calculating protein requirement 306, 307
  calculating fat intake 307
  estimating calorie needs 303–4
  estimating resting metabolic rate (RMR) 303–4
  fluid intake guidelines 305
  macronutrient guidelines 304, 307
  non-vegetarian meal plan – 2000 to 5000 kcal 309–15
  physical activity level (PAL) 304, 306
  vegetarian meal plans – 2000 to 5000 kcal 316–22
phosphates 16, 22
phosphocreatine 22, 23
physical activity level (PAL) 5–6, 249, 282, 304, 306
phytochemicals 104, 105, 265
planned drinking 153–4, 166–7, 294
plant-based athletes see vegan and vegetarian diets
polyphenols 138–9, 232, 233, 248, 265
polyunsaturated fatty acids 86, 87
positive nitrogen balance 202
pre-exercise meals and snacks 7–8, 11, 39–43, 64, 83
pro-hormone supplements 109, 143–4
probiotics and prebiotics 139–40, 232, 233, 238, 243–4, 248
progesterone 178, 214, 225, 227, 279, 288
prostaglandins 87
protein 9, 13, 17, 18, 19, 21, 22, 26, 27, 39, 53–5, 60, 64, 65, 67, 68, 69, 72–4, 78, 81, 82, 183, 185, 209, 241
  'Athlete's Plate' 13–14
  effect on endurance training 67–8, 69–70, 82

effect on resistance training 54–5, 69, 71, 72–3, 75, 82
milk-based 72–4, 76–7, 82, 205–6, 207
optimising MPS 4, 9, 70–8, 82, 202, 203–6, 207
oxidation 41, 182, 185
recommended intake 9, 11, 69–70, 78–81, 82, 254, 261, 266, 268, 283–4
supplements 11, 140–3, 206, 269, 276
weight loss and consumption 70, 82
when to consume 9, 11, 42, 70–1, 75–6, 82, 283–4
see also amino acids; creatine
pyruvate 23

quercetin 245

rapid weight loss 6, 180–1, 207
reactive oxygen species (ROS) 104–5, 111, 231
Reference Nutrient Intake (RNI) 93
rehydration 12, 77
  see sports drinks; water consumption
relative energy deficiency in sport (RED-S) 5, 177, 185, 208–9, 227, 300
  eating disorders and disordered eating 215, 216, 218–24, 227
  energy availability 209, 214–15, 217–18, 227
  gastrointestinal issues 215
  health consequences 213–16
  identifying 211, 213
  impact on bone health 208, 209, 214
  impact on cardiovascular system 215
  impact on endocrine system 214
  impact on growth and development 215
  impact on immune system 215
  impact on menstrual function 208, 209, 213, 214

iron deficiency 215
low energy availability (LEA) 208, 209–11, 214, 215, 216–17, 227
metabolic rate 214–15, 300
people at risk 211, 227
performance consequences 216–17
performance related symptoms 213
physiological symptoms 213
prevention 217
psychological symptoms 213, 215
risk of injury and illness 216, 218
risk stratification table 212
risk to young athletes 253
treatment 217–18
resting metabolic rate (RMR) 5, 6, 17, 181–2, 185, 191, 197, 207, 214–15, 282, 300, 303–4

sarcopenia 278, 279, 280
saturated fatty acids 10, 85–6, 91
sex-specific fat 175, 179
short chain fatty acids (SCFA) 229, 230, 232, 238
skinfold measurements 173–4
sodium bicarbonate 11
sodium 10, 155–6, 161–2, 258
soya protein 72, 73, 74
sports drinks 8, 10, 11, 12, 36, 38, 43, 44, 48–9, 130, 134–5, 156, 157, 158
  'lite' hypotonic drinks 164
  caffeine content 118, 121, 164, 167
  carbohydrate content 162–3, 167
  vs ordinary soft drinks and juices 163–4
  sodium in 161–2, 164, 167
  still vs sparkling 163
  stomach discomfort 159
  tooth decay and 37, 161
  types of 159–60
  when to choose 160–1, 167
  for young athletes 258–9
sports gels 11, 12, 37, 48–9, 118, 121, 130, 162, 236

sports supplements *see* individual supplements by name
sports/dilutional anaemia 102
steroid precursors 143
steroids 109, 110
stimulants 110, 130–1, 132
  see also caffeine
storage fat 175, 176, 179
stress fractures 97, 181, 214, 223, 226
sucrose 35–6, 47, 48–9
sugar and health 37–8
supplements, dietary 10–11, 94, 95–6, 97, 98, 101, 102–4, 105, 110, 206, 207, 227, 241–2, 243–4, 245, 253, 254, 259–60, 261, 268, 269–75, 287–8
supplements, sports 107–46
  see also individual products by name
sweat 10, 147–8, 155, 156, 158, 162, 286, 294
sweat rate, calculating 153, 154
sweatsuits, use of 151–2

taurine 144
testosterone 54, 77, 83, 109, 143, 171, 178–9, 181, 200, 277
  boosters 143–6
thermic effect of food (TEF) 17, 183
thermogenic supplements 130–1
thyroid hormone 179, 216, 274
time-restricted eating (TRE) 188
tooth decay 37, 161
total daily energy expenditure (TDEE) 17, 181, 303, 304
train high, sleep low protocol 62–3
training low 8, 44, 55–63, 64, 286
  protocols summarised 62
trans fatty acids 84, 90, 91
Tribulus terrestris 144–5
triglycerides 85

underwater weighing/ hydro densitometry 172
unsaturated fatty acids 10, 84, 86, 91, 123–4

urine monitoring/tests 150–1, 152, 166
URT infections 97–8, 125, 139, 140, 239, 241–2, 243, 244, 245

valine 66, 68, 112
vegan and vegetarian diets 23, 67, 91, 98, 259
  dietary supplements 268, 269–75, 276
  health benefits 262–3, 275, 276
  pitfalls for athletes 268–9
  protein requirements 266, 268, 276
  supporting athletic performance 263, 275
  supporting recovery 264–5
very low-carbohydrate diets (VLCDs) 185, 186
very low-fat diets (VLFDs) 187
vitamins 92, 229, 238
  as antioxidants 104
  deficiencies 223, 241, 248, 269, 276
  exercise and increased requirement 94–5, 105
  high doses and imbalances 102–4, 105
  nutritional requirements 92–3, 105
  supplements 10–11, 94, 95–6, 97, 98, 101–4, 105, 110, 206, 227, 241–2, 243
  vitamin A 9, 103, 105, 187
  vitamin B_1 (thiamine) 98
  vitamin B_{12} 98, 259, 273–4, 276
  vitamin B_2 (riboflavin) 98, 229
  vitamin B_3 (niacin) 98
  vitamin B_6 103, 105, 145, 273
  vitamin C 13, 96, 103, 111, 243, 248, 270–1
  vitamin D 4, 9, 10, 96–8, 103, 105, 187, 227, 241–2, 248, 259, 287–8
  vitamin E 9, 94, 95–6, 111, 187
  vitamin K 229

water/fluid consumption 152–6, 157, 159, 160–1, 162, 164, 167

see also sports drinks
weight management 180
  cardiovascular exercise 198–9
  creatine and weight gain 205
  diet psychology 192
  dieting and performance 180–1
  eating disorders 181
  high-calorie, nutrient-dense foods 206
  high-intensity interval training (HIIT) 199
  increasing energy intake 201, 202–6, 207
  influences on resting metabolic rate (RMR) 181–3, 185, 208
  lifestyle changes 196–7
  losing fat and keeping or gaining muscle 183–4, 195
  masters athletes 285–6
  menopause 280
  nutrient timing 203–5
  nutrition and muscle gain 201, 202–6, 207
  post-workout snacks 204
  rapid weight loss strategies 6, 180–1, 207
  reducing sugar 194
  repeated weight loss/yo-yo dieting 181, 207
  resistance exercise 197–8, 199–200
  skipping breakfast 196
  steps for an effective weight loss strategy 189–93, 195–9, 207
  training and weight loss diets 184–5
  types of weight loss diet 185–9
  weight gain supplements 206, 207
  weight loss 6, 41, 132, 152, 180–1, 185–99, 207
  weight/muscle gain 6, 199–206, 207
  see also body composition; relative energy deficiency in sport (RED-S)
whey 9, 72, 73, 74, 75, 206
  supplements 141

young athletes
  energy requirements 249–52, 261
  fluid intake 257–8, 261
  fuel consumption in 253–5
  recommended carbohydrate intake 254–5
  recommended protein intake 254, 261
  recovery snacks 256, 261
  risk of hypohydration 257, 261
  strength training 260–1
  supplements 253, 254, 259–60, 261
  tips for encouraging healthy eating 253
  weight loss and sport 253, 261
  what to eat after exercise 256, 261
  what to eat before exercise 255
  what to eat during exercise 255–6, 261

ZMA (zinc monomethionine aspartate and magnesium aspartate) 145–6

RECIPES

Breakfasts

athlete's porridge 323
breakfast muffins 324
fruit muesli 323
Greek yoghurt with banana and honey 325
yoghurt with dried fruit compote 324

Desserts

baked apples 344
banana pancakes 343
exotic fruit with lime 346
oat apple crumble 345
roasted peaches and plums with yoghurt 346
spiced fruit skewers 345
wholemeal bread and butter pudding 344

Main meals (non-vegetarian)

chicken and broccoli pasta 327
chicken and lentil salad 331
chicken and vegetable stir-fry 327
chicken with butternut squash 329
fish tagine with chickpeas 326
Moroccan chicken with rice 330
Moroccan fish stew 328
noodles with prawns and green beans 332
one-pot turkey and chickpea pilau 328
pilaff with plaice 332
potato and fish pie 333
quinoa and chicken salad with beetroot yoghurt 326
salmon and bean salad 330
salmon and vegetable pasta 325
spicy chicken with rice 329
sweet and sour chicken with mango 331

Main meals (vegetarian)

baked eggs with roasted Mediterranean vegetables 333
bean burgers 343
chickpeas with butternut squash and tomatoes 337
lentil and vegetable lasagne 342
mixed bean hotpot 342
pasta with chickpeas and spinach 340
potato, pea and spinach frittata 337
rice, bean and vegetable stir-fry 341
roasted vegetables with marinated tofu 338
spicy couscous 338
stir-fried vegetable omelette 336
sweet potato and lentil curry 334
sweet potato Spanish tortilla 335
tofu with noodles 336
vegetable risotto with cashew nuts 339
vegetable stir-fry with sesame noodles 340
vegetable tagine with chickpeas 334
vegetarian chilli 341
vegetarian shepherd's pie with sweet potato mash 335

Snacks

apple and cinnamon oat bars 349
banana and walnut loaf 350
banana muffins 348
blueberry muffins 350
cherry, almond and oat cookies 351
fruit Scotch pancakes 347
hummus with pine nuts 347
raisin bread 348
raspberry muffins 351
sultana flapjacks 349